Methods in Molecular Biology

Series Editor
John M. Walker
School of Life and Medical Sciences
University of Hertfordshire
Hatfield, Hertfordshire, AL10 9AB, UK

For further volumes:
http://www.springer.com/series/7651

Genetic Epidemiology

Methods and Protocols

Edited by

Evangelos Evangelou

Department of Hygiene and Epidemiology, University of Ioannina Medical School, Ioannina, Greece
Department of Epidemiology and Biostatistics, Imperial College London, London, UK

Humana Press

Editor
Evangelos Evangelou
Department of Hygiene and Epidemiology
University of Ioannina Medical School
Ioannina, Greece

Department of Epidemiology and Biostatistics
Imperial College London
London, UK

ISSN 1064-3745 ISSN 1940-6029 (electronic)
Methods in Molecular Biology
ISBN 978-1-4939-7867-0 ISBN 978-1-4939-7868-7 (eBook)
https://doi.org/10.1007/978-1-4939-7868-7

Library of Congress Control Number: 2018942871

Printed on acid-free paper

This Humana Press imprint is published by the registered company Springer Science+Business Media, LLC part of Springer Nature.
The registered company address is: 233 Spring Street, New York, NY 10013, U.S.A.

Preface

Genetic epidemiology is a relatively new field of epidemiology that studies the role of genetic factors in health and diseases and has witnessed some exciting findings in our quest to understand the nature of genetic inheritance. It is an amalgam of methods and approaches applied in traditional epidemiology, statistics, genetics, and bioinformatics and it brings together several scientific disciplines. In the last few years, scientists have been able to map thousands of genetic variants contributing to complex diseases helping to unravel the genetic causes of diseases on a population scale.

This book is a broad overview written at a level that should be accessible to a wide range of interested scientists including epidemiologists, genetic statisticians, human geneticists, clinicians, and bioinformaticians. I hope that this book will be also helpful for graduate students pursuing research in related fields. Some chapters of the book assume a basic level of competence with regard to statistic and probabilistic reasoning; however it was written and edited having in mind that a noncompetent reader will be able to follow, if not all, most of the text. For many scientists, genetic epidemiology is too convoluted to understand; however I hope to persuade the reader that this view is not correct. My goal was to provide a unifying overview of a fast-moving research while providing a description in some depth of the techniques and data that are helping us to understand our genome and how it is related to mainly complex diseases.

Chapter 1 provides an introduction to basic terms of epidemiology whereas Chapter 2 introduces the reader to the key principles of genetic epidemiology including genetic models of inheritance and associations. The next three chapters describe the process of quality control (Chapter 3), the analysis and the detection of common (Chapter 4) and rare variation (Chapter 5) whereas Chapter 6 outlines state-of-the-art meta-analyses approaches for the synthesis of such data. Chapter 7 outlines methods for detecting both gene-gene and gene-environment interactions as well as approaches for increasing statistical power.

The next seven chapters cover novel, state-of-the-art methods that go beyond the conventional approaches for the detection of common variation including analysis in the HLA region (Chapter 8), novel family-based approaches (Chapter 9), approaches for polygenic traits (Chapter 10), multivariate methods for meta-analysis of genetic associations and meta-analysis of gene expression data (Chapters 11 and 12). Chapter 13 covers the rapidly evolving method of Mendelian Randomization that is used for the estimation of causal effects of an exposure on an outcome, whereas computational methods for the analysis of Copy Number Variation are presented in Chapter 14. We conclude in the last two chapters by assessing the functional role of the identified variants (Chapter 15) and the challenges we are facing to use human genetics to identify and validate novel drug targets (Chapter 16).

I thank sincerely all those who have helped to bring this book together and I am grateful to the coauthors who accepted my invitation and contributed to this book, devoting valuable time and effort.

Ioannina, Greece *Evangelos Evangelou*

Preface

Contents

Contributors

EMIL VINCENT ROSENBAUM APPEL • *Section for Metabolic Genetics, Faculty of Health Sciences, Novo Nordisk Foundation Center for Basic Metabolic Research, University of Copenhagen, Copenhagen, Denmark*

PANTELIS G. BAGOS • *Department of Computer Science and Biomedical Informatics, University of Thessaly, Lamia, Greece*

LAZAROS BELBASIS • *Department of Hygiene and Epidemiology, University of Ioannina Medical School, Ioannina, Greece*

VANESA BELLOU • *Department of Hygiene and Epidemiology, University of Ioannina Medical School, Ioannina, Greece*

ANTONIO J. BERLANGA-TAYLOR • *Department of Epidemiology and Biostatistics, Faculty of Medicine, School of Public Health, MRC-PHE Centre for Environment and Health, Imperial College London, London, UK*

GEORGIA G. BRALIOU • *Department of Computer Science and Biomedical Informatics, University of Thessaly, Lamia, Greece*

ABBAS DEHGHAN • *Department of Epidemiology and Biostatistics, Imperial College London, London, UK*

ANDREW T. DEWAN • *Department of Chronic Disease Epidemiology, Yale School of Public Health, New Haven, CT, USA*

NIKI L. DIMOU • *Department of Computer Science and Biomedical Informatics, University of Thessaly, Lamia, Greece; Department of Hygiene and Epidemiology, University of Ioannina School of Medicine, Ioannina, Greece*

KAROL ESTRADA • *Translational Genome Sciences, Biogen, Cambridge, MA, USA*

JAVIER GUTIERREZ-ACHURY • *The Wellcome Trust Sanger Institute, Cambridgeshire, UK*

PANAGIOTA I. KONTOU • *Department of Computer Science and Biomedical Informatics, University of Thessaly, Lamia, Greece*

KAROLINE KUCHENBAECKER • *Wellcome Trust Sanger Institute, Cambridge, UK; University College London, London, UK*

ZOLTÁN KUTALIK • *Institute of Social and Preventive Medicine, University Hospital of Lausanne, Lausanne, Switzerland; Swiss Institute of Bioinformatics, Lausanne, Switzerland*

AURÉLIEN MACÉ • *Institute of Social and Preventive Medicine, University Hospital of Lausanne, Lausanne, Switzerland; Department of Computational Biology, University of Lausanne, Lausanne, Switzerland; Swiss Institute of Bioinformatics, Lausanne, Switzerland*

KYRIAKI MICHAILIDOU • *Department of Electron Microscopy/Molecular Pathology, The Cyprus Institute of Neurology and Genetics, Nicosia, Cyprus*

LOUKAS MOUTSIANAS • *The Wellcome Trust Sanger Institute, Cambridgeshire, UK*

KALLIOPE PANOUTSOPOULOU • *Wellcome Sanger Institute, Wellcome Genome Campus, Cambridgeshire, UK*

KATERINA G. PANTAVOU • *Department of Computer Science and Biomedical Informatics, University of Thessaly, Lamia, Greece*

ATHANASIA PAVLOPOULOU • *Department of Computer Science and Biomedical Informatics, University of Thessaly, Lamia, Greece; International Biomedicine and Genome Institute (iBG-Izmir), Dokuz Eylul University, Konak, Turkey*

RAHA PAZOKI • *Department of Epidemiology and Biostatistics (inc MRC-HPA Centre), School of Public Health, Imperial College London, London, UK*

KONSTANTINOS K. TSILIDIS • *Department of Hygiene and Epidemiology, University of Ioannina School of Medicine, Ioannina, Greece; Department of Epidemiology and Biostatistics, School of Public Health, Imperial College London, London, UK*

ARMAND VALSESIA • *Nestlé Institute of Health Sciences, Lausanne, Switzerland*

KLAUDIA WALTER • *Wellcome Sanger Institute, Wellcome Genome Campus, Cambridgeshire, UK*

ELEANOR WHEELER • *Wellcome Sanger Institute, Wellcome Genome Campus, Cambridgeshire, UK*

QI YAN • *Division of Pulmonary Medicine, Allergy and Immunology, Department of Pediatrics, Children's Hospital of Pittsburgh of UPMC, University of Pittsburgh, Pittsburgh, PA, USA*

Chapter 1

Introduction to Epidemiological Studies

Lazaros Belbasis and Vanesa Bellou

Abstract

The basic epidemiological study designs are cross-sectional, case-control, and cohort studies. Cross-sectional studies provide a snapshot of a population by determining both exposures and outcomes at one time point. Cohort studies identify the study groups based on the exposure and, then, the researchers follow up study participants to measure outcomes. Case-control studies identify the study groups based on the outcome, and the researchers retrospectively collect the exposure of interest. The present chapter discusses the basic concepts, the advantages, and disadvantages of epidemiological study designs and their systematic biases, including selection bias, information bias, and confounding.

Key words Bias, Case-control study, Cohort study, Confounding, Information bias, Observational studies, Selection bias, Study design

1 Definition of Epidemiology

Epidemiology is defined as "the study of the occurrence and distribution of health-related events, states, and processes in specified populations, including the study of the determinants influencing such processes, and the application of this knowledge to control relevant health problems" [1]. It is apparent that the scope of Epidemiology is very wide and mainly includes the study of incidence and prevalence of health conditions and traits, the study of their determinants (i.e., risk and protective factors), and the design of potential strategies for disease prevention.

Many subfields of Epidemiology have been developed, including environmental epidemiology, genetic epidemiology, and nutritional epidemiology. An early definition of *Genetic Epidemiology* defined it as "the field that addresses the etiology, distribution, and control of disease in groups of related individuals and the inherited causes of diseases in population [2, 3]. Later, this definition was broadened to include the role of interaction between the environment and the genetic factors in the occurrence of diseases [3]. Also, the term *Human Genome Epidemiology* was coined to

Evangelos Evangelou (ed.), *Genetic Epidemiology: Methods and Protocols*, Methods in Molecular Biology, vol. 1793,
https://doi.org/10.1007/978-1-4939-7868-7_1, © Springer Science+Business Media, LLC, part of Springer Nature 2018

describe "the field that uses systematic applications of epidemiologic methods and approaches to the human genome to assess the impact of human genetic variation on health and disease" [4]. The present chapter constitutes a brief introduction to epidemiologic study designs for Genetic Epidemiology.

2 Cross-Sectional Studies

The defining characteristic of cross-sectional studies is that both exposure and outcome are ascertained at the same time. The temporal sequence is often impossible to work out, because exposure and outcome are identified at one time point. However, cross-sectional studies are useful in Genetic Epidemiology, because genetic exposures cannot change over time and unquestionably preceded the outcome [5, 6].

3 Cohort Studies

A cohort study is "an observational epidemiological study in which subsets of a defined population can be identified who are, have been, or in the future may be exposed or not exposed to a factor or factors hypothesized to influence the occurrence of a given outcome" [1].

A cohort study tracks two or more groups forward from exposure to outcome. This type of study can be done by going ahead in time from the present (prospective cohort study) or by going back in time to identify the cohorts and following them up to the present (retrospective cohort study) [7]. In both prospective and retrospective designs, a cohort study moves in the same direction, although data gathering might not. The exposure of interest is measured at the beginning of the study, and the two groups are defined based on the exposure or the level of exposure to a specific factor.

Prospective cohort studies constitute the most reliable type of observational studies, and they present many advantages. The temporal sequence between putative cause and outcome is usually clear, given that the exposed and unexposed can often be seen to be free of the outcome at the beginning of the study [7]. Also, cohort studies are useful in the investigation of multiple outcomes that might arise after a single exposure [7]. For example, a cohort study can be designed to assess the association between birth weight and multiple health outcomes or traits. However, in this case, publication bias and reporting bias are often observed when the researchers publish or report only the statistically significant findings [8]. - Furthermore, testing multiple associations may lead to many false-positive findings due to chance. To avoid reporting and publication bias, several approaches have been proposed. Study registration and pre-specification of the project design and the analysis plan are important initiatives to avoid post-hoc secondary analyses seeking additional statistically significant findings [8]. To reduce the rate of false-positive findings in the field of Genetic Epidemiology, several statistical approaches for multiple testing have been suggested, including a more stringent P-value, q-values, or false discovery rate [9].

The cohort studies are also useful in the study of rare exposures [7]. For example, they are the appropriate study design to examine the health effects of occupational exposures, such as ionising radiation and chemicals. Moreover, cohort studies reduce the risk of survivor bias, i.e., diseases that are rapidly fatal are difficult to study because of this factor [7]. Finally, cohort studies allow the calculation of incidence rates, risk ratios, and other outcome measures, such as survival curves and hazard ratios [7].

However, cohort studies also have important shortcomings. Ideally, both cases and controls should be the same in all important aspects, except for the exposure of interest [7]. This seldom occurs, and the absence of comparability between groups being studied results in *selection bias* [10]. Also, cohort study is not the optimum study design for rare diseases or diseases that take a long time to develop, such as cancer [7]. Moreover, loss to follow-up can be an important issue in this study design, especially for longitudinal studies that have a long follow-up period. In this case, differential losses to follow-up between exposed and unexposed can bias results [7]. Another drawback is the potential change of the exposure status of study participants during the follow-up period [7].

One of the most frequent variations of cohort studies is the *nested case-control study*, which is "a type of case-control study in which cases and controls are drawn from the population in a cohort study" [1]. The rational for designing a case-control study nested in a cohort study is that some exposure variables are too expensive to determine on the full cohort [7]. Nested case-control studies can be designed to examine genetic associations for a specific health-related outcome. The variable of interest is measured in the cases group, and then the investigator chooses a random sample of all participants who did not develop the outcome. This approach minimizes the cost of measuring the variable of interest and ensures that the exposure was present before the development of the outcome. During the study design, a matching process is used and the controls are matched to cases by important characteristics, such as age and sex [7].

4 Case-Control Studies

A case-control study is an observational epidemiological study of persons with the disease of interest and a suitable control group of persons without the disease [1]. In this study design, study groups are defined by outcome, and the study population is divided into two groups, cases and controls, based on whether the outcome of interest has occurred [11, 12]. Case-control studies cannot yield incidence rates, but they provide an odds ratio, derived from the proportion of individuals exposed in each of the case and control groups [12]. When the incidence rate of a particular outcome in the population of interest is low (*rare disease assumption*), the odds ratio from a case-control study is considered a good approximation of risk ratio [12].

Case-control studies are considered an efficient study design in terms of time, money, and effort. Specifically, this study design is appropriate to investigate diseases with a low incident rate and diseases that have a long latency period, such as cancer [12]. However, case-control studies have also some disadvantages and, in these cases, cohort studies are considered a more efficient design. If the frequency of exposure is low, case-control studies quickly become inefficient, because researchers would have to examine many cases and controls to find one who had been exposed [12]. A simplified rule has been proposed indicating that cohort studies are more efficient in settings in which the incidence of outcome is higher than the prevalence of exposure [12]. Also, selection of a control group and obtaining exposure history [12] are two main methodological issues affecting the validity of the results of case-control studies and are discussed in more detail.

The term "*selection bias*" is used to describe "the bias in the estimated association or effect of an exposure on an outcome that arises from the procedures used to select individuals into the study or the analysis" [1]. Investigators can reduce selection bias by minimizing judgement in the selection process, and the selection process should be defined and described in detail for both case and control group [12]. Often only a sample of cases from a population is included as participants in a case-control study. During the selection process, investigators should focus on incident cases rather than prevalent cases, since diagnostic patterns change over time and this can affect the consistency of diagnosis between incident and prevalent cases [12]. Controls should be free of the disease being studied, but they should also be representative of those individuals who would have been selected as cases had they developed the disease. For example, if the case group included all affected individuals in a specified region, then the control group could be chosen at random from the general population of the same area [12].

The term "*information bias*" is used to describe "a flaw in measuring exposure, covariate, or outcome variables that results in different quality of information between comparison groups" [1]. A type of information bias is recall bias, which is "a systematic error due to differences in accuracy or completeness of recall to memory of past events or experiences" [1]. For example, in a case-control study for risk factors of melanoma, when information for past history of sun exposure, sunburns and solarium use is retrospectively collected, melanoma cases are more prone to report an increased exposure to these factors [13]. Also, information bias could be caused by data gatherers using different techniques to elicit information based on the case or control status. Thus, data gatherers should be unaware of the case or control status of the respondents, to minimize the risk for information bias [12].

Another important issue in the design of case-control studies is the *matching ratio* of controls to cases. There is usually little marginal increase in precision from increasing the ratio of controls to cases beyond four, except when the effect of exposure is large [14]. In general, the best way to increase precision in a case-control study is to increase the number of cases by widening the base geographically or temporally rather than by increasing the number of controls, because the marginal increase in precision from an additional case is greater than from an additional control [14].

5 Confounding

Selection bias and information bias have already been discussed in the section above. Another important issue in epidemiological studies is confounding. Three criteria should be fulfilled for a variable to be a confounder [15]. First, the confounding factor must be an extraneous risk factor for the disease. Second, a confounding factor must be associated with the exposure under study in the source population. Third, a confounding factor must not be affected by the exposure or the disease, and it cannot be an intermediate step in the causal path between the exposure and the disease of interest.

Several approaches have been suggested to control for confounding [10]. These methods can be applied either during the selection of cases and controls or during the statistical analyses. The simplest approach is restriction, i.e., during recruitment period researchers exclude individuals having the exposure that is suspected to be a confounding factor. Another way is pairwise matching. In a case-control study, during the selection of controls, cases and controls can be matched by the confounding factor. However, matching can be proven challenging if it is done on several potential confounding factors. Moreover, control for confounding can be done after a study has been completed. One approach is stratification which can be considered a post hoc restriction, done during the analysis [10]. Multivariate techniques (e.g., multivariate logistic regression) have also been proposed to examine the effect of one variable while controlling for the effect of many other factors [10].

References

1. Porta M (ed) (2014) A dictionary of epidemiology. Oxford University Press, Oxford
2. Morton NE (1997) Genetic epidemiology. Ann Hum Genet 61:1–13
3. Boslaugh SE (2007) Genetic epidemiology. In: Boslaugh SE (ed) Encyclopedia of epidemiology. SAGE Publications, Thousand Oaks, pp 417–420
4. Khoury M, Little J, Burke W (2004) Human genome epidemiology: scope and strategies. In: Human genome epidemiology. Oxford University Press, New York, pp 3–16
5. Cordell HJ, Clayton DG (2005) Genetic association studies. Lancet 366:1121–1131
6. Grimes DA, Schulz KF (2002) Descriptive studies: what they can and cannot do. Lancet (London, England). 359:145–149
7. Grimes DA, Schulz KF (2002) Cohort studies: marching towards outcomes. Lancet (London, England). 359:341–345
8. Ioannidis JPA, Munafò MR, Fusar-Poli P et al (2014) Publication and other reporting biases in cognitive sciences: detection, prevalence, and prevention. Trends Cogn Sci 18:235–241
9. Evangelou E, Ioannidis JPA (2013) Meta-analysis methods for genome-wide association studies and beyond. Nat Rev Genet 14:379–389
10. Grimes DA, Schulz KF (2002) Bias and causal associations in observational research. Lancet (London, England) 359:248–252
11. Gordis L (2014) Case-control and other study designs. In: Epidemiology. Saunders, Philadelphia, pp 189–214
12. Schulz KF, Grimes DA (2002) Case-control studies: research in reverse. Lancet (London, England). 359:431–434
13. Parr CL, Hjartåker A, Laake P et al (2009) Recall bias in melanoma risk factors and measurement error effects: a nested case-control study within the Norwegian women and Cancer study. Am J Epidemiol 169:257–266
14. Wacholder S, Silverman DT, McLaughlin JK et al (1992) Selection of controls in case-control studies. III. Design options. Am J Epidemiol 135:1042–1050
15. Rothman K, Greenland S, Lash T (2008) Validity in epidemiologic studies. In: Modern epidemiology. Lippincott Williams & Wilkins, Philadelphia, pp 128–148

Chapter 2

Key Concepts in Genetic Epidemiology

Kalliope Panoutsopoulou and Eleanor Wheeler

Abstract

Genetic epidemiology is a discipline closely allied to traditional epidemiology that deals with the analysis of the familial distribution of traits. It emerged in the mid-1980s bringing together approaches and techniques developed in mathematical and quantitative genetics, medical and population genetics, statistics and epidemiology. The purpose of this chapter is to familiarize the reader with key concepts in genetic epidemiology as applied at present to unveil the familial and genetic determinants of disease and the joint effects of genes and environmental exposures.

Key words Genetic epidemiology, Mendelian genetics, Genes, Deoxyribonucleic acid, Alleles, Single nucleotide polymorphism, Recombination, Linkage disequilibrium, Population genetics, Kinship, Identity-by-descent, Identity-by-state, Hardy-Weinberg equilibrium, Heritability, Association, Odds ratio

1 Introduction to Genetic Epidemiology

Genetic epidemiology is the scientific discipline that aims to unravel the role of the genetic determinants in health and disease and their complex interplay with environmental factors. In the past, genetic epidemiology has been particularly successful in mapping genes with large effect sizes at the individual level, for example in monogenic disorders where familial recurrence follows the laws of mendelian inheritance. With the advent of more high-throughput genotyping technologies and the development of more sophisticated bioinformatics and statistical genetics methodologies, the field of genetic epidemiology has recently focused its attention on dissecting the genetic architecture of common complex diseases. Unlike monogenic diseases, common complex diseases are caused by a large number of genes with small to modest effect sizes and their complex interplay with environmental factors. Large-scale genome-wide and whole genome sequencing association studies (GWAS and WGS) have catalogued a large number of genetic variations that are implicated in complex traits and diseases. It is

Evangelos Evangelou (ed.), *Genetic Epidemiology: Methods and Protocols*, Methods in Molecular Biology, vol. 1793, https://doi.org/10.1007/978-1-4939-7868-7_2, © Springer Science+Business Media, LLC, part of Springer Nature 2018

anticipated that subsequent translational efforts will transform the way medicine will be practised in the near future. This chapter introduces the reader to key concepts in molecular genetics, mendelian genetics, population genetics, and the fusion of these disciplines with epidemiology that has led to the science of genetic epidemiology.

2 Molecular Genetics and Variation

Genetics is the study of genes and heredity, the process by which characteristics are passed on from one generation to another. The carrier molecule of an organism's genetic information is called deoxyribonucleic acid (DNA). In this section, we describe the central dogma of biology to explain the flow of genetic information from DNA sequence to protein product and introduce the consequences of DNA variation in health and disease.

2.1 From DNA to RNA to Proteins

DNA is a large molecule consisting of two single strands, and each strand is composed of smaller molecules called nucleotides (Fig. 1). The nucleotides are composed of a sugar residue (deoxyribose),

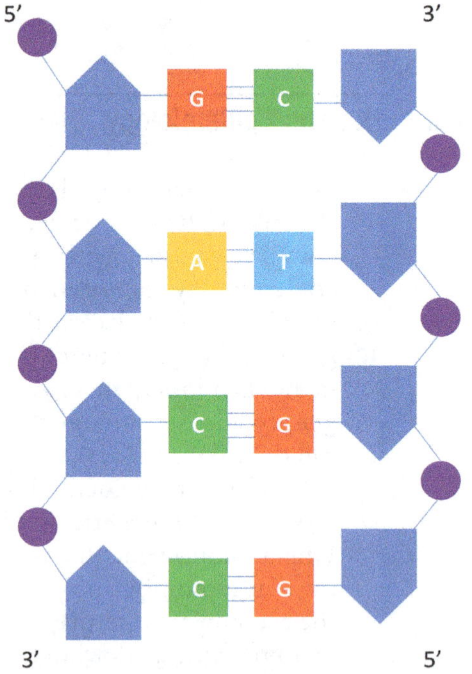

Fig. 1 Structure of a DNA molecule. Basic representation of an unwound DNA double helix segment depicting the phosphate group (purple circle), the sugar residue (blue pentagon), and the four different chemical bases (differentially colored squares). Complementary base pairing occurs between guanine (G) and cytosine (C) and between adenine (A) and thymine (T)

a phosphate group and a nitrogenous base which can be any of four types: adenine (A), cytosine (C), guanine (G), and thymine (T). The sugar residue and the phosphate group together form the nucleoside and alternating nucleosides form the DNA backbone. Covalent bonds bind bases to the nucleoside in one single strand. Weaker hydrogen bonds bind specifically A with T and G with C (also known as complementary bases) between the two single DNA strands resulting in the formation of a twisted double-stranded (dsDNA) molecule also known as the DNA double helix. Each single strand has different ends oriented in opposite directions termed five primed (5′) and three primed (3′) ends. The DNA sequence is essentially the order of the four bases across the genome and it is written down as letters for one strand only in the 5′ to 3′ direction, in this example GACC. This linear sequence of DNA is also known as its primary structure. The complementary strand in this case, written in the 3′ to 5′ direction, would be CTGG (Fig. 1). The length of the DNA is measured in base pairs (bp) so the DNA fragment in the example shown is 4 bp long. As we will describe below it is the order of these four chemical bases in the DNA that determines the proteins that are synthesized and carry out all the important functions in human organisms.

The process of protein synthesis can be summarized in two steps: transcription of a DNA sequence into ribonucleic acid (RNA) and translation of RNA into amino acids which form proteins. During the process of transcription the DNA double helix is unzipped into single strands. A single DNA strand acts as a template for the synthesis of a complementary strand of RNA in the 5′ to 3′ direction which is catalyzed by the RNA polymerase enzyme. The structure of RNA is similar to the single stranded DNA except that its backbone is composed of a sugar residue called ribose and the chemical base uracil (U) is present instead of T. RNA transcription that leads to proteins occurs in certain regions of the DNA which are transcribed to messenger RNA (mRNA). These regions are known as genes and typically contain alternating segments of sequence called exons, the protein coding sequences, separated by segments of noncoding DNA called introns. mRNA is further edited to make mature mRNA where introns are cut out and exons are spliced. Differential or alternative splicing of exons gives rise to different gene transcripts ensuring that multiple proteins can be coded by one gene.

The genetic information that is now contained in mRNA is translated into proteins according to the genetic code (Table 1). The genetic code defines how specific base triplets known as codons are combined to form amino acids, the building blocks of proteins. The combination of the four different bases (A, G, C, U) into triplets can make $4^3=64$ different codons which encode 20 different amino acids. Because several amino acids can be encoded by more than one codon the code is said to be degenerate and codons that

Table 1
The genetic code

	U		C		A		G		
U	UUU	Phe	UCU	Ser	UAU	Tyr	UGU	Cys	U
	UUC	Phe	UCC	Ser	UAC	Tyr	UGC	Cys	C
	UUA	Leu	UCA	Ser	UAA	'Stop'	UGA	'Stop'	A
	UUG	Leu	UCG	Ser	UAG	'Stop'	UGG	Trp	G
C	CUU	Leu	CCU	Pro	CAU	His	CGU	Arg	U
	CUC	Leu	CCC	Pro	CAC	His	CGC	Arg	C
	CUA	Leu	CCA	Pro	CAA	Gln	CGA	Arg	A
	CUG	Leu	CCG	Pro	CAG	Gln	CGG	Arg	G
A	AUU	Ile	ACU	Thr	AAU	Asn	AGU	Ser	U
	AUC	Ile	ACC	Thr	AAC	Asn	AGC	Ser	C
	AUA	Ile	ACA	Thr	AAA	Lys	AGA	Arg	A
	AUG	Met	ACG	Thr	AAG	Lys	AGG	Arg	G
G	GUU	Val	GCU	Ala	GAU	Asp	GGU	Gly	U
	GUC	Val	GCC	Ala	GAC	Asp	GGC	Gly	C
	GUA	Val	GCA	Ala	GAA	Glu	GGA	Gly	A
	GUG	Val	GCG	Ala	GAG	Glu	GGG	Gly	G

Table of codons showing the corresponding amino acid encoded by each base triplet
Ala Alanine, *Arg* Arginine, *Asp* Aspartate, *Asn* Asparagine, *Cys* Cysteine, *Gln* Glutamine, *Glu* Glutamate, *Gly* Glycine, *His* Histidine, *Ile* Isoleucine, *Leu* Leucine, *Lys* Lysine, *Met* Methionine, *Phe* Phenylalanine, *Pro* Proline, *Ser* Serine, *Thr* Threonine, *Trp* Tryptophan, *Tyr* Tyrosine, *Val* Valine

correspond to the same amino acid are called synonymous. Start (methionine codon) and stop codons signal the initiation and termination of the RNA translation into long chains of amino acid residues (polypeptides) a process that occurs in the cell plasma, at organelles called ribosomes. This process involves two more classes of RNA molecules: ribosomal RNA (rRNA) molecules that form the core of a cell's ribosome and transfer RNA (tRNA) molecules that carry amino acids to the ribosomes during protein synthesis. Proteins consist of one or more chains of amino acid residues folded into a 3D structure that determines their function and activity.

2.2 Human Genome and Variation

Nuclear DNA (nDNA) is found in the nucleus of almost every human cell (except for red blood cells) tightly packed in structures called chromosomes. Mitochondrial DNA (mtDNA) which is found in the cell structures known as mitochondria is responsible for providing the energy that the cell needs to function. nDNA encodes for the majority of the genome in eukaryotes; in humans it is 3.3 billion bp long and contains approximately 20,000 genes [1].

nDNA is distributed in 22 pairs of autosomes and in one pair of sex chromosomes which is XY in males and XX in females. One of the pair is derived from the mother and one from the father. All human cells contain two copies of each chromosome and are thus called diploid, except for gametes (sperm and ova) which are haploid. Because autosomal chromosome pairs contain the same genes at the same position they are called homologous chromosomes. However, because each chromosome from a homologous pair is derived from a different individual (mother or father) variations at certain DNA locations can be present. There are several classes of variation but the most frequent are single nucleotide polymorphisms (SNPs) which are variations in a single DNA base. Thus, at a given locus (region) in a homologous pair of chromosomes an individual can have either the same DNA base between the members of the pair (i.e., AA), or a different base, i.e., (AT). At that same position another individual may have TT. AA, AT, or TT denote the genotype of an individual at this site. Because of this variation, the site is said to be polymorphic and A and T are called alleles. The individual who carries AA at that locus is said to be homozygous for the A allele, AT heterozygous, and TT is homozygous for the T allele. The series of alleles along a single chromosome is called haplotype.

One of the two alleles will be present at a lower frequency in the population than the other allele; the less frequent is called the minor allele and the most frequent is called the major allele. A DNA variation is said to be rare when the minor allele frequency (MAF) is less than 0.01 (1%) meaning that the minor allele is observed in 10 or less individuals out of 1000. For rare variants the term single nucleotide variation (SNV) is used instead of SNP.

If $f(\text{AA})$, $f(\text{AB})$, and $f(\text{BB})$ are the frequencies of the three genotypes at a biallelic locus, then the frequency p of the A allele and the frequency q of the B allele in the population are obtained by counting alleles.

$$p = f(\text{AA}) + 1/2f(\text{AB}) = \text{frequency of A}$$
$$q = f(\text{BB}) + 1/2f(\text{AT}) = \text{frequency of B}$$

Because p and q are the frequencies of the only two alleles present at that locus, they must sum to 1.

$$p + q = f(\text{AA}) + f(\text{BB}) + f(\text{AB}) = 1$$
$$q = 1 - p \text{ } and \text{ } p = 1 - q$$

SNPs are the simplest form of DNA variation among individuals and are the focus of current research to unravel the genetic aetiology of common, complex diseases. There are several other forms of genetic variation such as microsatellites (typically nucleotide repeats that exist in variable numbers), insertions/deletions (one or several bases are duplicated/lost), duplications and translocations (usually large sequences that are cut from one site in the genome and inserted in another site). These are called structural variations and are covered in more detail elsewhere in this book (*see* Chapter 14).

2.3 The Impact of DNA Variation in Health and Disease

DNA sequence variations are the result of genetic mutations that may be introduced during DNA replication or due to DNA exposure to damaging agents. Hereditary mutations are passed on from parent to offspring. Mutations are essential for our evolution and our long-term survival. However, a very small percentage of all mutations can also lead to medical conditions of various severities.

For variants that fall in protein-coding genes it is easier to make predictions about their effect on gene function. There is a wide range of databases that describe these functional consequences such as Ensembl [2] and UCSC [3]. For example, non-synonymous variants, i.e., those that cause amino acid changes may introduce a premature stop codon leading to a shortened transcript; small insertion/deletions (indels) can change the translational reading frame. These belong to the category of loss of function (LoF) variants that comprise highly deleterious variants responsible for severe diseases. Non-synonymous, missense variants where the length is preserved can sometimes, but not always, affect the structure or function of the protein. A very well-known example is sickle-cell anaemia, caused by a missense mutation, A to T, in the gene coding for the beta-globin chain constituent of hemoglobin. This mutation results in the substitution of glutamic acid to valine (GAG codon changes to GTG); the disease is manifested in homozygous individuals and is caused by aggregation and precipitation of hemoglobin. In heterozygous individuals (known as carriers) 50% of the hemoglobin is still produced so the symptoms are far less severe. Interestingly, the mutation has thought to have arisen because it provides protection to malaria.

The protein-coding part of the genome represents approximately 1% of the genome. Base variations outside gene regions are typically implicated in common complex diseases. The exact mechanisms by which changes in the DNA sequence outside genes and their complex interplay with environmental factors can cause disease are the subject of extensive research in the current era [4]. We will briefly introduce some terms in order to understand how variations in the DNA outside of protein-coding regions can affect tightly controlled dynamic processes that govern transcription and translation of the primary sequence to genes and proteins respectively.

Transcription and translation are complex processes regulated by many factors [5, 6]. Briefly, the initiation of transcription is controlled by promoters, which are DNA elements upstream of the gene where different forms of RNA polymerase and other associated transcription factors bind. Transcription factors are broadly divided into activators and repressors that bind to enhancers (noncoding DNA sequences 200–1000 bp long containing multiple activator and repressor binding sites) and can activate and/or repress a wide repertoire of target genes. Enhancers can be found near the regulated gene (5′ upstream of the promoter or within the first intron of the gene they affect) or they can be distal, found in introns of neighboring genes or intergenic regions, i.e., between genes. The configuration of the genome called DNA looping brings together promoters, enhancers, activators, repressors, and other RNA processing factors to achieve the tight regulation at the gene expression level. The process of translation involves several components of the translational machinery and is also tightly regulated by several factors for example short oligonucleotides called microRNAs (miRNAs). Therefore, variants falling outside protein-coding regions that affect the tight regulation or alter the dynamics of these processes can increase susceptibility to a certain disease.

Transcriptional regulation also occurs at the level of chromatin structure by controlling the accessibility of the DNA to polymerase and other complexes. Histone modification, DNA methylation, and noncoding RNAs are epigenetic changes (heritable changes in gene expression not involving changes in the underlying DNA sequence). Epigenetic change is a natural process that can silence genes but can also be influenced by age, lifestyle, other environmental factors, and disease state. The crosstalk between genetics and epigenetics may also explain the impact of variants outside promoters or protein-coding sequences in health and disease.

3 DNA Transmission

The first step in the process by which genetic information is transmitted from generation to generation is called meiosis. During this process a single cell divides to produce four cells containing half the original amount of genetic information. This section gives an overview of the process of meiosis and describes the patterns of DNA transmission first introduced by Mendel and how these relate to modern genetics.

3.1 Meiosis and Recombination

Meiosis is the process of cell division that leads to gametes, sperm, and ovum. A simplistic description of this process is depicted in Fig. 2 for one homologous chromosome.

In a diploid cell the maternally derived and paternally derived dsDNA of a chromosome undergoes DNA replication (it is duplicated) to produce two identical dsDNA molecules, the sister chromatids, held together by the centromere. The resulting homologous chromosomes pair up. At this stage it is possible to exchange different segments of genetic material between homologous chromosomes leading to the formation of recombinant chromosomes. In the first meiotic division event that follows non-sister chromatids are separated and distributed in two diploid cells. In the second meiotic division the sister chromatids are separated and

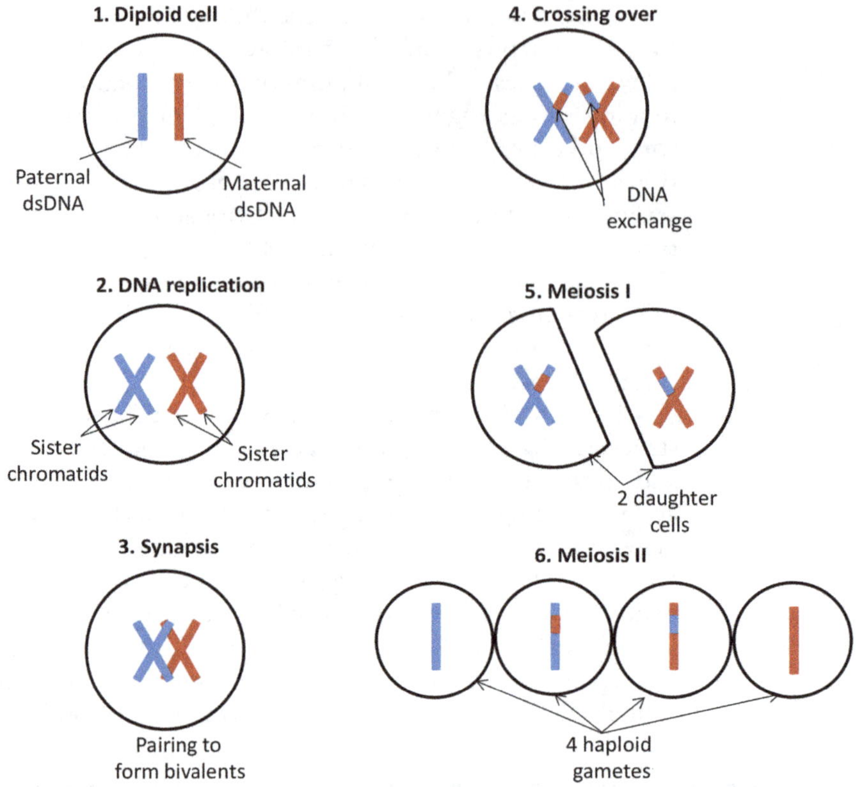

Fig. 2 An overview of meiosis. (1) A homologous chromosome of a diploid cell which contains the maternally derived and paternally derived double-stranded DNA (dsDNA). (2) DNA replication to produce two identical dsDNA molecules, the sister chromatids. (3) Pairing up of homologous chromosomes. (4) Crossing over and exchange of DNA segments between homologous chromosomes. (5) First meiotic division—separation of non-sister chromatids to two diploid cells. (6) Second meiotic division—separation of sister chromatids to four haploid gametes

distributed in four haploid gametes. Gametes (sperm and ova) fuse together during reproduction to form a zygote diploid cell.

An important aspect of meiosis is that homologous chromosomes are distributed randomly and independently to the gametes. So there is a 50% probability that a gamete will receive one chromosome from the mother rather than the father and there are 2^{23} distinct gametes that a mother or father will produce.

Furthermore, crossing over accounts for further shuffling of genetic material because the sister chromatids held together by the centromere are not identical. Figure 2 shows one recombination event between two chromosomal segments but in reality the mean number per cell is ~55 in males and double as much in females. The further apart two genes are, the more likely it is that there will be recombination between DNA segments. The probability of recombination is termed the recombination fraction (θ) and forms the key to linkage analysis as discussed in Subheading 4.1.

3.2 Mendelian Genetics and Relevance to Modern Genetics

Modern genetics originated with Gregor Mendel, an Augustinian monk living in Czech Republic in the mid-eighteenth century, long before it was known that genes are the basic units of heredity. Mendel carried out a lengthy series of cross-breeding experiments with garden peas and observed the transmission of seven easily distinguishable traits including stem height (tall versus short), flower color (violet versus white), and pea morphology (round versus wrinkled). By describing the inheritance patterns mathematically he was able to demonstrate that heredity was transmitted by what he described as "factors" in a predictable and logical manner that could be studied by experimental means. He proposed three laws that are known today as Mendel laws: The law of dominance, the law of segregation, and the law of independent assortment.

The first two laws were derived as a result of cross-fertilizing plants with distinct traits in monohybrid, reciprocal crosses. For example, Mendel pollinated a male white flower pea plant with pollen from a female violet flower plant and noted that all plants in the first generation (F1) had violet flowers (Fig. 3a). He then repeated the cross reciprocally, i.e., with male violet and female white flowered plants and noted the same result. When members of F1 were self-fertilized the second generation (F2) comprised 705 plants with violet petals and 224 plants with white petals. Additional experiments with tall and short-stemmed plants or yellow and green peas demonstrated that the ratio of plants with one characteristic over another in the F2 generation approximated 3:1. Mendel reached his first conclusion: each trait (flower color) is controlled by a unit factor (gene) with each unit factor existing in more than one form (pair of alleles) responsible for the appearance of different characteristics (phenotype). The second conclusion from his experiment was that at the phenotypic level one of the alleles (the V allele) was dominant over the other allele (the v allele that is conversely termed recessive); this explained why plants in F1 appeared violet but were all heterozygotes (Vv). We now know that during sexual reproduction when an organism produces gametes the two alleles of each parent segregate (separate) randomly so that each gamete receives one allele. They then fuse together to produce the pair of alleles that is carried over in the next generation. The resulting genotype ratio in F2 is 1 homozygote for the dominant allele (VV): 2 heterozygotes (Vv): 1 homozygote for the recessive allele (vv). At the phenotypic level this produces a 3:1 ratio of violet versus white flowers (Fig. 3a).

The third law of independent assortment was established as a result of Mendel's dihybrid crosses looking at the inheritance pattern of two traits at the same time, for example crosses between plants with round or wrinkled peas that were either yellow or green (Fig. 3b). At the phenotypic level the round shape is dominant over the wrinkled shape so we denote the alleles as R and r for each of these distinct traits respectively. Yellow color is dominant over

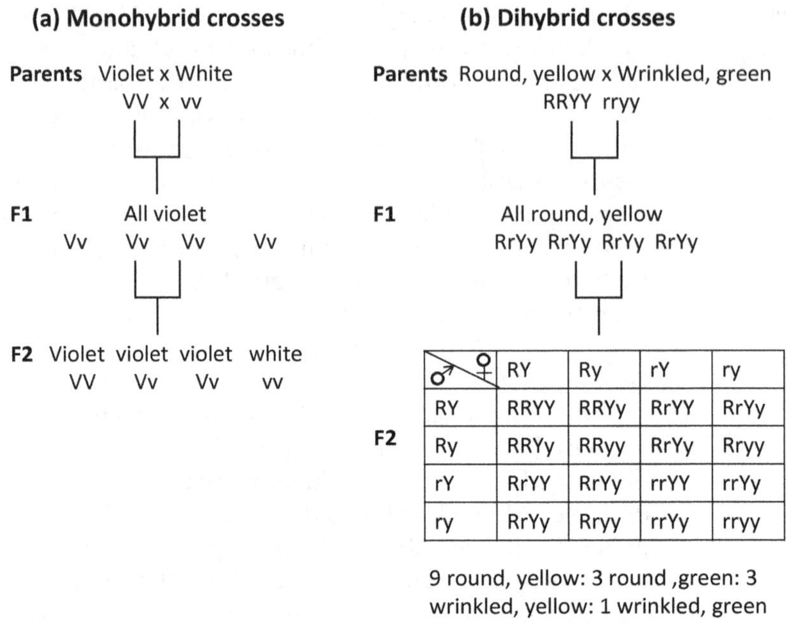

Fig. 3 Mendel's monohybrid and dihybrid crosses. (**a**) An example of monohybrid crosses between peas with violet flowers and white flowers. In the first generation (F1) all heterozygous (Vv) flowers appear violet because of the dominance of the V allele (violet color) over the v allele (white color). In the second generation (F2) the ratio of flowers is 3 violet (VV, Vv, Vv): 1 white (vv). (**b**) An example of dihybrid crosses between round, yellow peas with wrinkled, green peas. In F1 all heterozygous flowers for both characteristics (RrYy) appear round and yellow because of the dominance of the R allele (round shape) over the r allele (wrinkled shape) and the dominance of the Y allele (yellow color) over the (y) allele green color. In F2 several possible genotypes that can arise for these unlinked loci are shown in the Punnett square. Parental and non-parental trait combinations appear at a ratio of 9 round yellow peas: 3 round, green peas: 3 wrinkled, yellow peas: 1 wrinkled green pea

green color so we denote the alleles as Y and y respectively. When round, yellow peas (RRYY) were crossed with wrinkled, green peas (rryy) all the plants in F1 were double heterozygotes (RrYy) and appeared as round, yellow peas. In F2 however, parental and non-parental combinations appeared at a regular ratio—9 round yellow peas: 3 round, green peas: 3 wrinkled, yellow peas: 1 wrinkled green pea. The Punnett square table in Fig. 3b shows all the possible genotypes that can arise in F2 that lead to this phenotypic ratio. The first conclusion from this experiment is that the parental traits are not linked; they can be split and give rise to non-parental trait combinations. The second conclusion is that for the 9:3:3:1 ratio to arise different pairs of alleles must segregate independently.

We now know that Mendel studied traits for genes that were in different chromosomes. The third law is generally true for loci that are found in different chromosomes and are thus unlinked.

3.3 Phenotype Transmission in Families

Mendel's monohybrid crosses on pea plants revealed patterns of phenotype transmission that formed the basis of further clinical research unraveling various inheritance patterns in families. Examination of disease transmission in large family pedigrees revealed five basic patterns categorized based on dominant or recessive mode of inheritance and whether the phenotype is transmitted by autosomes or sex chromosomes.

A disease is said to be transmitted in an autosomal dominant fashion if one allele present in autosomal chromosomes is sufficient to cause the affected status. Autosomal recessive inherited disorders require the presence of two disease-causing alleles in autosomes for disease manifestation. Diseases transmitted in a X-chromosomal dominant pattern are infrequent. If the disease-causing allele is inherited from the paternal X chromosome, all daughters will be affected whereas if the disease-causing allele is inherited from the maternal X chromosome roughly half of the children will be affected irrespective of their gender. Diseases transmitted in a X-chromosomal recessive pattern will almost exclusively affect males if the mutation is passed on by the mother. Females will be affected only if they inherit both disease-causing alleles from each of the parents. Y-chromosomal inheritance affects only males, both fathers and sons. Few diseases follow a straightforward Mendelian inheritance pattern and in most cases this is due to incomplete penetrance (*see* Subheading 5.2).

4 Population Genetics

A basic concept in population genetics is the principle of *Hardy-Weinberg Equilibrium* (HWE), identified independently by Godfrey Hardy and Wilhelm Weinberg in 1908, describing the relationship between allele and genotype frequencies. As above, consider a biallelic autosomal locus (a locus with just two alleles) with alleles A and B whose allele frequencies are p and q (where $q = 1-p$) respectively. If the locus is under Hardy-Weinberg Equilibrium, then in a large, randomly mating population, the genotype frequencies of the genotypes AA, AB, and BB are expected to be in the proportions p^2, $2pq$, and q^2, where $p^2 + 2pq + q^2 = 1$. These proportions do not vary from one generation to the next, and even if the frequencies are not in those proportions in a given generation, they will return to the expected proportions after a single generation. This assumes the absence of selection (occurring through the preferential advantage of a particular genotype over another, or migration of individuals with a particular genotype), mutations or population stratification. The presence of HWE is usually used as a quality check in genetic studies, but significant deviations from HWE can also indicate the presence of selection or inbreeding.

4.1 Linkage and Linkage Disequilibrium

Mendel's third law of independent assortment means that every gene is transmitted from parent to offspring independently from all other genes. However, genes located close to each other on the chromosome are less likely to be separated by a recombination event, and are more likely to be inherited together. This concept is called *linkage*. The probability of recombination is represented by the recombination fraction θ, $0 \leq \theta \leq 0.5$. Alleles at loci on different chromosomes are unlinked and have a 50:50 chance of being inherited together ($\theta = 0.5$), and alleles are linked if θ is less than 0.5. These deviations from independent assortment form the basis of linkage mapping in families [7].

At the population level, we use the term *linkage disequilibrium (LD)* [8] to refer to the residual correlation between specific alleles at SNPs on a chromosome that has not been broken down by historical recombination. For SNPs, the most commonly used measure of LD is r^2 [9], which ranges between 0 and 1, where $r^2 = 1$ implies the SNP alleles are perfectly correlated.

The combination of alleles on a chromosome are called *haplotypes*, and regions of high LD bounded by regions of preferential recombination (*recombination hotspots*) are called *haplotype blocks* [10]. There are typically a limited number of distinct haplotypes in a short segment of the chromosome, so we can select SNPs to represent the haplotypes in the region, and infer the genotypes at the other SNPs which were not directly genotyped. This haplotype-tagging approach has led to the era of whole-genome association studies (*see* Chapter 4).

4.2 Identity by Descent (IBD) and Identity by State (IBS)

Two genes (or DNA fragments) are defined as being *identical by descent* if one is a copy of another, or if they are both copies of the same ancestral gene. Two genes are identical by state if they represent the same allele. For example, if we consider the first simple pedigree (also known as a nuclear family) in Fig. 4, the parents have different alleles at the locus, so both offspring must have inherited the *a* allele from their father and the *c* allele from their mother, meaning they share 2 alleles IBD. In the second pedigree, the parents have the same alleles, although under the assumption of

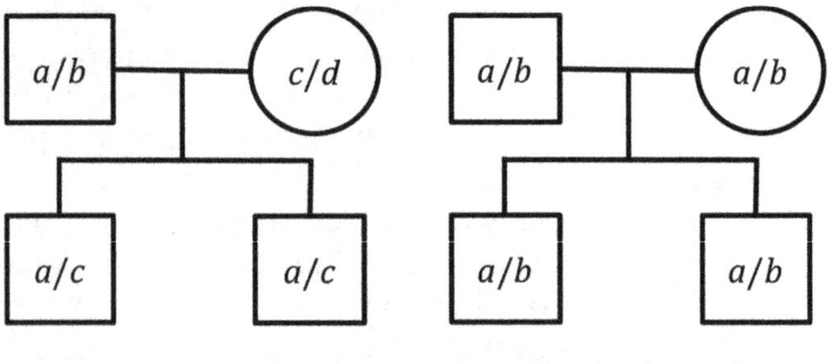

Fig. 4 Example pedigrees with parents and two offspring. Genotypes at a marker (alleles *a,b,c,d*) are shown. The parents are assumed to be unrelated (i.e., no inbreeding)

Table 2
Kinship coefficients and IBD sharing probabilities for relative pairs assuming no inbreeding

	IBD sharing probabilities			Kinship coefficient
Relationship of relative pair	2 (z_2)	1 (z_1)	0 (z_0)	($\Phi = 1/2\ z_2 + 1/4\ z_1$)
Monozygotic twins	1	0	0	1/2
Parent-offspring	0	1	0	1/4
Full siblings	1/4	1/2	1/4	1/4
Half siblings	0	1/2	1/2	1/8
First cousins	0	1/4	3/4	1/16
Second cousins	0	1/16	15/16	1/64
Uncle-nephew	0	1/2	1/2	1/8

no inbreeding, they will not be from the same common ancestor. Therefore, the offspring will share two alleles IBD if they inherited both alleles from the same parents (e.g., *a* from the father and *b* from the mother, or zero alleles IBD if they inherited their alleles from different parents). If they share zero alleles IBD, we can say that they share two alleles *identical by state* (the same alleles, but not inherited from the same common ancestor). Excess sharing of alleles IBD can be used to identify related individuals, and estimate their relationship. This is also particularly relevant for population-based association studies that assume all individuals are independent (*see* Subheading 5.2).

4.3 Kinship and Inbreeding

If we consider an autosomal locus where each individual carries two copies of a gene, the *kinship coefficient* between two individuals is the probability that genes selected at random, one from each individual, are IBD. The *inbreeding coefficient* is defined as the probability that the two genes carried by an individual are IBD, which is equivalent to the kinship coefficient for the individual's parents. Under the assumption of no inbreeding, Table 2 shows the kinship coefficients and IBD sharing probabilities for relative pairs.

5 Where Genetics Meets Epidemiology

The aggregation of disease phenotypes (such as diabetes status) or similarity in quantitative traits (such as height) in families is an indication that the phenotype may have a genetic component. For binary traits, we use a measure called the *recurrence risk ratio*, λ_R, to define the risk of disease for a relative of an affected family member of type R, compared to the population prevalence of disease [11]. For example, we denote the recurrence risk ratio of disease in siblings as λ_S, and offspring as λ_O. As for traditional epidemiological studies, the *disease prevalence* is defined as the proportion of cases in the population at a particular time. *The disease incidence* is the rate of new cases in a given time-period.

5.1 Variance Components Models and Heritability

The estimated genetic contribution to a phenotype is called the *heritability*. In 1918, R. A. Fisher introduced the concept of variance, and the *analysis of variance* method [12]. For a trait, X, which we assume to be normally distributed, the total phenotypic variance (V_P) is made up of both environmental (V_E) and genetic components (V_G). We can further subdivide the genetic variance into additive (average effects of loci summed additively across loci), dominance (interactions between alleles at a locus), and epistatic (interactions of alleles between different loci) variances:

$$V_P = V_A + V_D + V_I + V_E$$

Similarly, the environmental variance can be divided into pure environmental variance affecting the individual or the population and variance due to gene-environment interactions.

Broad-sense heritability (H^2) is the proportion of phenotypic variance (V_P) attributable to all genetic effects (V_G) including dominance and epistatic effects:

$$H^2 = V_G/V_P$$

Narrow-sense heritability is most commonly used, and represents the proportion of the phenotypic variance determined by only the additive genetic effects:

$$h^2 = V_G/V_A$$

Although variance component methods were designed for quantitative traits, we can extend the model to binary traits by assuming that a normally distributed quantitative trait called the *liability* underlies the binary trait. A threshold is set such that the proportion of the liability distribution above the threshold is equal to the disease prevalence. For common diseases, estimates of heritability are often used to determine whether genetic approaches will be sufficiently powered to identify genetic variants contributing to risk of disease.

5.2 Genetic Models and Association

At a SNP with two alleles A and B there are three possible unordered genotypes, AA, AB and BB. In epidemiological terms, we can treat the SNP as the exposure variable. *Penetrance* reflects the risk of disease in an individual with respect to the genotype. For a disease trait, there are a number of penetrance models (or *modes of inheritance*) used to define the relationship between genotype and disease, including *multiplicative*, *additive*, *recessive*, and *dominant*.

Table 3
Penetrances under standard genetic models

	Genetic model			
Genotype	**Genotype (general)**	**Recessive**	**Dominant**	**Additive**
AA (reference)	f_0	0	0	0
AB	f_1	0	1	1
BB	f_2	1	1	2

Table 4
Genotype relative risks (GRR) for genotypes AB, BB (where B is the risk allele) compared to the baseline genotype AA under standard genetic models

	Genetic model				
Genotype	**GRR**	**Dominant** $\gamma_1 = \gamma_2 = \gamma$	**Recessive** $\gamma_1 = 1$ $\gamma_2 = \gamma,$ $\gamma > 1$	**Multiplicative** $\gamma_1 = \gamma, \gamma > 1$ $\gamma_2 = \gamma_1^2$	**Additive** $\gamma_1 = \gamma,$ $\gamma > 1$ $\gamma_2 = 2\gamma_1$
AB	γ_1	γ	1	γ	γ
BB	γ_2	γ	γ	γ^2	2γ

Under the additive model, γ_2 can also be expressed as $2\gamma_1 - 1$ [17], although $\gamma_2 = 2\gamma_1$ is commonly used [18]

Define, f_0, f_1 and f_2, as the probability of disease given the genotypes AA, AB, BB respectively where the B allele is assumed to be the *risk (increasing) allele*. The penetrances under the models above can be represented as shown in Table 3. For example, under a dominant model, an individual with genotype AB or BB will have disease, whereas under a recessive model, only individuals carrying two copies of the risk allele (BB) will have disease. Well-known examples are Huntington's disease (dominant), and cystic fibrosis (recessive, both parents are required to be "carriers" of the risk allele). The *genotype relative risks* found by comparing the genotypes AB and BB to the reference genotype AA (containing no disease-causing alleles) can be defined as follows:

$$\gamma_1 = \frac{f_1}{f_0}, \quad \gamma_2 = \frac{f_2}{f_0}$$

The relationships between γ_1 and γ_2 under standard genetic models are described in Table 4.

A key concept in genetic epidemiology is that of *association*, the statistical relationship between a genetic variant and a phenotype of interest [13]. In a way that resembles traditional epidemiological approaches, we test whether a particular allele at a SNP is more frequent in people with disease than people without disease than would be expected by chance. Alleles associated with disease are not necessarily causal for disease (or similarly for influencing a quantitative trait). It is possible to detect association at a SNP due to linkage disequilibrium between that SNP and the causal SNP, also known as *indirect association*.

The most common design for association analysis of disease traits in the population is a case-control study, where a sample of unrelated affected cases and unaffected controls are recruited. The case control design is *retrospective*, given that the individuals are collected and information on their genotype (exposure) is obtained retrospectively. Relative risks (as described above) can only be estimated from the data in *prospective* cohort studies, where individuals are selected into the study on the basis of their exposure (genotype), and followed for a specified time period to see who develops disease. In retrospective studies we can use the *odds ratio* (OR), the ratio of the odds of disease in the exposed group compared to the non-exposed, where exposure is defined by carrying a particular allele at a SNP locus and an OR of one indicates independence between the SNP and disease.

Conventional X^2 tests of association using contingency tables can be used to test for association between a SNP and disease. Table 5a shows the genotype counts for cases and controls at a SNP with alleles A and B, where allele B is assumed to be the risk allele. The chi-square test statistic, measuring deviation from the expected genotype counts, follows a chi-squared distribution with two degrees of freedom (2 d.f.). This model makes no assumptions on the ordering of the genotypes and each genotype is assumed to have an independent association with disease. The tables can be simplified under standard genetic models described above. For example, under a recessive model, two copies of allele B are required for a γ-fold risk of disease and the contingency table can be summarized as a 2×2 table (1 d.f.) by pooling the AA and AB

Table 5
Contingency tables for the full genotype model and the multiplicative model

(a) Genotype model				
Genotype	**AA**	**AB**	**BB**	X^2 (2 d.f.)
Cases	a	b	c	OR (AB relative to AA) $= \frac{bd}{ae}$
Controls	d	e	f	
				OR (BB relative to AA) $= \frac{cd}{af}$
(b) Multiplicative model				
Genotype	**A**	**B**	X^2 (1 d.f.)	
Cases	$2a + b$	$b + 2c$	Allelic OR $= \frac{(b+2c)(2d+e)}{(2a+b)(e+2f)}$	
Controls	$2d + e$	$e + 2f$		

genotypes. The additive model, where there is a γ-fold increased risk of disease for the AB genotype and a 2γ-fold increased risk of disease for the BB genotype, can be tested using the Cochran-Armitage trend test. A commonly used test is the allelic case control test, where the numbers of A and B alleles are pooled ignoring which genotype they came from resulting in a 2×2 table (1 d.f.) as shown in Table 5b. This test is more powerful than the general genotype model under a multiplicative model, but assumes Hardy-Weinberg Equilibrium in the cases and controls. To adjust for covariates such as age and sex or additional SNPs logistic regression in standard statistical software can be used.

In Table 5a, the odds of being a case and having genotype AB is b/e. Similarly, the odds of being a case and having genotype AA is a/d. The OR of genotype AB relative to genotype AA is therefore

$$\frac{b/e}{a/d} = \frac{bd}{ae}$$

The OR for genotype BB relative to AA, and the allelic OR under a multiplicative model can similarly be calculated (Table 5).

For a quantitative trait, tests of association are usually performed in a cohort of unrelated individuals, randomly selected from the population. Assuming additive SNP effects, where the effect of the SNP on the trait increases linearly with the number of copies of the effect allele, the SNP genotypes AA, AB, BB can be coded as 0, 1, 2 and tests of association can be performed using standard linear regression.

It is important to remember that the significance threshold for any test of association needs to be adjusted for the number of independent tests performed. In genome-wide association analyses for example, the number of independent tests in European populations is estimated to be 1 million, and $p = 5 \times 10^{-8}$ (0.05/1,000,000) has become the widely accepted "genome-wide significance" threshold.

Population studies can be susceptible confounding by *population stratification*. This can arise when cases and controls are sampled from populations with different proportions of underlying subpopulations. An extreme example would be when cases and controls are sampled from distinct ethnic groups leading to spurious associations with SNP alleles due to differences in allele frequency between the ethnic groups [14]. Family studies using related controls can control for this problem, in addition to methods designed to deal with known/cryptic relatedness [15, 16].

References

1. ENCODE Project Consortium (2012) An integrated encyclopedia of DNA elements in the human genome. Nature 489:57–74. https://doi.org/10.1038/nature11247
2. Flicek P, Ahmed I, Amode MR et al (2013) Ensembl 2013. Nucleic Acids Res 41: D48–D55. https://doi.org/10.1093/nar/gks1236

3. Meyer LR, Zweig AS, Hinrichs AS et al (2013) The UCSC genome browser database: extensions and updates 2013. Nucleic Acids Res 41: D64–D69. https://doi.org/10.1093/nar/gks1048
4. Ritchie GR, Flicek P (2014) Computational approaches to interpreting genomic sequence variation. Genome Med 6:87. https://doi.org/10.1186/s13073-014-0087-1
5. Carlberg C, Molnár F (2016) Mechanisms of gene regulation. Springer, Netherlands. https://doi.org/10.1007/978-94-007-7905-1
6. Sonenberg N, Hinnebusch AG (2009) Regulation of translation initiation in eukaryotes: mechanisms and biological targets. Cell 136:731–745. https://doi.org/10.1016/j.cell.2009.01.042
7. Teare MD (2011) Genetic epidemiology. Humana Press, New York
8. Pritchard JK, Przeworski M (2001) Linkage disequilibrium in humans: models and data. Am J Hum Genet 69:1–14. https://doi.org/10.1086/321275
9. Hill WG, Robertson A (1968) Linkage disequilibrium in finite populations. Theor Appl Genet 38:226–231. https://doi.org/10.1007/BF01245622
10. Cardon LR, Abecasis GR (2003) Using haplotype blocks to map human complex trait loci. Trends Genet 19:135–140. https://doi.org/10.1016/S0168-9525(03)00022-2
11. Risch N (1990) Linkage strategies for genetically complex traits. I. Multilocus models. Am J Hum Genet 46:222–228
12. Fisher RA (1918) The correlation between relatives on the supposition of Mendelian inheritance. Trans R Soc Edinburgh 52:399–433
13. Cordell HJ, Clayton DG (2005) Genetic association studies. Lancet 366:1121–1131. https://doi.org/10.1016/S0140-6736(05)67424-7
14. Cardon LR, Palmer LJ (2003) Population stratification and spurious allelic association. Lancet 361:598–604. https://doi.org/10.1016/S0140-6736(03)12520-2
15. Anderson CA, Pettersson FH, Clarke GM et al (2010) Data quality control in genetic case-control association studies. Nat Protoc 5:1564–1573. https://doi.org/10.1038/nprot.2010.116
16. Price AL, Zaitlen NA, Reich D et al (2010) New approaches to population stratification in genome-wide association studies. Nat Rev Genet 11:459–463. https://doi.org/10.1038/nrg2813
17. Schaid DJ (1999) Likelihoods and TDT for the case-parents design. Genet Epidemiol 16:250–260. https://doi.org/10.1002/(SICI)1098-2272(1999)16:3<250::AID-GEPI2>3.0.CO;2-T
18. Camp NJ (1997) Genomewide transmission/disequilibrium testing—consideration of the genotypic relative risks at disease loci. Am J Hum Genet 61:1424–1430. https://doi.org/10.1086/301648

Chapter 3

Quality Control of Common and Rare Variants

Kalliope Panoutsopoulou and Klaudia Walter

Abstract

Thorough data quality control (QC) is a key step to the success of high-throughput genotyping approaches. Following extensive research several criteria and thresholds have been established for data QC at the sample and variant level. Sample QC is aimed at the identification and removal (when appropriate) of individuals with (1) low call rate, (2) discrepant sex or other identity-related information, (3) excess genome-wide heterozygosity and homozygosity, (4) relations to other samples, (5) ethnicity differences, (6) batch effects, and (7) contamination. Variant QC is aimed at identification and removal or refinement of variants with (1) low call rate, (2) call rate differences by phenotypic status, (3) gross deviation from Hardy-Weinberg Equilibrium (HWE), (4) bad genotype intensity plots, (5) batch effects, (6) differences in allele frequencies with published data sets, (7) very low minor allele counts (MAC), (8) low imputation quality score, (9) low variant quality score log-odds, and (10) few or low quality reads.

Key words Genome-wide association study, Whole genome sequencing, Sample quality control, Variant quality control

1 Introduction

High-throughput approaches such as genome-wide association scans (GWAS) and whole genome sequencing (WGS) technologies are used to interrogate the genotypes of tens of thousands of individuals at hundreds of thousands or millions of sites across the genome for association with diseases or other complex traits. Rigorous quality control (QC) at the sample and variant level is crucial to the success of the study because it can dramatically reduce the number of false positive or false negative findings down the line. Extensive research over the past 10 years in the field of GWAS has established several commonly accepted criteria and thresholds for sample and variant QC after the genotype calling process [1, 2]. Most of these QC steps are applicable to sequencing data but additional filters have, and will constantly be developed as these technologies evolve. Here, we describe the most commonly applied sample and variant QC steps in datasets from GWAS and low-depth WGS studies. We recommend that most of the QC steps, and in

Evangelos Evangelou (ed.), *Genetic Epidemiology: Methods and Protocols*, Methods in Molecular Biology, vol. 1793, https://doi.org/10.1007/978-1-4939-7868-7_3,

particular the example thresholds that are presented here based on previous research are tested for suitability and adapted to each study.

2 Sample QC

The aim of performing sample QC is to remove low quality samples often caused by poor DNA quality and/or insufficient quantity and/or contamination; and to identify individuals with discordant information based on other sources, accidental swaps, samples that show batch effects, duplicated and related samples and ethnic outliers. It is recommended that QC at the sample level is best carried out before variant QC because it can adversely influence variant QC metrics. In addition, sample QC metrics can also be influenced by bad quality variants so variants with high missing genotype rates should not be taken into consideration when calculating these metrics. This can be achieved by pre-filtering the dataset for bad quality variants before proceeding to sample QC. With the exception of the sex determination QC all other sample QC steps are carried out using autosomal variants only.

2.1 Sample Call Rate

The proportion of missing genotypes per sample is a good indicator of DNA quality. Samples with high proportion of missing genotypes (i.e., low call rate) will typically fail other sample QC metrics and if they are not removed from the data they could lead to spurious associations. Previous GWAS studies have excluded subjects with missing genotype rate greater than 2%–5%. However, because this threshold depends on several study-specific factors an empirical threshold should be determined by examining the distribution of the missing genotype proportion per individual across all study samples.

2.2 Sex Discrepancies and Other Identity Checks

Self-reported sex is usually available from subject enrolment but the sex of an individual can also be inferred from X chromosome genetic data. Discrepancies between these two sources of information may indicate sample swaps, sample contamination or incorrect data entry for self-reported sex. These can be investigated further by feeding back conflicting sex information to the collection centers. Having the correct sex information is also important in studies where sex is included as a covariate in the analysis or to stratify males and females for calculating effect sizes in separate in studies of sexual dimorphic traits.

Before a genotyping or sequencing experiment takes place, some labs run small-scale marker assays in Sequenom MassARRAY iPLEX and Fluidigm platforms. Sex determination markers contained in these platforms can be used to estimate genetic sex and this can serve as a basic concordance test between genetically estimated and self-reported sex information. However, typically in GWAS or WGS experiments sex is inferred by calculating mean homozygosity across all variants on the X chromosome. Women have two copies of the X chromosome whereas males have only one copy so they cannot be heterozygous for typed variants on this chromosome. The most commonly used QC software (PLINK) [3, 4] will call a sample male if the X chromosome homozygosity rate is more than 0.8; a female call is made if this estimate is less than 0.2. Samples that fall between these two thresholds are ambiguous and often this correlates with poor call rate and/or contamination. In rare instances this can be attributed to chromosomal abnormalities.

Further checks for sample identity can be performed by checking concordance of genotypes for the same individuals at a set of variants genotyped in more than one platform. For example, genotype concordance of a panel of variants from Sequenom/Fluidigm platforms can be checked against genotypes derived from GWAS or WGS for the same individuals at these markers. Genotypes derived from a sequencing experiment can be compared against genotypes derived from a GWAS experiment if these exist for the same or a subset of common individuals. When enough overlapping markers are available the degree of relatedness between samples can be estimated by calculating genome-wide identity-by-descent (IBD) as described in the relatedness QC section (*See* Subheading 2.4).

2.3 Heterozygosity

Excess genome-wide heterozygosity is also a very good indicator of poor DNA quality and/or sample contamination. In the case of rare variants typically defined as having a minor allele frequency (MAF) <1%, excess heterozygosity can also be caused by differences in ethnicity of the samples assayed. On the other hand, excess genome-wide homozygosity may indicate some degree of inbreeding.

The mean genome-wide heterozygosity of a sample is the fraction or the proportion of non-missing genotypes that are heterozygous in relation to all the genotypes. This metric is platform- and sample-specific; it varies according to the marker content, the proportion of rare to common variants that have been assayed and the population examined. The threshold is therefore best determined by examining the distribution of mean genome-wide heterozygosity of all samples separately for common and rare variants. A reasonable approach is to remove samples that are plus or minus 3 standard deviations (SD) from the mean as shown in Fig. 1.

2.4 Relatedness

Having related individuals in the data may be desirable due to the study design (for example family-based studies or isolated populations) but it can also be introduced accidentally (cryptically related and/or duplicated samples). Estimating relatedness with genetic data is an important step in the QC process; the goal is to validate

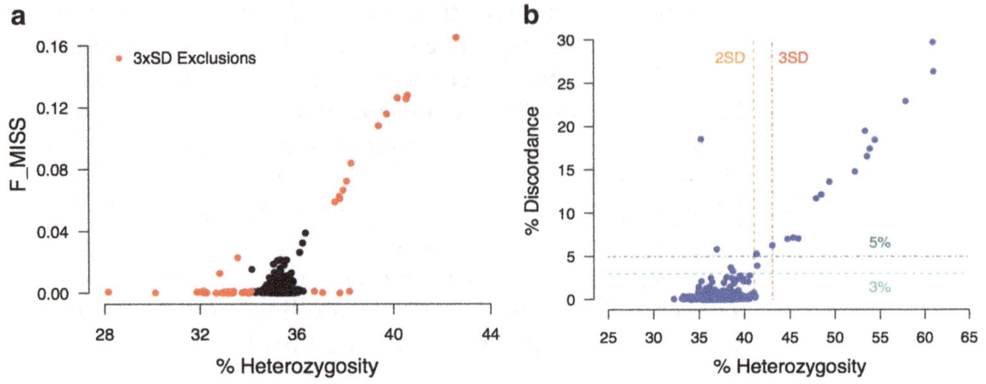

Fig. 1 (**a**) Heterozygosity versus call rate. Individuals with mean heterozygosity more or less than three standard deviations (SD) from the mean are labeled in red. (**b**) Discordance is strongly correlated with heterozygosity, where discordance (in %) is calculated from a comparison between sequenced and genotyped variants (modified from the UK10K cohorts study). The lines at 2SD and 3SD mark the two times and three times standard deviation from the sample mean of the heterozygous rate and the lines at 3% and 5% show cutoffs for the discordance rate. A threshold at 3SD would capture more or less samples with a discordance rate of >5%

known (recorded) relationships, to identify pedigree errors, to decide on the analysis strategy that correctly accounts for related/duplicated samples, or to remove the related/duplicated pairs (usually one individual from a related pair) from downstream analysis. For family-based studies differences between recorded and estimated relationships could indicate sample swaps or adoption, misattributed paternity, etc. For case-control and population-based cohorts cryptically related or accidentally duplicated individuals can significantly inflate the significance of the association study results. These individuals are either removed from the analysis or kept in, but the data will then require analysis with approaches that appropriately account for relatedness, for example linear mixed models (LMMs).

In a homogeneous sample, the degree of relatedness between samples can be estimated by calculating genome-wide IBD given identity-by-state (IBS) information. IBS is a term used to describe two identical alleles or two identical segments or sequences of DNA. An IBS segment is IBD in two or more individuals if they have inherited it from a common ancestor without recombination. Duplicated samples and monozygotic twins are expected to share 2 alleles at every locus so the proportion of IBD equals 1, for parent-offspring pairs IBD is 0.5 and this value halves for second-degree (0.25), third-degree relatives (0.125), and so on. IBS/IBD calculations are affected by linkage disequilibrium (LD) so it is recommended to remove highly correlated markers by a method called LD-pruning as well as complex regions such as the Major Histocompatibility Complex (MHC) region before the IBD calculations take place. In practice, because of fluctuations that can be introduced by the LD structure and by genotyping/sequencing errors the threshold of the proportion of IBD > 0.9 is used to identify individuals that are duplicated and the threshold of the proportion of IBD > 0.2 is used to identify individuals that are second-degree or closer relatives. In outbred populations, samples may show an unexpectedly large number of relationships with other samples at even lower IBD thresholds which may indicate subtle contamination.

2.5 Ethnicity

Population stratification can be a major confounding factor in genetic association studies. If undetected, it can lead to inflation of the test statistic and false positive associations due to the differences in allele frequency between the different populations. To guard against it, studies in outbred populations try to match individuals for broad ethnic background upon recruitment and then rely on statistical approaches to remove ethnic outliers or to correct for subtle population stratification. We present below two of the most commonly used approaches to identify and remove ethnic outliers and admixed individuals.

Ethnic outliers can be identified by principal component analysis (PCA) [5] or multidimensional scaling approaches (MDS) [3] which cluster individuals depending on their genetic similarity. Genetic data from sampled individuals can be analyzed alone or merged with genetic data from samples of known ethnicity from source populations or publically available datasets. Publically available datasets comprising samples with known ethnicities are getting larger and more diverse; the widely used 1000 Genomes Project data contains genotypes of 2504 individuals from 26 populations [6]. Clustering of samples can be visualized onto a two-dimensional projection on axes of genetic variation termed principal components. Ethnic outliers are typically removed from the dataset but more subtle population stratification may not be picked up during this step; however, it can be corrected or accounted for downstream of the QC process. For example, including principal components as covariates in the association analysis, genomic control, linear mixed models, and LD score regression are approaches that can correct for subtle population stratification.

For WGS data the number of singletons per sample can also be used to identify samples with different ancestry. In general, there is a positive correlation between the number of singletons called and the read coverage (or depth) of the sequenced fragments, where read coverage or depth means how many sequenced fragments overlap each nucleotide on average after alignment to a reference genome. However, samples from different ancestries will appear as outliers when plotting the number of singletons versus average read depth for each sample (Fig. 2).

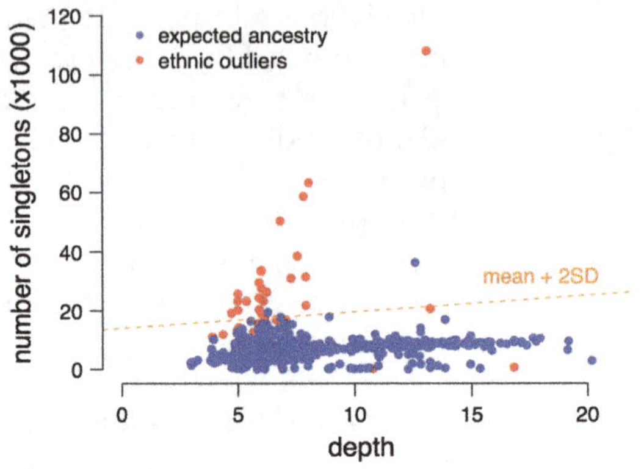

Fig. 2 Depth versus number of singletons. Samples with different ancestries, depending on the population, might be distinguished by a higher number of singletons, i.e., variants that are not shared with other samples in the cohort (modified from the UK10K cohorts study)

2.6 Batch Effects

Batch effects between samples in a single experiment can introduce bias in the analysis and lead to noise and false positive associations. Batch effects can be introduced by several sources, for example due to different sources of DNA (saliva versus blood), different collections, DNA extraction, genotyping or sequencing centers, as well as different chips and sequencing platforms available. Batch effects are highly undesirable and best avoided by careful planning at the start of the study. Often, studies combine samples post-hoc and genotyping/sequencing processes are carried out in batches over a period of time making the introduction of these effects unavoidable. QC fails partitioned per plate can identify batch effects for samples on different plates. Fortunately, gross batch effects are picked up by PCA or MDS; the principal components that are capturing this can be used as covariates in the analysis to eliminate some of this variation. Samples that have been genotyped/sequenced in duplicate could be useful to detect suspected batch effects particularly if these are more subtle. It is also possible to identify a subset of genotypes that cause this bias and remove these markers from further analysis as described in the variant QC section (*see* Subheading 3.5).

2.7 Sequence-Specific Checks for Sample Contamination

Additional checks for sample contamination can be performed for WGS data. For example, if GWAS genotypes are available, it is possible to estimate the degree of the sample contamination and even to detect the source of the contamination by calculating likelihoods based on two-sample mixture models with the publicly available software VerifyBamID (http://genome.sph.umich.edu/wiki/VerifyBamID) [7]. VerifyBamID requires two input files, a file in VCF format that contains external genotypes or allele frequency information, and a file in BAM format that contains the sequenced reads. There are two options available, free-mix and chip-mix. The first option, free-mix, can be used for estimating contamination if only sequence data are available, and the second option, chip-mix, can be used for estimating contamination or sample swaps when also GWAS genotype data are available. If CHIPMIX $\gg$ 0.02 and/or FREEMIX $\gg$ 0.02, it means that 2% or more of non-reference bases are observed in reference sites. In those cases, it is recommended to inspect the data more carefully for potential contamination.

An alternative way to check for sample contamination is to compare the genotypes from the sequence data with the genotypes from existing GWAS data. If the overall discordance or the non-reference discordance (NRD) appears to be high between the two data sources, then this also points to sample contamination (Fig. 1). The NRD is calculated only from the non-reference (or alternative) genotypes, which usually represent the minor alleles, but not exclusively. In a variant call set based on sequenced reads the reference allele (REF) and the alternative allele (ALT) are clearly allocated, since reference genomes are being used for aligning the sequenced reads from next generation sequencing platforms. Mostly ALT will be the minor allele, but in some cases it will be the major allele. Often a few samples will be contaminated and they will appear as outliers. However, if the outliers appear as a smear or as a long tail of the main distribution, it might reveal a widespread low level sample contamination which should be examined more closely.

3 Variant QC

Variant QC usually follows after the individuals that fail sample QC have been removed from the dataset. As with sample QC, variant QC is performed to ensure that only high quality variants are included in downstream analysis. The main steps are described below.

3.1 Genotype Call Rate

As with sample call rate, variants with high degree of missingness across study samples constitute low quality variants that can introduce false positive associations and hinder the identification of truly associated variants. To determine an appropriate threshold, the distribution of missing data proportion for each variant should be examined. Typically, GWAS studies exclude variants with missing call rate above 2%–5%. For low-frequency or rare variants a more stringent threshold is recommended and this is typically set at > 1%.

3.2 Call Rate Differences by Phenotypic Status

Spurious associations can be introduced when call rate differs significantly by case/control status [8]. This can be examined with a chi-square test of non-random missingness in cases versus controls. Removal of variants with $p < 10^{-4}$ has been reported in the literature.

3.3 Deviation from Hardy-Weinberg Equilibrium (HWE)

In a relatively homogeneous population, gross departures from HWE can be indicative of genotyping error. This is evaluated by calculating Hardy-Weinberg test statistics for each variant using an exact test. However, departures from HWE may also be due to selection and therefore, in a case-control study this QC step is usually performed in controls. Various HWE p-value exact thresholds have been employed in GWAS ranging from less stringent to more stringent ($p < 5 \times 10^{-12}$ to $p < 0.0001$) and studies have chosen to either remove the variants that fail this filter or flag them for further scrutiny.

3.4 Genotype Cluster Plots

Genotype calling algorithms vary in their ability to call common and rare variants correctly. Therefore, for each associated variant one needs to scrutinize its genotype cluster plots. These are scatter plots of normalized probe intensities for each individual. For a biallelic common variant a good quality cluster plot is expected to show three clearly distinct clusters: one for the individuals who are homozygotes for the major allele, one for the heterozygotes and one for the homozygotes for the minor allele (Fig. 3). Upon visual

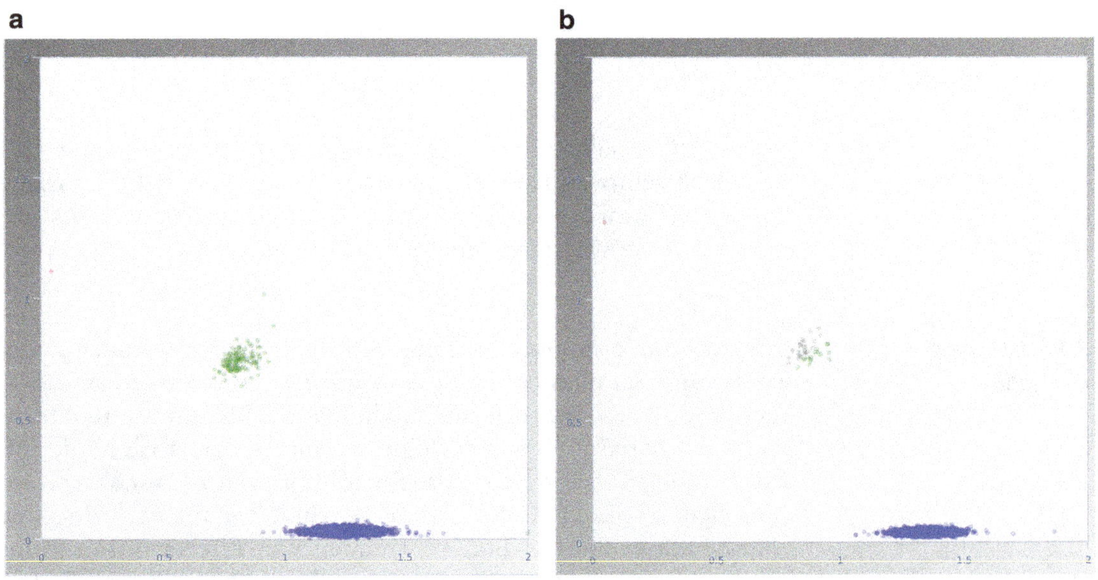

Fig. 3 Genotype intensity (cluster) plots for a rare variant. Depicted in blue are the individuals that are homozygotes for the major allele (AA), in green are the heterozygotes (AB), and in red is the homozygote for the minor allele (BB). Missing calls are depicted in gray. (**a**) Shows a good cluster plot (**b**) shows a bad cluster plot where several heterozygotes have not been called

inspection variants with overlapping clusters and/or samples that have not been called or have been incorrectly assigned to a cluster should be removed from the analysis. Genotype calling is even more problematic for rare variants. The minor allele cluster may be composed of none or a few calls and any missing or incorrectly assigned calls for rare variants will have a bigger effect on the apparent association with a trait or disease. Therefore, it is recommended that removal of rare variants based on imperfect clustering is more stringent than for common variants.

3.5 Variants Causing Batch Effects

As discussed in the sample QC section there are instances where batch effects could be alleviated by removing the variants that cause them, obviating the need for correcting for batch effects on a genome-wide scale. As examples we present two different approaches that were used to remove batch effects in two high profile GWAS and WGS studies, the African Genome Variation Project [9] and the UK10K project [10]. In the former, principal component analysis showed clear batch effects between samples that were typed on two versions of the Illumina HumanOmni 2.5 M platform, the octo and the quad Beadchips. The principal components that captured this separation were identified and variant loadings were calculated along these principal components in order to remove highly weighted variants. The authors checked the correlation of variant weights and genotype discrepancy between a subset of samples that were typed on both platforms and found this to be highly correlated. Subtle chip effects and/or chip effects at rare variants may not be picked up by the PCA approach. For example, panel A of Fig. 3 shows the genotype calls of cases that were typed on one version of the Illumina Human CoreExome Beadchip (v1.0) and panel B shows the genotype calls of controls that were typed on the next version of the same chip (v1.1). In panel B several heterozygotes have not been called. A genotype concordance test where missing calls are not taken into account will not pick this up this either. A stringent threshold for call rate differences by case/control status in this instance would remove most of these variants but the best way to ensure that variants have been accurately called is by examining their genotype intensity plots.

In the UK10K project [10] where ~4000 samples from two cohorts were sequenced in two different centers batch effects were visualized in a multidimensional scaling analysis by labeling the samples by cohort and sequencing center (Fig. 4). Then logistic regression models were fitted using sequencing center as the case/control status to test for allele frequency differences between the two centers and by treating the cohort of origin as a covariate. Variants that showed a significant association with sequencing center were removed from further analysis. However, this approach can be only used for variants that are not too very rare (e.g., MAF $>$ 1%).

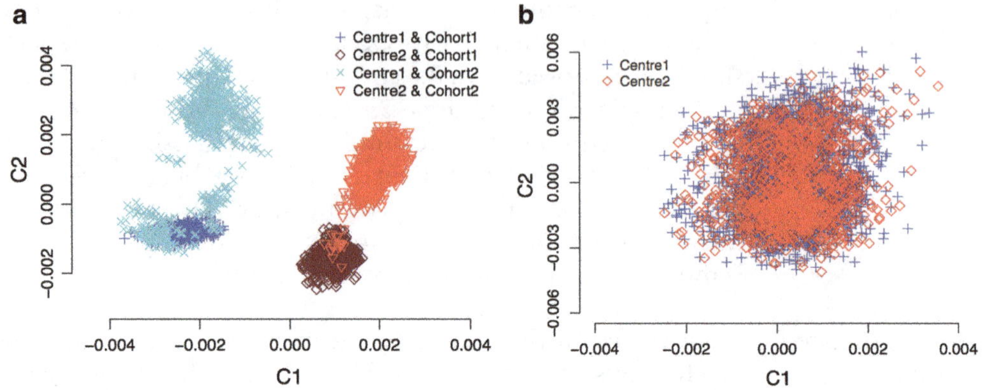

Fig. 4 Sample batch effects. (**a**) A multi-dimensional scaling analysis (MDS) highlights the sample batch effects for two cohorts sequenced at two different centers over some period of time by plotting the first component against the second component. (**b**) The first two MDS components after removing the batch effect. Both panels show data adapted from the UK10K cohorts study

3.6 Allele Frequency Comparisons with 1000 Genomes and UK10K Projects

To analyze the overall quality of the variant calling, the allele frequencies of the call set can be compared to an existing published data set such as the 1000 Genomes Project [6] or the UK10K Project [10] in a case-control analysis manner. Variant sites that differ greatly in allele frequencies could be removed to boost the quality of the call set. Additionally, common variants with allele frequency greater than 5% should be mostly shared with those large-scale sequencing data sets.

3.7 MAF and Minor Allele Count (MAC) Filters

MAF filters are optional but they can eliminate a lot of noise in the data. This is particularly important for studies that have been typed on older genotyping platforms and called with earlier versions of genotype calling algorithms with poor performance at calling rare variants. Imposing a MAF filter of less than 1% across all samples is strongly recommended if the data is to be used for imputation. MAC filters for cases and controls in separate are more robust to study sample size and are more effective filters for particularly unbalanced case/control designs. In an unbalanced study design the MAC but not necessarily the MAF will be different in cases and controls which can invalidate the assumptions of the association test, inflate the test statistic, and lead to spurious associations at low frequency or rare variants [11].

3.8 Imputation to Fill in Missing Genotypes and Post Imputation QC

A large proportion of the genotypes that will be removed by the variant QC steps will be captured by genotype imputation. Imputation refers to the statistical inference of unobserved genotypes which is achieved by combining the study sample genotypes with haplotypes from publically-available sources such as the HapMap, 1000 Genomes Project, UK10K Project and more recently the Haplotype Reference Consortium [12–14]. Imputation using the latest reference panel by the Haplotype Reference Consortium (comprising 64,976 haplotypes at 39,235,157 variants constructed using WGS data from 20 studies of mainly European ancestry) will lead to accurate genotype imputation at MAFs as low as 0.1%. Imputation is a probabilistic approach and the accuracy depends on many factors including the density and content of the platform used to genotype the SNPs, as well as the ethnicity of the study population. The most widely used metric for imputation accuracy is the imputation information score which ranges from 0 to 1. Variants with imputation information score <0.3–0.4 are considered low quality and are typically removed from downstream analysis. In practise these filters are best determined by sequential filtering and examination of the inflation in a quantile-quantile (QQ) plot.

3.9 Sequence-Based Variant Quality Score QC

The procedure of the variant quality score recalibration (VQSR) aims at calculating a new quality score called VQSLOD (variant quality score log-odds) that is supposed to be well calibrated and therefore allows fine-tuning of the specificity and sensitivity of the variant call set (https://software.broadinstitute.org/gatk). In other words, fine-tuning the specificity and sensitivity means maximizing the number of variants called and minimizing the false positive rate at the same time. The VQSR method uses machine learning algorithms, i.e., Gaussian mixture models, to help distinguish between true and false variants by combining annotations from several sources (e.g., read depth, mapping quality, and inbreeding coefficient) and by training them against a trustworthy set of variants. This approach results in determining a threshold for the VQSLOD score from the sensitivity/specificity of the variant call set against the training set to filter out the low quality variants.

3.10 Imputation Refinement for Low-Depth Sequencing Data

For cost reasons most WGS studies so far have been performed at low read depth, i.e., less than ~10× (a read depth of 10× means that each nucleotide was covered on average by 10 sequenced reads). It is possible to improve the quality of variants in regions that are covered only by a few or low quality reads by borrowing information from other samples. Therefore, it is customary to add a genotype imputation step, which helps in refining the genotypes by phasing them into haplotypes first and then filling in missing or low quality genotypes by searching for similar haplotypes. This approach is based on Hidden Markov Models (HMM) that calculate a probability of each genotype for each of the missing genotypes [12–14].

References

1. The Wellcome Trust Case Control Consortium (2007) Genome-wide association study of 14,000 cases of seven common diseases and 3,000 shared controls. Nature 447 (7145):661–678. https://doi.org/10.1038/nature05911
2. Anderson CA, Pettersson FH, Clarke GM et al (2010) Data quality control in genetic case-

control association studies. Nat Protoc 5 (9):1564–1573. https://doi.org/10.1038/nprot.2010.116
3. Purcell S, Neale B, Todd-Brown K et al (2007) PLINK: a tool set for whole-genome association and population-based linkage analyses. Am J Hum Genet 81(3):559–575. https://doi.org/10.1086/519795
4. Chang CC, Chow CC, Tellier LC et al (2015) Second-generation PLINK: rising to the challenge of larger and richer datasets. Gigascience 4:7. https://doi.org/10.1186/s13742-015-0047-8
5. Reich D, Price AL, Patterson N (2008) Principal component analysis of genetic data. Nat Genet 40(5):491–492. https://doi.org/10.1038/ng0508-491
6. 1000 Genomes Project Consortium, Auton A, Brooks LD et al (2015) A global reference for human genetic variation. Nature 526 (7571):68–74. https://doi.org/10.1038/nature15393
7. Jun G, Flickinger M, Hetrick KN et al (2012) Detecting and estimating contamination of human DNA samples in sequencing and array-based genotype data. Am J Hum Genet 91(5):839–848. https://doi.org/10.1016/j.ajhg.2012.09.004
8. Clayton DG, Walker NM, Smyth DJ et al (2005) Population structure, differential bias and genomic control in a large-scale, case-control association study. Nat Genet 37 (11):1243–1246. https://doi.org/10.1038/ng1653
9. Gurdasani D, Carstensen T, Tekola-Ayele F et al (2015) The African genome variation project shapes medical genetics in Africa. Nature 517(7534):327–332. https://doi.org/10.1038/nature13997
10. Walter K, Min JL, Huang J et al (2015) The UK10K project identifies rare variants in health and disease. Nature 526(7571):82–90. https://doi.org/10.1038/nature14962
11. Ma C, Blackwell T, Boehnke M et al (2013) Recommended joint and meta-analysis strategies for case-control association testing of single low-count variants. Genet Epidemiol 37 (6):539–550. https://doi.org/10.1002/gepi.21742
12. Browning BL, Browning SR (2009) A unified approach to genotype imputation and haplotype-phase inference for large data sets of trios and unrelated individuals. Am J Hum Genet 84(2):210–223. https://doi.org/10.1016/j.ajhg.2009.01.005
13. Fuchsberger C, Abecasis GR, Hinds DA (2015) minimac2: faster genotype imputation. Bioinformatics 31(5):782–784. https://doi.org/10.1093/bioinformatics/btu704
14. Howie B, Marchini J, Stephens M (2011) Genotype imputation with thousands of genomes. G3 (Bethesda) 1(6):457–470. https://doi.org/10.1534/g3.111.001198

Chapter 4

Genome-Wide Association Studies

Abbas Dehghan

Abstract

Genetic association studies have made a major contribution to our understanding of the genetics of complex disorders over the last 10 years through genome-wide association studies (GWAS). In this chapter, we review the key concepts that underlie the GWAS approach. We will describe the "common disease, common variant" theory, and will review how we finally afforded to capture the common variance in genome to make GWAS possible. Finally, we will go over technical aspects of GWAS such as genotype imputation, epidemiologic designs, analysis methods, and considerations such as genomic inflation, multiple testing, and replication.

Key words Genome-wide association studies, Genetic association, Genotype imputation, Linkage disequilibrium

1 Introduction

It has long been known that the risk of complex disorders such as cardiovascular diseases, type 2 diabetes, or cancer is highly affected by the genetic background of the individual, however, the exact genetic structures that convey the risk were unknown. Researchers have applied different approaches in recent decades to pinpoint the genes that predispose individuals to complex disorders. In this chapter we focus on the genome-wide association study or GWAS, a novel approach that has revolutionized the study of genetics of complex disorders. This approach examines the whole genome in an agnostic system for regions where DNA sequence variations regulate a complex trait or affect the risk of the disease.

The findings of GWAS could have several implications. It could either be used to identify individuals who are at a higher risk of the disease or to shed light on pathways that underlie complex disease. The latter not only enhances our knowledge of the disease, but may also contribute to developing novel medications. Alternatively, this information could be used in the context of precision medicine to tailor the medication for better effects or less adverse effects. In this

Evangelos Evangelou (ed.), *Genetic Epidemiology: Methods and Protocols*, Methods in Molecular Biology, vol. 1793, https://doi.org/10.1007/978-1-4939-7868-7_4,

chapter, we will briefly review the technology, study design, and analytical methods that are used in GWAS.

2 Genetic Association Versus Linkage Study

2.1 Genetic Variants

The genome or the totality of the genetic material of a cell varies from individual to individual. The variations could be existence of an excess piece of DNA (insertion), missing pieces (delete), or single nucleotide mutations [1]. When mutations are present in more than 1% of the population, they are called single nucleotide polymorphism or SNP. However, in recent years, mutations are referred to as rare or low-frequency SNPs in the literature. Given their simplicity, abundance, and dispersion across the whole genome, SNPs were the first and yet are the most common type of variation that is studied in GWAS. Insertion and deletions (Indel)s are also studied in recent GWAS next to SNPs.

2.2 Common or Rare Variants

Variants have different frequencies. Some are present in a small proportion of the population and some others are very common. There are also private variants that are only identified in one individual. So far millions of variants are discovered in humans and sequencing further individuals will discover more novel variants. The novel variants, of course, are likely to be rare variants in general population. However, any rare or low-frequency variant may be common in a specific ethnic group or an isolated population.

The frequency of the variants is commonly expressed by minor allele frequency (MAF). The fraction indicates the abundance of the less common variant in the pool of alleles in the reference population. For instance, a MAF of 0.3 means that 30% of the alleles carried by the populations are the one that is less common in the reference population. The frequencies could be different in study population than the reference population. As a result, MAF in a sample may sometimes exceed 0.5.

2.3 Common Disease Common Variant Hypothesis

Common disease, common variant hypothesis, is one of the foundations of GWAS. This hypothesis states that common disorders are likely to be influenced by common genetic variants. On one hand, given that common diseases occur in a large proportion of the population, the causal genes could not be rare. On the other hand, the causal variants should, in comparison with rare variants, have a small effect. Otherwise, nearly all who have inherited the deleterious variants should develop the disease which is in contrast to the multifactorial nature of the complex diseases. For instance, a single high penetrance variant with a MAF of 0.30 should lead to a disease that happens in nearly 30% of the population. Therefore, common variants by definition cannot have high penetrance. However, genetic studies have shown that complex disorders such as cardiovascular diseases and cancer are highly heritable. The conclusion is that common diseases are caused by multiple genetic variants.

In recent decade GWAS has tested the common disease, common variant hypothesis for a wide range of traits and diseases [2]. Although the variants that are identified are continuously increasing, the small effect of genetic variants has led to small percentage of variance explained by these variants. This supports the common disease common variant hypothesis, although this does not exclude the role of rare variants in developing common diseases next to common variants.

2.4 Genome-Wide Approaches for Monogenic and Complex Disorders

Genome-wide search for genetic risk factors has been done in two methods: genome-wide linkage study (GWLS) and GWAS. GWLS looks for physical segments of the genome that is linked to a given trait or disease. It compares the inheritance of traits or diseases with inheritance of DNA segments in a pedigree. GWLS was applied successfully to identify rare genetic variants that contribute to monogenic disorders or highly penetrant traits. It was also applied to multifactorial traits and diseases to map their regulating locus. Nevertheless, it had limited success when it was applied to common disorders like coronary artery disease, asthma, diabetes, or psychiatric disorders. Therefore, it was concluded that the genetic architecture of common disorders is different from rare disorders and will require different investigation approaches [3].

GWAS, however, is based on use of a large number of SNPs or other markers that are genotyped in known linkage regions and is studied in unrelated individuals. Compared to GWLS, GWAS have several advantages. First, it has a better genetic resolution. The resolution is in centimorgan range for GWLS and in kilobases for GWAS. Therefore, GWAS pinpoints the causal gene in a better way. In fact, the most significant SNP in GWAS is either the causal variant or is located in its vicinity. GWLS, however, highlights a large region that may include up to hundreds of genes. GLWS are also difficult to be used for late-onset diseases. A researcher should find family pedigrees including a couple of generations. However, GWAS could be applied to general populations with different age distributions. Finally, GWLS is the most efficient when one gene is inherited in a family but when it comes to multiple genes in general population, GWAS provide a better statistical power [4].

In conclusion, the most efficient approach to study genetics of a trait or disorder depends on the magnitude of effect and allele frequency of the variants that will be used. The variants with large effects are not likely to be common. Common variants with small effect are the ones that are targeted by GWAS and rare variants with large effect are best studied by GWLS. Rare variants with small effects are a real challenge to study and are not investigated much in recent years. Sequencing in large sample sizes may be an approach for this type of genetic effects.

3 Capturing the Common Variation in Genome

3.1 Linkage Disequilibrium

Genetic variants that are located on a chromosome are inherited together. However, this tie is broken apart through generations by genetic recombination. Genetic recombination involves the pairing of homologous chromosomes during meiosis. In a population with random mating, recombination events decrease the correlation between genetic variants and eventually all alleles in the population become independent. When two variants are inherited independent of each other, they are called "in linkage equilibrium." Likewise, the correlation that may remain between two variants is referred to as "linkage disequilibrium" or LD. LD describes the degree to which a genetic variant is inherited together with another genetic variant in a population over time. LD between two genetic variants could be different from one population to another depending on the distance from the founder population, and mating patterns. For instance, the genome of African and African-descent populations, due to being the oldest human population, have gone through more recombination events and therefore include smaller correlated regions compared to other ethnic groups such as Caucasians or Asians.

The level of linkage disequilibrium between two genes is measured by various indices [5]. The coefficient of linkage disequilibrium (D) is defined as

$$D = P_{\mathrm{AB}} - (P_{\mathrm{A}} \times P_{\mathrm{B}})$$

where P_{A} and P_{B} are the allele frequency at two loci and PAB is the frequency of A and B occurring together (AB haplotype). D is a difficult coefficient to interpret since its range of possible values depends on the frequencies of the two alleles. As an alternative, D' is defined as D divided by the maximum difference between the observed and expected allele frequencies ($D' = D/D_{\min}$). D' varies between -1 and 1. A D' of 1 or -1 means that there is no evidence for recombination between the markers. If allele frequencies are the same, the two variants give the same information and could be used as surrogates for each other. A D' of 0 indicates that the two variants are inherited independent of each other (in perfect equilibrium).

An alternative to D' is the correlation coefficient (r^2) that is expressed as

$$r^2 = {}^{D}\Big/\sqrt{P_{\mathrm{A}}(1-P_{\mathrm{A}})P_{\mathrm{B}}(1-P_{\mathrm{B}})}$$

Correlation coefficient or r^2 is between 0 and 1. Higher values indicate that the genetic variants are highly correlated and in essence include the same genetic variance. The implication of a high LD for genetic studies is that genotyping and study of only one of the variants may be enough and the second variant includes redundant information.

Given that LD is usually high between close by variants in a region, the genome could be broken down into pieces with high LD. These pieces are called LD blocks. By use of this concept, one can study a limited number of variants and yet capture the whole genetic variation of the genome. The short listed genetic variants that are used in such an approach are called "tagging" variants.

3.2 Human HapMap Project

In order to achieve a shortlist of SNPs that could represent the whole genome, we needed a comprehensive set of information on the LD pattern of the genome. The HapMap international Project was an effort to draw the inheritance pattern of LD blocks in different ethnic groups and to interrogate the common variation in human genome [6]. The project conducted whole genome sequencing techniques to identify common SNPs and characterize their LD pattern. It was done primarily in a number of European descent populations, the Yoruba population of African origin, Han Chinese individuals from Beijing, and Japanese individuals from Tokyo. The data from the HapMap project indicated that more than 80% of the common variation in human genome could be captured by studying approximately 500,000–1,000,000 SNPs across the genome. The first wave of the GWAS were based on nearly 2,500,000 SNPs that were introduced by the HapMap project. Later, other sequencing projects such as the 1000 Genomes project or local sequencing efforts were used as a backbone for GWAS.

Although the HapMap project played a crucial role in making GWAS possible, its data browser is not available since June 2016. This is mainly due to the fact that more recent projects such as the 1000 Genomes project are becoming the standard for research in population genetics and genomics.

3.3 Aiming for Indirect Associations

GWAS were aiming to look up the whole genome for variants that modify the physiology of human body and regulate a trait or affect the risk of a disease. To this end, one should take a challenging and exhaustive effort of studying all genetic variants across the genome. However, the shortlist of SNPs provided by projects such as HapMap allowed us to study the association of such biologically functional variants even if the variant was not present in the shortlist. The LD between the HapMap chosen SNP and the functional variant allowed indirect examination of the association between the variant and the trait or disease of interest [7]. Although this approach increases the coverage of the genome, one should be careful when it comes to interpreting the results of a GWAS. The identified SNPs in GWAS are in most cases not the main functional variant that regulates the trait or causes the disease. It is in fact a tagging SNP that is in high LD with the functional variant in the region.

4 How Did We Afford to Cover the Whole Genome?

4.1 Genotyping Technologies

Although the HapMap project introduced a short list of few hundred thousand SNPs to cover the common variance of the genome, genotyping so many SNPs with low-throughput methods that was available in 1990s was a real challenge. In fact, the availability of microarray technology for high-throughput genotyping with a reasonable pricing gave birth to GWAS. Most of genotyping arrays are manufactured by two companies, Illumina (San Diego, CA) and Affymetrix (Santa Clara, CA). Illumina and Affymetrix use two different platforms. The first generations of these arrays were mainly designed for European descent populations. Therefore, their coverage of the common variation was better in Caucasians than in Asians or African descent populations [8].

4.2 Imputations

When genome-wide association studies became a possibility, it was soon clear that the sample sizes that are available at every center are not large enough to address the small effects of common variants for complex disorders and traits. Therefore, studies started to form consortia to combine their data in meta-analyses. One major challenge, however, was the differences between platforms. This meant that every study had a different set of SNPs and the overlapping SNPs were limited. It was known, however, that once the LD patterns are clear, the alleles for untyped variants could be estimated based on genotyped variants. This process was named genotype imputation since it estimates the missing variants that are not genotyped by the genotyping array. In early days, HapMap was the only reference panel that was available and the data imputed based on this reference panel gave birth to the first wave of GWAS. HapMap included nearly 2,500,000 SNPs and this set were the list of SNPs that all studies imputed their data. A few years later, the 1000 Genomes project provided an alternative imputation platform including a much larger set of SNPs as well as Indels [9]. Recently, the Haplotype Reference Consortium (HRC) has collected a large reference panel of human haplotypes by combining sequencing data from various populations. The HRC reference panels include a comprehensive bank of genetic variants and their haplotypes which not only increases the number of variants that could be imputed but also adds to the accuracy of the genotype imputation (especially for low-frequency variants) [10].

Genotype imputation is based on information provided by haplotypes. In the first step, the variants are linked together based on the most common haplotypes (phasing). Second, the haplotypes are compared to the reference panel. The haplotypes available at the reference panel are normally denser and include more variants compared to the genotyped data. The missing variants in the study population are filled out using the data from the reference panel. In many instances, however, several haplotypes from the reference panel matches the data set. Several solutions could be applied in such instances. A simple method is to use the most likely allele. Such data is called "best guess" imputed data and is expressed as discrete numbers as 0, 1, or 2 (number of the coded alleles). An alternative is to form the data as a combination of the number of alleles and their probabilities, thus take the uncertainty into account. This data is expressed on a continuous scale from 0 to 2 and called "dosage data."

Every population should primarily be imputed using a reference panel with a similar ethnic background. However, a cosmopolitan reference panel that includes haplotypes from various ethnic groups may also improve the imputation quality since every individual may carry small haplotypes from a far ancestor from a different ethnic group.

5 Epidemiologic Design of GWAS

GWAS could be done in different epidemiologic designs depending on the characteristics of the phenotype and data. Phenotypes could either be quantitative (e.g., height) or categorical (often dichotomous, e.g., diseased/healthy). Quantitative traits could also be broken down into categorical variables (e.g., recoding BMI into normal weight, overweight, and obese), however, this is not recommended from a statistical perspective since information is lost due to the categorization and statistical power is reduced. Quantitative traits could be studied in a cross-sectional design. Given that genetic data is constant over time. It is yet acceptable if DNA samples were collected in a different round of the study than phenotype measurement. Nevertheless, the potential effect of survival between the two rounds on the results, if relevant, should not be overlooked. Binary outcomes are commonly studied in a case-control design. Such designs are popular since they allow the investigator to collect a large number of diseased cases from disease registries, hospital admissions, or large epidemiologic studies. A relevant set of individuals are used as controls. Such designs, however, mostly rely on cross-sectional identification of the diseased cases which are called "prevalent cases." The downside of using prevalent cases is that they do not represent all those who have developed the disease in a population. For instance, prevalent cases of coronary artery disease do not include cases of sudden cardiac death or under represent those who have passed away shortly after MI due to arrhythmias. If the survival after the disease is affected by genetic factors, a GWAS on prevalent cases could be misleading. In such an instance, the alleles that are associated with a better survival after disease could be mistakenly picked up as risk allele for the disease since they are enriched in prevalent cases. This is known as

Neyman's bias or incidence-prevalence bias [11]. To avoid this bias, a prospective setting suits the study best to ensure that a representative set of cases are included in the study.

6 Statistical Analysis of GWAS

6.1 Genetic Model

One of the first assumptions that should be made for a GWAS is the genetic inheritance model. Single variants could affect the phenotype or disease in an additive, recessive/dominant, or multiplicative model. The additive model assumes that there is a linear uniform increase in the risk by adding further copies of the risk allele. In GWAS the additive model is most commonly used model since the exact inheritance model is not known the variants and additive model has reasonable power to detect variants that have additive or dominant effect [12]. The power of this approach, however, is limited if the inheritance model is recessive. Moreover, applying an additive model does not allow identifying the underlying genetic model. Some GWAS examine the best inheritance model fit of their findings in a secondary analysis. Alternatively, some studies repeat their analysis based on several inheritance models but adjust their significance threshold for the number of tests.

6.2 Univariate Analysis

The main analysis in GWAS is normally a regression model. Depending on the nature of the phenotype, a linear, logistic, or Cox regression model is applied. Quantitative phenotypes are commonly analyzed using linear regression models. The genetic variants are the independent factors and the quantitative trait is the dependent variable in the model. Normal distribution is not a strict prerequisite for a linear regression model. However, transformations are used when the phenotype is severely skewed. Although transformation will make the beta estimates difficult to interpret, it helps in avoiding the results to be driven by outliers. Dichotomous phenotypes such as diseases are analyzed either using logistic regression models or if time to event data is provided, a Cox regression model.

GWAS are mainly done primarily in an age and sex adjusted model. Further adjustment, if applicable, could be done for study site or population substructure. Given that genetic variants are inherited randomly, confounding by environmental risk factors is not a major issue. However, confounding by population substructure should be evaluated and adjusted. Every population may be composed of people with different ancestral backgrounds and therefore allele frequencies could vary across subpopulations. When the phenotype or the risk of disease is different among these subpopulations, the test statistics will be inflated across the genome. To illustrate this inflation QQ-plots are used to plot the distribution of the observed test statistics against the distribution of the test statistics under a null hypothesis. The deviation of the observed test statistics could be measured and expressed as λ. This index is equal to 1, when there is no genomic inflation. Measures above 1.05 are commonly unacceptable in HapMap imputed data and are dealt with either by adjusting for principle components representing population stratification in the regression model or correcting the test statistics for the genomic inflation.

6.3 Multivariate Adjustments

Although the findings in an age and sex adjusted model are not likely to be driven by confounding bias, researchers are sometimes interested in examining the effect of adjustment for certain factors mainly, aiming to examine their potential mediatory role. It should be noted that adjustment comes at the cost of higher degrees of freedom and may negatively affect the statistical power.

6.4 GWIS

Next to the single variant analysis, researchers are sometimes interested in studying the interaction effect between genetic variants or between the variants and environmental risk factors. Such an analysis for the whole genome is called genome-wide interaction analysis or GWIS. Although valid interaction could be valuable and may have clinical and public health implications, the very small interaction effects have so far hampered the efforts to identify robust interactions. Significant, validated, and robust interactions are very scarce. Applying GWIS to study gene-gene interaction has an extra challenge. Given that every GWAS includes hundreds of thousands of genetic variants, the interaction between all variants will include billions of tests which is computationally exhaustive and statistically underpowered. To prune the list of SNPs some investigators use single variant analysis results and pick up the most significant variants, presumably with an arbitrary significance threshold. However, this approach has the downside of overlooking variants that are purely epistatic, i.e., the effect is only shown in the presence of a certain allele of the other interaction genetic variant. Such associations are likely to be overlooked in single variant analysis. Another approach is to limit the analysis to a specific pathway or make a short list of the variants based on their biological relevance.

6.5 Conditional Analysis

In GWAS, commonly, every identified locus is represented by the most significant genetic variant in a genomic region. It is assumed that either the other genetic variants are showing a signal due to their correlation with the sentinel variant or the sentinel SNP is capturing the largest amount of variance from the functional variant in the region. In practice, however, there could be multiple causal variants and the variants in the array could capture different fractions of the variance of the causal variant. Therefore, multiple variants could represent different associations that are independent of each other. Identifying independent variants in a region could help to increase the proportion of variance that could be explained by the genetic variants.

Conditional analysis is the conventional analytical method to identify independent associations in one locus. To this end, the analysis is repeated for all variants in that locus, adjusted for the sentinel SNP. If the statistical power is large enough, further genetic variants could be identified. This procedure should be conducted over and over to identify further independent associations. Although this procedure is straightforward when it is done for a single study, it would be administratively cumbersome and time consuming when a large meta-analysis of summary statistics is done. The researcher needs to contact the participating studies to conduct the analysis, collect the data, run the meta-analysis, and perform the cycle over and over to make sure that no further signals are left. An alternative approach is introduced where summary-level statistical data and a LD reference panel is used to identify multivariant loci. The method is implemented in GCTA statistical software that is nowadays used for this purpose [13, 14].

6.6 Multiple Testing

Statistical tests are considered significant in classic epidemiology when the p value is smaller than 0.05. This threshold, however, should be adjusted when the hypothesis is examined using multiple tests since the chances of false positive or spurious findings increase by the number of tests. Therefore, adjustment for multiple testing is very crucial to the validity of the findings. Although conservative approaches toward multiple testing could ensure the validity of the findings, an ultimate approach should not hamper the statistical power of the study to identify genetic variants with small effects.

The most commonly applied method to deal with multiple testing is the Bonferroni correction where the significance threshold is divided by the number of tests. In GWAS, millions of variants are tested to identify the one that is associated with the phenotype of interest. In a GWAS where 500,000 variants were genotyped, the significance threshold will be $0.05/500{,}000 = 1 \times 10^{-7}$. The HapMap imputed GWAS, however, are commonly using 5×10^{-8} as the genome-wide significant threshold. This threshold is justified based on an assumption that the contemporary arrays include correlated variants and effectively include one million tests [15]. Although GWAS based on extended reference panels such as 1000 Genomes should consider more stringent significance threshold, many of them are yet using 5×10^{-8}.

An alternative approach to take care of multiple testing is false discovery rate (FDR). The FDR estimates the rate of type I error and enables the investigator to set a threshold where the proportion of false positive results are under a certain limit. In practice it is very common to choose an FDR of 5%. This means that 5% of the associations above this threshold are likely to be false positive (null hypothesis wrongly rejected) [16].

A third option is to perform permutation. To this end, the phenotype of interest is shuffled hundreds or thousands of times across the population to produce databases where the genotype and phenotype are distributed similar to the original dataset but they are not associated with each other. The analysis is repeated each time and the test statistics represent an empirical distribution of the test statistics under null hypothesis. The test statistic is compared to the null distribution and significance is deduced. Permutation could be done by several statistical packages including PLINK which is popular in running GWAS [17].

6.7 Replication

GWAS are hypothesis free studies that examine the whole genome in an agnostic approach. The function of GWAS could therefore be considered hypothesis generating. To test this hypothesis, the association should be validated in an independent sample. This step is known as replication. Although the value of the replication for GWAS findings is widely appreciated, there are inconsistencies in identifying the associations that deserve replication, defining a proper replication study and criterion for refuting the finding based on the replication results.

Any replication effort should be done under the same circumstances as in the discovery. The inheritance model, definition of the phenotype, and covariate adjustment should be identical. One major challenge, however, is to provide sufficient sample size. Associations are commonly stronger in GWAS than replication studies, a phenomenon known as the winner's curse that complicates the sample size estimation for replication studies [18]. Lack of replication in a small population set is always difficult to interpret. It is not possible to find out whether the association is absent due to the false positive association in discovery panel or lack of power in the replication set.

The replication study should also be done in an identical sample that is independent of the discovery set. Once the finding is replicated in a similar population, the association could be extended to other ethnic groups by replicating it in those populations. Some studies use the latter both as a mean for replication and generalization. Although replicated associations could be considered replicated and generalized, lack of association, for instance in a different ethnic group, is difficult to interpret. It may be due to a difference in LD pattern across populations or false positive finding in the discovery panel.

7 Concluding Note

It is no exaggeration to say that GWAS have revolutionized the field of human genetics. Thousands of genetic loci are introduced in association with various complex traits and disorders in recent decade using GWAS. Many of the findings refer to pathways and mechanisms that were not in the radar due to our limited biological knowledge. The discoveries are expected to continue as larger sample sizes and better imputation platforms are becoming available. At the same time, next generation sequencing seems to move GWAS one step forward by providing a comprehensive DNA sequence readout of the genome. Despite this advancement, genotyping technologies are likely to keep their role as a valid technique for GWAS due to their cheaper prices, larger available sample sizes, and simpler analytical methods. In fact, sequencing further individuals may improve current imputation reference panels and help the microarray genotyping technology as a rival for sequencing technologies by advancing the imputation quality of low-frequency variants.

References

1. 1000 Genomes Project Consortium, Abecasis GR, Altshuler D et al (2010) A map of human genome variation from population-scale sequencing. Nature 467(7319):1061–1073. https://doi.org/10.1038/nature09534
2. Hindorff LA, Sethupathy P, Junkins HA et al (2009) Potential etiologic and functional implications of genome-wide association loci for human diseases and traits. Proc Natl Acad Sci U S A 106(23):9362–9367. https://doi.org/10.1073/pnas.0903103106
3. Hirschhorn JN, Daly MJ (2005) Genome-wide association studies for common diseases and complex traits. Nat Rev Genet 6(2):95–108. https://doi.org/10.1038/nrg1521
4. Risch N, Merikangas K (1996) The future of genetic studies of complex human diseases. Science 273(5281):1516–1517
5. Guo SW (1997) Linkage disequilibrium measures for fine-scale mapping: a comparison. Hum Hered 47(6):301–314
6. International HapMap Consortium (2005) A haplotype map of the human genome. Nature 437(7063):1299–1320. https://doi.org/10.1038/nature04226
7. Wang DG, Fan JB, Siao CJ et al (1998) Large-scale identification, mapping, and genotyping of single-nucleotide polymorphisms in the human genome. Science 280 (5366):1077–1082
8. Li M, Li C, Guan W (2008) Evaluation of coverage variation of SNP chips for genome-wide association studies. Eur J Hum Genet 16 (5):635–643. https://doi.org/10.1038/sj.ejhg.5202007
9. 1000 Genomes Project Consortium, Abecasis GR, Auton A et al (2012) An integrated map of genetic variation from 1,092 human genomes. Nature 491(7422):56–65. https://doi.org/10.1038/nature11632
10. McCarthy S, Das S, Kretzschmar W et al (2016) A reference panel of 64,976 haplotypes for genotype imputation. Nat Genet 48 (10):1279–1283. https://doi.org/10.1038/ng.3643
11. Hill G, Connelly J, Hebert R et al (2003) Neyman's bias re-visited. J Clin Epidemiol 56 (4):293–296
12. Lettre G, Lange C, Hirschhorn JN (2007) Genetic model testing and statistical power in population-based association studies of quantitative traits. Genet Epidemiol 31(4):358–362. https://doi.org/10.1002/gepi.20217
13. Yang J, Lee SH, Goddard ME et al (2011) GCTA: a tool for genome-wide complex trait analysis. Am J Hum Genet 88(1):76–82. https://doi.org/10.1016/j.ajhg.2010.11.011
14. Yang J, Ferreira T, Morris AP et al (2012) Conditional and joint multiple-SNP analysis of GWAS summary statistics identifies additional variants influencing complex traits. Nat Genet 44(4):369–375., S361-363. https://doi.org/10.1038/ng.2213
15. Pe'er I, Yelensky R, Altshuler D et al (2008) Estimation of the multiple testing burden for genomewide association studies of nearly all common variants. Genet Epidemiol 32 (4):381–385. https://doi.org/10.1002/gepi.20303

16. van den Oord EJ (2008) Controlling false discoveries in genetic studies. American journal of medical genetics part B, neuropsychiatric genetics: the official publication of the international society of. Psychiatr Genet 147B (5):637–644. https://doi.org/10.1002/ajmg.b.30650

17. Purcell S, Neale B, Todd-Brown K et al (2007) PLINK: a tool set for whole-genome association and population-based linkage analyses. Am J Hum Genet 81(3):559–575. https://doi.org/10.1086/519795

18. Zollner S, Pritchard JK (2007) Overcoming the winner's curse: estimating penetrance parameters from case-control data. Am J Hum Genet 80(4):605–615. https://doi.org/10.1086/512821

Chapter 5

Assessing Rare Variation in Complex Traits

Karoline Kuchenbaecker and Emil Vincent Rosenbaum Appel

Abstract

While genome-wide association studies have been very successful in identifying associations of common genetic variants with many different traits, the rarer frequency spectrum of the genome has not yet been comprehensively explored. Technological developments increasingly lift restrictions to access rare genetic variation. Dense reference panels enable improved genotype imputation for rarer variants in studies using DNA microarrays. Moreover, the decreasing cost of next generation sequencing makes whole exome and genome sequencing increasingly affordable for large samples. Large-scale efforts based on sequencing, such as ExAC, 100,000 Genomes, and TopMed, are likely to significantly advance this field.

The main challenge in evaluating complex trait associations of rare variants is statistical power. The choice of population should be considered carefully because allele frequencies and linkage disequilibrium structure differ between populations. Genetically isolated populations can have favorable genomic characteristics for the study of rare variants.

One strategy to increase power is to assess the combined effect of multiple rare variants within a region, known as aggregate testing. A range of methods have been developed for this. Model performance depends on the genetic architecture of the region of interest.

Key words Low frequency variants, Rare variants, Sequencing, Association study, Aggregate test, Burden test, Isolated population

1 Background

The discovery of genetic variants contributing to the heritability of complex traits has boomed in recent years. Hundreds of associations, mostly of common variants with small effects, have been identified for outcomes such as anthropometric measures, blood biomarkers, and common diseases. However, rare variants are likely to play an important role in the genetics of many of these traits. Identifying variants with large effects could be particularly useful from a clinical perspective. In the context of disease, the accuracy of predicted risks of carriers of such variants can significantly improve. Furthermore, trait associations with such variants could lead to important biological insights and novel treatments for diseases.

Evangelos Evangelou (ed.), *Genetic Epidemiology: Methods and Protocols*, Methods in Molecular Biology, vol. 1793, https://doi.org/10.1007/978-1-4939-7868-7_5, © Springer Science+Business Media, LLC, part of Springer Nature 2018

A number of empirical findings demonstrate the importance of rare variants and illustrate their clinical potential. Several of these success stories relate to lipid traits. For example, targeted sequencing of data from the Dallas Heart Study revealed an association between low-density lipoprotein (LDL) cholesterol and rare nonsense mutations in *PCSK9* [1]. This gene encodes a protein that is involved in the regulation of LDL cholesterol levels. These LDL-decreasing mutations were also shown to lead to a significant reduction in risk of coronary heart disease (CHD) [2]. Monoclonal antibodies targeting this molecule were developed to reduce CHD risk and these lowered LDL levels beyond what could be achieved by statins alone [3, 4]. As another example, a study using samples from a cosmopolitan UK population [5], as well as studies in isolated populations [6–8], identified several rare variants in the apolipoprotein C-III (APOC3) gene affecting levels of triglycerides in blood with evidence for a cardioprotective effect of these alleles [8–10]. An antisense oligonucleotide was developed to lower APOC3 levels and it also led to decreased triglycerides in patients with high-baseline levels [11].

One of the main technical challenges for the discovery of rare variant associations has been the limited coverage of rare variation by DNA microarrays commonly used in genome-wide association studies (GWAS) (*see* Subheading 3). However, the decreasing cost of whole exome and whole genome sequencing make these technologies increasingly affordable for larger sample sizes (Table 1). The first large genome sequencing project was the 1000 Genomes Project [12], followed by the UK10K Project [13]. These efforts have significantly advanced the field of genomics. Large numbers of additional variants were discovered and insights into population genetics gained. These projects enabled hundreds of other studies to operate in a very cost-effective way by using DNA microarray genotyping and carrying out genotype imputation with the haplotypes from the sequencing efforts as reference panels. Recognizing the potential of genomics for medicine, governments in the UK and USA seized the opportunity of more affordable sequencing. The precision medicine initiative, launched by US President Barack Obama in 2015, aims to advance personalized medicine through the Trans-Omics for Precision Medicine (TOPMed) programme which involves whole-genome sequencing of 62,000 individuals, possibly up to 100,000 at a later stage [14]. The focus of this programme is on heart, lung, blood, and sleep disorders. There is also a large-scale initiative in the UK, the 100,000 Genomes Project [15]. It involves whole-genome sequencing of germline and tumor DNA of 25,000 cancer patients and also of DNA of 50,000 individuals to study rare diseases. The aim of this programme is to implement genomic medicine in routine clinical practice for rare diseases and cancer [16]. The maximum potential of such initiatives can be realized when data from different sequencing projects are combined. This has recently been done for whole exome sequencing studies. The Exome Aggregation Consortium (ExAC) project, a collection of exome data from more than 60,000 individuals, yielded important findings with implications for the pathogenicity of mutations in coding regions [17]. These large sequencing projects could significantly advance our understanding of the role of rare genetic variation.

In the next section, we discuss differences between populations with respect to variant frequency and linkage disequilibrium patterns and how these affect design considerations for studying rare variants. The subsequent part is devoted to the measurement of rare variants and compares DNA microarray genotyping with DNA sequencing technologies. The final part describes different statistical analysis techniques to assess trait associations of rare variants. The focus lies on aggregate tests that assess the combined effect of multiple variants in order to improve statistical power.

While rare structural variants play an important role for some complex traits, this chapter only covers single nucleotide variants. The term "low frequency" is used for variants with minor allele frequencies (MAF) between 1% and 5% and "rare" for variants with MAF less than 1%.

2 Population-Specific Differences in Genetic Variation

Genetic diversity and linkage disequilibrium (LD) structure differ between populations. Some alleles are common in one and rare in another population and some variants are only present in some populations. It is vital to put consideration into the choice of population for a given study, especially for rare variant association studies. Differences in LD structure mean that tagging properties of variants on GWAS arrays can differ greatly between populations resulting in differences in the accuracy with which the signal of a variant can be captured. Variant frequency and imputation accuracy affect statistical power to detect an association. The effect of a variant might also differ between populations due to different environments or epistasis. Several genetic associations with complex traits were found to be population-specific, such as the association of the *MTNR1B* locus with glucose metabolism in European populations but not in East Asian populations [18].

A number of factors shape the genetic make-up of a population including population size, historical bottlenecks, and natural selection [19]. The effects of a bottleneck are long lasting. After a bottleneck the genetic make-up of the population is composed exclusively of the genetic variation from the lineages that survived the bottleneck while some variants present in the original population are lost. When the population starts expanding again, the variation from the surviving lineages will remain frequent to a much higher extent than variation introduced into the population after the bottleneck. The underlying LD pattern in the surviving linages will be maintained in the expanding population, only broken up by new recombination events [19].

As a consequence, genetic diversity and LD structure are markedly different between Sub-Saharan African and European populations, for example, with higher levels of genetic diversity in the African populations and longer spans of LD in the European populations [20]. European populations share a historic bottleneck, the migration out of Africa, while the populations of Africa consist of several smaller populations, without a common historic event, that continuously admixed, splitting up the LD blocks and allowing for more genetic diversity [20].

2.1 The Special Case of Isolated Populations

An isolated population is a small population that has undergone a bottleneck in its history and remained isolated from other populations after the bottleneck. Due to the genetic drift some variants have risen in frequency and there are higher levels of relatedness and longer LD blocks compared to non-isolated population [21]. Greater environmental and phenotypic homogeneity are often observed as well. Taken together, this gives rise to greater statistical power to detect associations of alleles that have drifted to higher frequency, which makes isolated populations particularly attractive for studying rare variants. However, note that in isolated populations only a subset of the rare variants seen in the general population, from which the isolate was derived, will be present, limiting the association testing to those variants.

A number of recent locus discoveries in population isolates have highlighted these properties [7, 22–25]. As an example, the Greenlandic population is a small isolated population with high degrees of relatedness, large LD blocks, fewer rare variants in total, but with higher allele frequency in the average for observed variants [26]. These features were exploited by Moltke et al. who found an association between the nonsense p.Arg684Ter variant in *TBC1D4* and postprandial hyperglycemia, impaired glucose tolerance, and risk of type II diabetes [27]. This variant is extremely rare in cosmopolitan populations (only one allele was found in the 1092 individuals of the 1000 Genome project), but common in the Greenlandic population (MAF = 17%). To observe the same number of alleles seen in the Greenlandic cohort in the 1000 Genomes populations, one would have had to sample over 400,000 individuals. This highlights important considerations regarding the study of rare variants in isolated populations. Rare variants can rise to higher frequencies leading to increased statistical power for discovery, but observed associations may be limited to the isolated population because the variant may not be present or may be extremely rare in other populations. This does not diminish the relevance of the locus discovery, however, as these findings can point to biological pathways involved in complex traits that would otherwise have been overlooked.

3 Genotyping Technologies and Rare Variants

Here, we discuss two types of genotyping technologies, DNA microarrays, and sequencing. We explore the pros and cons of applying these technologies when investigating rare variants. We further differentiate between whole exome sequencing (WES) and whole genome sequencing (WGS).

3.1 DNA Microarray Genotyping

DNA microarray genotyping, also known as chip genotyping, is a comparably cheap and versatile technology, with prices down to $50 per sample for a genome-wide chip. The technology has been widely used and advanced software has been designed to ease the workload of bioinformatics (Table 1).

DNA microarrays are based on known variants and use a calling algorithm based on clustering. Clustering is a method to automatically draw clusters around similar genotype calls, based on the intensity of the colored light used by the high-throughput microarray genotyping machine. Clustering is dependent on the total number of samples in each cluster. This means that the clustering algorithms perform best for common variants where the three clusters, homozygotes wild-type, heterozygote, and homozygote derived, are of similar size. Clustering often performs poorly when only a few samples can be gathered into one cluster which is the case for rare variants.

Genome-wide DNA microarrays are designed on the basis of tagging which exploits the fact that variants are inherited through

Table 1
Overview of essential features of different genotyping technologies

	GWAS Chip	Exome Chip	WES	Low depth WGS	High depth WGS
Region covered	Genome	Mostly exome	Exome	Genome	Genome
Discovery of novel variants	No	No	Yes	Yes	Yes
Bioinformatics and QC workload	Comparably low	Comparably low	Medium	Large	Large
Cost compared to of a full genome[a]	4%	6%	20%	30%	100%

WES whole exome sequencing; *WGS* whole genome sequencing
[a]The price of a genome ($1245 in October 2016) was estimated from [28]. The fraction represents an approximate estimation from prices in our laboratory

haplotypes. Variants are selected for inclusion on the chip in such a way that each LD block is represented. Tagging reduces the number of variants needed to adequately cover the majority of genetic variation down to thousands. Using genotype imputation one can then make use of the information contained in multiple typed variants to infer the genotypes of the variants missing from the array. This requires a reference panel of genomes that contain the variants missing on the chip, so that their relation to typed variants can be inferred. There are general GWAS chips that were designed to capture maximal genetic information with a limited number of variants. There are also custom arrays that were designed to target regions of the genome that are of interest to a specific disease or trait, such as the MetaboChip or OncoArray.

GWAS arrays generally have very good coverage of common genetic variation. However, rare variants are on average in lesser LD with other variants than common variants, resulting in lower coverage. In the context of single SNP association analysis, Yang et al. showed empirically that 81% of common and 25% of rare (MAF $\leq$ 1%) variation can be captured by the best tagging SNP using the CoreExome array in combination with imputation to the 1000 Genomes Project reference panel [29]. Recently, large reference panels from the UK10K study [14] and The Haplotype Reference Consortium [30] have become available and have increased the power to impute low frequency and rare variants from DNA microarrays [29].

There are several strategies to improve access to rare variation through chip genotyping. The Exome Chip [31] was designed to capture rare coding variants based on exome sequencing and has since been used to genotype millions of samples in different association studies which identified rare variant associations with various traits and diseases [26, 32, 33]. The Exome Chip offers a very cost-effective solution for large-scale genotyping of rare variants in exons (Table 1). However, the focus on rare exonic variants also represents an important limitation because the majority of complex trait associations identified so far were with noncoding variants. Furthermore, the array is targeted to European populations and is not suited to discover de novo mutations. For this, exome sequencing is a better option.

3.2 Next Generation Sequencing

Generally, genotype sequencing is more expensive than DNA microarrays, but has several advantages, especially in the context of low frequency and rare variants. Prices for whole exome sequencing are around three times cheaper than for whole genome sequencing at the time of writing this chapter. However, the costs have been decreasing continuously as the technology matures (Table 1). There are options to make sequencing more cost-effective. One common approach is to lower the depth, the average number of overlapping sequence fragments, called reads, mapped to the same position. Alternatively, one can opt to cover only specific regions, such as candidate genes.

Advanced software is available for researchers working with sequencing data. However, the bioinformatics workload involved in the quality control (QC) and analysis of sequencing data is more taxing than for DNA microarrays (Table 1).

3.2.1 Whole Exome Sequencing

Whole exome sequencing (WES) is a common strategy to investigate rare variants while keeping the cost down. This is done by limiting the regions that are sequenced to only the exome, without compromising the sequencing depth. This allows for accurate calling of rare variants in regions where they are likely to have an effect. WES also enables the detection of novel variants, which is not possible with DNA microarrays.

Focusing on the exome is motivated by the fact that variants found in an exon of a gene can be disruptive to the protein sequence and can therefore have an effect on the function of the protein. Mendelian diseases represent an extreme case of this where the disease can be caused by a single variant. Evolutionary conservation has therefore restricted the frequency of exonic variants with severe effects. WES is recommended when investigating the effects of rare variants on monogenic diseases. However, the majority of previously identified associations identified for complex traits were for noncoding variants [34].

3.2.2 Whole Genome Sequencing

Whole-genome sequencing (WGS) offers the potential to access the entire genetic information of an individual. It enables the discovery of novel variants, and makes it possible to access rare variants outside as well as within coding regions. As WGS covers the whole genome, it also enables the mapping of the underlying genetic architecture of complex polygenetic traits and the study of large structural variations, such as copy-number variations (CNV).

The amount of data generated per individual is considerably larger than for WES or chip genotyping. For example, in comparison with a chip-based GWAS, WGS requires about 1000 times more space to store the post-QC genotype information for chromosome 1 (~2 million WGS variants and ~ 58,000 GWAS tag-SNPs) for 1200 individuals (~13 GB, in a compressed VCF-file [12], for the WGS genotypes versus ~20 MB, in binary plink-files, for Omni Exome Chip genotypes of the same individuals). Processing of these files requires more computational resources, is more time consuming, and requires technical expertise. Furthermore, control of type I error requires consideration as a larger number of statistical tests are carried out (*see* Subheading 4.1.2).

The biggest drawback of WGS is its cost. It is considerably more expensive than WES and DNA Microarray genotyping.

While cost can be lowered by using a low read depth, this is at the expense of quality of the genotype calls. Using a low depth, e.g., an average depth of one read per position, known as 1 × WGS, will lead to more errors in calling variants. This can affect the discovery of novel variants in particular. One strategy to improve on this is by using imputation with large reference panels. A strict QC pipeline, especially when investigating novel rare variants, is needed to avoid type I errors. Overall, low depth WGS offers a cost effective method for studying rare variants.

While it is a significant advantage of WGS over WES to be able to access noncoding variation, the interpretation of the findings can be much less straightforward in comparison with associations of mutations affecting protein sequence. Understanding regulatory effects is complex and represents a very active area of research. One approach to ease interpretation of association findings is to use annotation scores that represent the likelihood of a given variant to affect protein expression. This has been done using different sources of information for coding as well as noncoding variants, e.g., for the Eigen [35], GWAVA [36], or CADD scores [37].

As the technology develops and genome annotations improve, the challenges involved in sequencing will become easier to meet, and WGS will become more feasible for increasingly large sample sets.

4 Association Analyses Methods for Rare Variants

4.1 Single Variant Association Tests

Fast and efficient estimation procedures have been developed to carry out association tests for large numbers of genetic variants. Most genetic association studies assume an additive genetic model where the SNP effect is estimated per copy of the effect allele. Usually, either linear or logistic regressions are used to estimate and test SNP associations for continuous or dichotomous outcomes, respectively. Increasingly, linear mixed models are applied which allow for the inclusion of relatives and account for possible population stratification by adjusting for genetic similarity between individuals. Details are described elsewhere is this book (*see* Chapters 3 and 4). These methods are also applicable to low frequency and rare variants. However, in case-control studies for variants with small numbers of carriers of the rare allele, the p-values of asymptotic logistic regression tests can be inaccurate [38, 39]. In this context, the minor allele count (MAC) has been established as a more useful metric than the minor allele frequency (MAF) because it is the absolute number of alleles that affects the performance of the test [38]. It has been shown that logistic regression tests can perform poorly for variants with MAC of less than 400 which can be used as a guidance for choosing an appropriate test.

One solution to the problem is to use Fisher's exact test instead which represents the gold standard to assess an association between categorical variables with small counts [40]. However, it is rarely used in this context because it cannot adjust for covariates. Alternative methods include Firth regression which is a penalized likelihood-based method that has been shown to perform well for rare variants [38, 41]. Permutation approaches have also been proposed [39]. Finally, a computationally efficient resampling approach for score tests has been developed [42].

4.1.1 Effect of Population Stratification, Non-normality and Outliers

Association testing for rare variants can be less robust to violations of assumptions. Rare variant association analyses (both single variant and aggregate tests) can be more strongly affected by non-normality, outliers and population stratification than association analyses for common variants [43]. With respect to outliers, it should be taken into account that extreme values of a trait could also be observed as the result of a rare high penetrance mutation, as seen in Mendelian diseases. Therefore, exclusions of outliers and variable transformations need to be considered carefully. Furthermore, association tests are particularly sensitive to population stratification because even small levels of stratification can lead to different frequencies of rare variants [44–49]. Therefore, quality control has to be particularly thorough. However, adjusting for fine-scale patterns of population stratification can be difficult with traditional methods when stratification for rare variants differs from that of common variants. For more details *see* Chapter 3.

4.1.2 Significance Threshold

For single variant association testing, multiple testing is an important consideration. In GWAS and sequencing studies, the associations of hundreds of thousands or even millions of genetic variants are evaluated, leading to a high multiple testing burden. Most of these variants are unlikely to causally affect the trait of interest so that the prior probability of association is small for each variant. The majority of previously published genetic association studies used an adjusted p-value threshold to account for the number of independent tests. Because many variants are in LD with each other and therefore not independent, a Bonferroni adjustment for the total number of variants tested would be too conservative. For chip-based genome-wide association studies, a p-value threshold of 5×10^{-8} has been established and is used routinely as it has been demonstrated to be valid for many GWAS arrays [50–52]. However, this threshold is not valid for whole exome or whole genome sequencing. The addition of many rare variants that tend to be in less strong LD with other variants leads to an increased number of independent tests.

The significance threshold for rare variant studies depends on the genotyping technology used, MAF threshold for variants considered (related to sequencing depth) and the population as that affects the genomic LD structure (*see* Subheading 2). For samples from cosmopolitan populations of European ancestry it has been demonstrated that a threshold of 1×10^{-8} for whole-genome and 3×10^{-7} for whole exome sequencing provide a level of adjustment for variants with MAF > 0.001 that is equivalent to the adjustment of the 5×10^{-8} threshold for common variants [53]. There is a higher burden of multiple testing for samples of African ancestry due to greater genetic diversity. Isolated populations on the other hand have longer shared haplotypes and therefore require adjustment for a smaller number of independent tests which renders them particularly suitable for the analysis of rare variation (*see* Subheading 2).

4.1.3 Statistical Power to Identify Novel Associations

Due to the high multiple testing burden, one of the main challenges for genetic association studies is to provide sufficient statistical power to detect novel associations with a trait of interest. For the identification of associations of low frequency and rare variants, statistical power is an even greater challenge. Factors impacting on the power to detect a trait association include frequency and effect size of a variant and how well it can be imputed in case it was not genotyped or sequenced directly [54]. As discussed in Subheading 3, in GWAS the average imputation accuracy for rare variants is lower than for common variants due to their reduced linkage disequilibrium. Therefore, the power to detect associations of rare variants can be low in GWAS.

Low frequency of variants can severely limit statistical power to find trait associations. For example, given a disease prevalence of 10%, a sample size of 10,000 cases and 10,000 controls, an OR of 1.2 per risk allele, the power to detect an association at $p < 5 \times 10^{-8}$ for a common variant with MAF = 0.4 is >98% whereas the power for a low frequency variant with MAF = 0.05 is <20%. As Fig. 1 demonstrates, given a moderate effect size (e.g., OR = 1.5) variants with MAF = 0.01 require more than 30,000 samples while variants with MAF = 0.001 require more than 300,000 samples to achieve sufficient discovery power (>80%). This demonstrates that in this setting, associations of rare variants are realistically discoverable only if the variants have moderate to large effect sizes.

Therefore, an important question concerns the effect size distribution of rare variants. If effect sizes are consistently small, then even large studies have limited power to detect rare variant associations. For many health-related complex traits it is now firmly established that almost all associated common variants have relatively small effects (i.e., OR < 1.5). Despite very high statistical power, common variants with large effects have not been discovered. Similar conclusions cannot be drawn with respect to the rare variants. As the power calculations demonstrate, larger sample might be needed to identify associations of rare variants. Moreover, all genetic association studies with more than 100,000 samples that have been published to-date used GWAS genotyping and had therefore limited coverage of rare variants (*see* Subheading 3). For

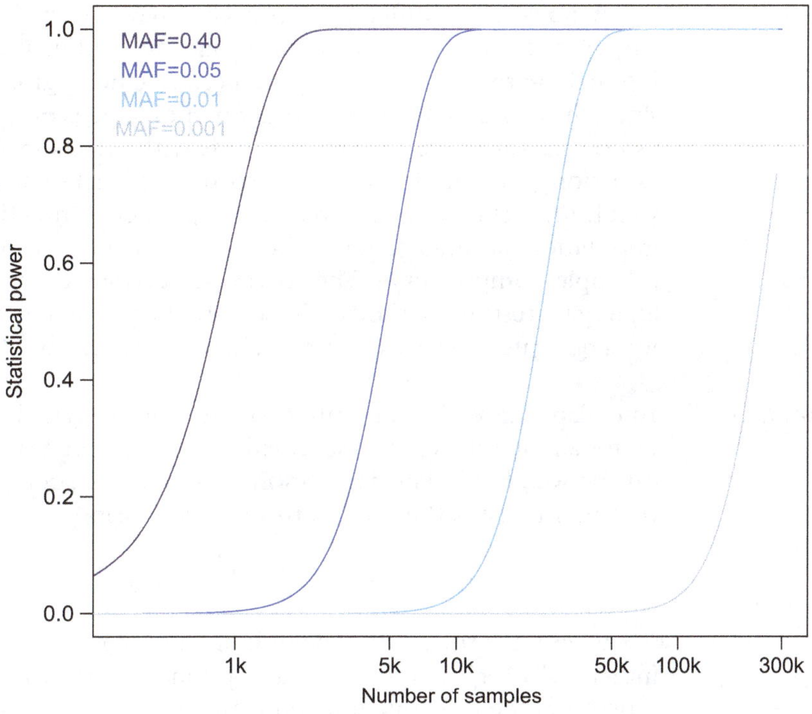

Fig. 1 Power to detect a variant association with OR= 1.5 at $p < 5 \times 10^{-8}$ in a case-control study with a 50:50 ratio of cases to controls and a disease prevalence of 10%

traits under selection, it is likely that variants of moderate to large effect are rare. In line with this, rare and low-frequency variants are strongly enriched for functional and deleterious variants [55–57]. However, genetic architecture differs between traits and is an ongoing field of research.

4.2 Aggregate Testing

In order to increase statistical power to detect rare variant associations, analysis methods have been developed to test the combined effect of several variants. These tests are known as aggregate or gene-based tests. There are several arguments supporting the use of aggregate methods. These include the observations that recent population expansion may have led to high numbers of functional variants, that a combination of variants can be necessary to create a phenotype, and that an increasing number of genes have been discovered with multiple common and/or rare associated variants. Finally, a number of previous successful discoveries from gene-based tests provide proof of principle [58]. Variants are usually combined within genes. An alternative unit can be sliding windows across the genome to assess the combined effect of variants located close to each other. Combining variants from genes in a common pathway has also been suggested [59].

A number of different approaches have been developed for aggregate testing. In general, decisions involved in aggregate testing include the unit of aggregation (e.g., gene, region of a certain size), the coding scheme for the genotypes (e.g., score, carrying any vs no rare alleles, recoding of variants with effects in the opposite direction), variant filtering (e.g., frequency, functional annotation), weighting scheme (e.g., frequency, predicted functional effect, imputation accuracy), and whether to include covariates (e.g., principle components). The following sections describe different aggregate testing methods. Please note that meta-analysis methods for aggregate tests are described elsewhere in this book.

4.2.1 Collapsing Tests

In collapsing tests the numbers of rare alleles carried are summed up for all variants within a specified region (e.g., gene). Each variant can be weighted. The association between this aggregate and the trait of interest is then tested through regression:

$$f(y_i) = \alpha + \beta \sum_j w_j g_{ij}$$

where y_i is the phenotype of individual i, g_{ij} is the genotype of individual i for variant j, w_j is an optional weight for variant j, $f()$ represents the link function and is the logit for dichotomous traits and linear for continuous traits. Note that there is just one regression coefficient β for the aggregate effect rather than separate ones for individual variants.

Several different implementations of the collapsing approach have been developed. RVT can be used for continuous as well as dichotomous outcomes [60]. It can estimate the effect per additional minor allele carried or compare individuals who carry at least one minor allele with those who do not. The Cohort Allelic Sums Test (CAST) [61], Combined Multivariate and Collapsing (CMC) [62], and Weighted Sum Statistic (WSS) [63] were designed specifically for dichotomous outcomes and differ in terms of their coding of the genotypes, variant filtering, and weighting. For regions that contain a mix of causal and non-causal variants, the CMC test had highest statistical power among these methods [62, 64].

It has been demonstrated that for studies based on GWAS chip genotyping, imputation of variants improves power to detect gene-based associations [65]. There are several modified versions of the collapsing tests that can use imputed variants and account for variant quality. The cumulative minor allele test (CMAT) [66] and GRANVIL [67], an implementation of RVT, can use dosages for imputed variants. The Accumulation of Rare variants Integrated and Extended Locus-specific test (ARIEL) is another adaptation of RVT that can also use weights to adjust for variant quality scores [68].

In order to overcome some of the limitations of collapsing tests, modifications have been developed that adapt to properties of the data. The data adaptive test (aSum) [64] involves two stages. Results from a marginal model evaluating single SNP associations are used to recode variants. An extension, the step-up test [69], can be used to filter variants if their marginal test provides little evidence for association. The estimated regression coefficient test (EREC) [70] is another two-stage procedure that uses the regression coefficients from the marginal test as weights for the collapsing test. It adds a small constant to each weight because regression coefficients from single variants tests tend to be unstable for rare variants. The Kernel-based adaptive cluster method (KBAC) [71] uses Kernel-based adaptive weighting in order to select likely causal variants. The variable threshold (VT) approach [72] changes the MAF thresholds for each region in order to identify the optimal variant selection.

Most of the original collapsing methods are less powerful when the associations of the rare alleles of different variants are in opposite directions [73–75]. In the presence of different directions of effect, the data-adaptive approach performed well while the VT method performed well in the case of consistent direction of effect but existence of non-causal variants [74, 76]. However, adaptive methods tend to be computationally intensive because most of them require permutation tests in order to obtain p-value estimates.

4.2.2 Variance-Component Methods

The most widely used variance-component method is SKAT [77]. It assumes a multiple regression model with variants as predictors and variant-specific regression coefficients so that the direction and magnitude of the association of each variant can vary. A mixed model is fitted assuming a random effect for genotype with $\beta_j \sim N(0, w_j\tau)$ where τ is the variance component. The overall effect of the variants can then be assessed by testing whether $\tau = 0$ via a variance-component score test. Covariates are incorporated as fixed effects. It is also possible to include interaction effects. For a dichotomous outcome without covariates SKAT and the C-alpha test [73] are equivalent. Without weights, SKAT reduces to the sum of squares of the marginal score statistics, SSU test [78].

There are a number of modified versions of SKAT. For example, C-SKAT was designed to estimate aggregate effects for both common and rare variants [79]. AP-SKAT is an implementation that avoids deriving p-values from an asymptotic distribution which can lead to bias while reducing the computational load from permutation [80].

4.2.3 Combined Tests

SKAT is a popular choice because it accounts for differences in direction and magnitude of effect between variants. Moreover, it outperforms most adaptive testing methods in terms of computational efficiency because it does not require permutation testing. However, which model has the highest statistical power depends on the underlying genetic architecture of the region and trait under consideration. Collapsing methods have higher power when the majority of variants are causal and have the same direction of effect [74, 77]. In practice, there usually is little prior knowledge about the genetic architecture. Therefore, SKAT-O [81] has been developed. It combines variance component and collapsing approaches in order to maximize power for different scenarios. Alternative unified approaches include MiST [82] and CCS for case control studies [83]. CCS models the variant distributions in cases and controls and can account for ascertainment by using a retrospective likelihood approach. It has been shown to perform favorably when samples sizes are small, variants are rare, and when there is a high proportion of non-causal variants [83]. In a recent simulation study, unified approaches had higher power than collapsing and variance component tests given a range of genetic architectures [84].

A general framework has been developed that enables combining any gene-based tests of choice into a unified approach [85]. This strategy provided higher statistical power than running tests separately and using Bonferroni correction.

One potential problem with both collapsing and variance component methods is that these tests can yield inflated type I error levels [86]. Therefore, inflation should be assessed.

4.2.4 Bayesian Approaches

Several Bayesian approaches have been developed. One advantage is that they can make use of prior information regarding variants [87, 88]. The exponential combination (EC) approach [89] uses a quadratic score term for the aggregate effect of variants and is particularly powerful when the proportion of causal variants is low. However, it requires permutation in order to estimate *p*-values and is therefore computationally demanding. The Variational Bayes discrete mixture test (VBDM) [90] on the other hand is very computationally efficient because it is based on Bayes approximate inference. VBDM explicitly models non-causal variant and therefore performs particularly well in a scenario with many non-causal variants.

4.2.5 Functional Data Analysis

In the framework of functional data analysis, the genomic region of interest is conceptualized as a sequence of variants which was the result of a stochastic process that depends on linkage and linkage disequilibrium and the genetic effects are therefore a function of variant location [91]. While variance component methods only account for LD between pairs of variants, this approach makes optimal use of the LD structure between multiple genetic variants in the region. Moreover, it is possible to include rare as well as common variants. Aggregate tests have been developed within this framework for continuous [91, 92] and dichotomous traits [93–95]. Using the same simulation setup as the original studies for variance component methods, these functional linear model approaches were shown to have higher statistical power than variance component methods in most of the tested scenarios [91, 92, 96, 97].

4.2.6 Relatedness

Most of the methods described so far assume that samples are independent. However, including relatives can increase statistical power to detect a genetic association [98]. For family-based studies with known pedigrees there are transmission-based tests [99, 100]. There is also a pedigree-based option for SKAT for continuous traits, famSKAT [101]. Other models use a genetic relatedness matrix rather than pedigree structures. This provides more flexibility for incorporating complex or unknown family structures. These methods are also applicable when there is a mix of related and unrelated individuals. Pedgene [102] offers rapid collapsing as well as variance-component tests for dichotomous and continuous traits and so do famrvtests for continuous traits [103]. There are other family-based modifications of SKAT, including FFBSKAT [104] and ASKAT [105]. MONSTER is a generalization of SKAT-O that accounts for relatedness [106]. Finally, there is also a modification of the functional linear model approach to use data from related individuals [107].

4.2.7 Survival Analysis

Some studies assess associations of genetic variants with time to an event within a survival analysis framework. A modified version of collapsing tests and SKAT, the CoxBT and CoxSKAT likelihood ratio tests were developed for this setting [108]. Other variance component implementations exist [109, 110]. There is also an extension of the functional linear model approach to assess region-based associations using Cox regression [111].

5 Conclusion

Method development for aggregate testing of rare variants is a dynamic area of research. One of the advantages is that tests have been developed for a variety of different study designs. On the other hand, it can be difficult to navigate this field and identify the optimal test for a given study. The statistical power of each method is dependent on the genetic architecture of the trait (and region) of interest and the ranking of tests changes for different scenarios. In situations with little prior knowledge regarding the genetic architecture of the trait of interest, unified approaches incorporating methods that perform well given high as well as low proportions of causal variants can be a good choice.

As in single variant association testing, hits from aggregate tests also require confirmation using an independent replication sample. However, the locus needs to be validated rather than a single variant. This that may require targeted sequencing of the locus [112].

References

1. Cohen J, Pertsemlidis A, Kotowski IK et al (2005) Low LDL cholesterol in African Americans resulting from frequent nonsense mutations in PCSK9. Nat Genet 37 (3):328–328. https://doi.org/10.1038/ng0305-328c
2. Cohen JC, Boerwinkle E, Mosley TH (2006) Sequence variations in PCSK9, low LDL, and protection against coronary heart disease. New Engl J Med 354(12):1264–1272. https://doi.org/10.1056/NEJMoa054013
3. Roth EM, McKenney JM, Hanotin C, Asset G, Stein EA (2012) Atorvastatin with or without an antibody to PCSK9 in primary hypercholesterolemia. New Engl J Med 367 (20):1891–1900. https://doi.org/10.1056/NEJMoa1201832
4. Koren MJ, Scott R, Kim JB et al (2012) Efficacy, safety, and tolerability of a monoclonal antibody to proprotein convertase subtilisin/kexin type 9 as monotherapy in patients with hypercholesterolaemia (MENDEL): a randomised, double-blind, placebo-controlled, phase 2 study. Lancet 380 (9858):1995–2006. https://doi.org/10.1016/S0140-6736(12)61771-1
5. Timpson NJ, Walter K, Min JL et al (2014) A rare variant in APOC3 is associated with plasma triglyceride and VLDL levels in Europeans. Nat Commun 5:4871. https://doi.org/10.1038/ncomms5871
6. Gilly A, Ritchie GR, Southam L (2016) Very low-depth sequencing in a founder population identifies a cardioprotective APOC3 signal missed by genome-wide imputation. Hum Mol Genet 25(11):2360–2365. https://doi.org/10.1093/hmg/ddw088
7. Tachmazidou I, Dedoussis G, Southam L et al (2013) A rare functional cardioprotective APOC3 variant has risen in frequency in distinct population isolates. Nat Commun 4:2872. https://doi.org/10.1038/ncomms3872
8. Pollin TI, Damcott CM, Shen HQ et al (2008) A null mutation in human APOC3 confers a favorable plasma lipid profile and apparent Cardioprotection. Science 322 (5908):1702–1705. https://doi.org/10.1126/science.1161524
9. Jorgensen A, Frikke-Schmidt R, Nordestgaard BG, Tybjaerg-Hansen A (2014) Loss-of-function mutations in Apoc3 and reduced risk of ischemic vascular disease. Atherosclerosis 235(2):E18–E18
10. Crosby J, Peloso GM, Auer PL et al (2014) Loss-of-function mutations in APOC3, triglycerides, and coronary disease. New Engl J Med 371(1):22–31. https://doi.org/10.1056/NEJMoa1307095
11. Gaudet D, Alexander VJ, Baker BF et al (2015) Antisense inhibition of apolipoprotein C-III in patients with hypertriglyceridemia. New Engl J Med 373(5):438–447. https://doi.org/10.1056/NEJMoa1400283
12. Altshuler DM, Durbin RM, Abecasis GR et al (2015) A global reference for human genetic variation. Nature 526(7571):68–74. https://doi.org/10.1038/nature15393
13. UK10K Consortium, Walter K, Min JL et al (2015) The UK10K project identifies rare variants in health and disease. Nature 526 (7571):82–90. https://doi.org/10.1038/nature14962
14. National Heart Lung and Blood Institute (2016) Trans-Omics for Precision Medicine (TOPMed) Program. https://www.nhlbi.nih.gov/research/resources/nhlbi-precision-medicine-initiative/topmed. Accessed 8 Nov 2016
15. Genomics England (2016) The 100,000 Genomes Project. https://www.genomicsengland.co.uk/the-100000-genomes-project/. Accessed 8 Nov 2016
16. Peplow M (2016) The 100 000 genomes project. BMJ 353. ARTN i1757. https://doi.org/10.1136/bmj.i1757
17. ExAC project pins down rare gene variants (2016). Nature 536(7616):249. https://doi.org/10.1038/536249a

18. Wang H, Liu L, Zhao J et al (2013) Large scale meta-analyses of fasting plasma glucose raising variants in GCK, GCKR, MTNR1B and G6PC2 and their impacts on type 2 diabetes mellitus risk. PLoS One 8(6):e67665. https://doi.org/10.1371/journal.pone.0067665
19. Gillespie JH (2010) Population genetics: a concise guide. Johns Hopkins University Press, Baltimore
20. Campbell MC, Tishkoff SA (2008) African genetic diversity: implications for human demographic history, modern human origins, and complex disease mapping. Annu Rev Genomics Hum Genet 9:403–433. https://doi.org/10.1146/annurev.genom.9.081307.164258
21. Varilo T, Peltonen L (2004) Isolates and their potential use in complex gene mapping efforts - commentary. Curr Opin Genet Dev 14 (3):316–323. https://doi.org/10.1016/j.gde.2004.04.008
22. Minster RL, Hawley NL, Su CT et al (2016) A thrifty variant in CREBRF strongly influences body mass index in Samoans. Nat Genet 48 (9):1049–1054. https://doi.org/10.1038/ng.3620
23. Steinthorsdottir V, Thorleifsson G, Reynisdottir I et al (2007) A variant in CDKAL1 influences insulin response and risk of type 2 diabetes. Nat Genet 39(6):770–775. https://doi.org/10.1038/ng2043
24. Holm H, Gudbjartsson DF, Sulem P et al (2011) A rare variant in MYH6 is associated with high risk of sick sinus syndrome. Nat Genet 43(4):316–320. https://doi.org/10.1038/ng.781
25. Huyghe JR, Jackson AU, Fogarty MP et al (2013) Exome array analysis identifies new loci and low-frequency variants influencing insulin processing and secretion. Nat Genet 45(2):197–201. https://doi.org/10.1038/ng.2507
26. Moltke I, Fumagalli M, Korneliussen TS et al (2015) Uncovering the genetic history of the present-day greenlandic population. Am J Hum Genet 96(1):54–69. https://doi.org/10.1016/j.ajhg.2014.11.012
27. Moltke I, Grarup N, Jorgensen ME et al (2014) A common Greenlandic TBC1D4 variant confers muscle insulin resistance and type 2 diabetes. Nature 512(7513):190–193. https://doi.org/10.1038/nature13425
28. Wetterstrand K (2016) DNA Sequencing Costs: Data from NHGRI Genome Sequencing Program (GSP). http://www.genome.gov/sequencingcostsdata. Accessed 28 Oct 2016
29. Yang J, Bakshi A, Zhu Z et al (2015) Genetic variance estimation with imputed variants finds negligible missing heritability for human height and body mass index. Nat Genet 47(10):1114–1120. https://doi.org/10.1038/ng.3390
30. McCarthy S, Das S, Kretzschmar W et al (2016) A reference panel of 64,976 haplotypes for genotype imputation. Nat Genet 48(10):1279–1283. https://doi.org/10.1038/ng.3643
31. Abecasis G, Altshuler D, Boehnke M, et al (2016) Exome Chip. http://genome.sph.umich.edu/wiki/Exome_Chip_Design. Accessed 31 Oct 2016
32. Wessel J, Chu AY, Willems SM et al (2015) Low-frequency and rare exome chip variants associate with fasting glucose and type 2 diabetes susceptibility. Nat Commun 6:5897. https://doi.org/10.1038/ncomms6897
33. Peloso GM, Auer PL, Bis JC et al (2014) Association of low-frequency and rare coding-sequence variants with blood lipids and coronary heart disease in 56,000 whites and blacks. Am J Hum Genet 94(2):223–232. https://doi.org/10.1016/j.ajhg.2014.01.009
34. Visscher PM, Brown MA, McCarthy MI et al (2012) Five years of GWAS discovery. Am J Hum Genet 90(1):7–24. https://doi.org/10.1016/j.ajhg.2011.11.029
35. Ionita-Laza I, McCallum K, Xu B et al (2016) A spectral approach integrating functional genomic annotations for coding and noncoding variants. Nat Genet 48(2):214–220. https://doi.org/10.1038/ng.3477
36. Ritchie GRS, Dunham I, Zeggini E et al (2014) Functional annotation of noncoding sequence variants. Nat Methods 11 (3):294–U351. https://doi.org/10.1038/nmeth.2832
37. Kircher M, Witten DM, Jain P et al (2014) A general framework for estimating the relative pathogenicity of human genetic variants. Nat Genet 46(3):310–315. https://doi.org/10.1038/ng.2892
38. Ma C, Blackwell T, Boehnke M et al (2013) Recommended joint and meta-analysis strategies for case-control association testing of single low-count variants. Genet Epidemiol 37 (6):539–550. https://doi.org/10.1002/gepi.21742
39. Bigdeli TB, Neale BM, Neale MC (2014) Statistical properties of single-marker tests for rare variants. Twin Res Hum Genet 17

(3):143–150. https://doi.org/10.1017/thg.2014.17

40. Fisher RA (1922) On the interpretation of chi-squared from contingency tables, and the calculation of P. J R Stat Soc 85(1):87–94. https://doi.org/10.2307/2340521
41. Wang X (2014) Firth logistic regression for rare variant association tests. Front Genet 5:187. https://doi.org/10.3389/fgene.2014.00187
42. Lee S, Fuchsberger C, Kim S et al (2016) An efficient resampling method for calibrating single and gene-based rare variant association analysis in case-control studies. Biostatistics 17(1):1–15. https://doi.org/10.1093/biostatistics/kxv033
43. Auer PL, Reiner AP, Leal SM (2016) The effect of phenotypic outliers and non-normality on rare-variant association testing. Eur J Hum Genet 24(8):1188–1194. https://doi.org/10.1038/ejhg.2015.270
44. O'Connor TD, Kiezun A, Bamshad M et al (2013) Fine-scale patterns of population stratification confound rare variant association tests. PLoS One 8(7):e65834. https://doi.org/10.1371/journal.pone.0065834
45. Zhang Y, Shen X, Pan W (2013) Adjusting for population stratification in a fine scale with principal components and sequencing data. Genet Epidemiol 37(8):787–801. https://doi.org/10.1002/gepi.21764
46. Babron MC, de Tayrac M, Rutledge DN et al (2012) Rare and low frequency variant stratification in the UK population: description and impact on association tests. PLoS One 7(10): e46519. https://doi.org/10.1371/journal.pone.0046519
47. Liu Q, Nicolae DL, Chen LS (2013) Marbled inflation from population structure in gene-based association studies with rare variants. Genet Epidemiol 37(3):286–292. https://doi.org/10.1002/gepi.21714
48. Mathieson I, McVean G (2012) Differential confounding of rare and common variants in spatially structured populations. Nat Genet 44(3):243–246. https://doi.org/10.1038/ng.1074
49. Tintle N, Aschard H, Hu I et al (2011) Inflated type I error rates when using aggregation methods to analyze rare variants in the 1000 genomes project exon sequencing data in unrelated individuals: summary results from group 7 at genetic analysis workshop 17. Genet Epidemiol 35 Suppl 1:S56–S60. https://doi.org/10.1002/gepi.20650
50. International HapMap Consortium (2005) A haplotype map of the human genome. Nature 437(7063):1299–1320. https://doi.org/10.1038/nature04226
51. Pe'er I, Yelensky R, Altshuler D et al (2008) Estimation of the multiple testing burden for genomewide association studies of nearly all common variants. Genet Epidemiol 32 (4):381–385. https://doi.org/10.1002/gepi.20303
52. Dudbridge F, Gusnanto A (2008) Estimation of significance thresholds for genomewide association scans. Genet Epidemiol 32 (3):227–234. https://doi.org/10.1002/gepi.20297
53. Fadista J, Manning AK, Florez JC et al (2016) The (in)famous GWAS P-value threshold revisited and updated for low-frequency variants. Eur J Hum Genet 24(8):1202–1205. https://doi.org/10.1038/ejhg.2015.269
54. Sham PC, Purcell SM (2014) Statistical power and significance testing in large-scale genetic studies. Nat Rev Genet 15(5):335–346. https://doi.org/10.1038/nrg3706
55. Kryukov GV, Pennacchio LA, Sunyaev SR (2007) Most rare missense alleles are deleterious in humans: implications for complex disease and association studies. Am J Hum Genet 80(4):727–739. https://doi.org/10.1086/513473
56. Nelson MR, Wegmann D, Ehm MG et al (2012) An abundance of rare functional variants in 202 drug target genes sequenced in 14,002 people. Science 337(6090):100–104. https://doi.org/10.1126/science.1217876
57. Fu W, O'Connor TD, Jun G et al (2013) Analysis of 6,515 exomes reveals the recent origin of most human protein-coding variants. Nature 493(7431):216–220. https://doi.org/10.1038/nature11690
58. Bansal V, Libiger O, Torkamani A et al (2010) Statistical analysis strategies for association studies involving rare variants. Nat Rev Genet 11(11):773–785. https://doi.org/10.1038/nrg2867
59. Wu G, Zhi D (2013) Pathway-based approaches for sequencing-based genome-wide association studies. Genet Epidemiol 37(5):478–494. https://doi.org/10.1002/gepi.21728
60. Morris AP, Zeggini E (2010) An evaluation of statistical approaches to rare variant analysis in genetic association studies. Genet Epidemiol 34(2):188–193. https://doi.org/10.1002/gepi.20450
61. Morgenthaler S, Thilly WG (2007) A strategy to discover genes that carry multi-allelic or

mono-allelic risk for common diseases: a cohort allelic sums test (CAST). Mutat Res 615(1–2):28–56. https://doi.org/10.1016/j.mrfmmm.2006.09.003

62. Li B, Leal SM (2008) Methods for detecting associations with rare variants for common diseases: application to analysis of sequence data. Am J Hum Genet 83(3):311–321. https://doi.org/10.1016/j.ajhg.2008.06.024
63. Madsen BE, Browning SR (2009) A groupwise association test for rare mutations using a weighted sum statistic. PLoS Genet 5(2): e1000384. https://doi.org/10.1371/journal.pgen.1000384
64. Han F, Pan W (2010) A data-adaptive sum test for disease association with multiple common or rare variants. Hum Hered 70 (1):42–54. https://doi.org/10.1159/000288704
65. Magi R, Asimit JL, Day-Williams AG et al (2012) Genome-wide association analysis of imputed rare variants: application to seven common complex diseases. Genet Epidemiol 36(8):785–796. https://doi.org/10.1002/gepi.21675
66. Zawistowski M, Gopalakrishnan S, Ding J et al (2010) Extending rare-variant testing strategies: analysis of noncoding sequence and imputed genotypes. Am J Hum Genet 87(5):604–617. https://doi.org/10.1016/j.ajhg.2010.10.012
67. Magi R, Kumar A, Morris AP (2011) Assessing the impact of missing genotype data in rare variant association analysis. BMC Proc 5 (Suppl 9):S107. https://doi.org/10.1186/1753-6561-5-S9-S107
68. Asimit JL, Day-Williams AG, Morris AP et al (2012) ARIEL and AMELIA: testing for an accumulation of rare variants using next-generation sequencing data. Hum Hered 73 (2):84–94. https://doi.org/10.1159/000336982
69. Hoffmann TJ, Marini NJ, Witte JS (2010) Comprehensive approach to analyzing rare genetic variants. PLoS One 5(11):e13584. https://doi.org/10.1371/journal.pone.0013584
70. Lin DY, Tang ZZ (2011) A general framework for detecting disease associations with rare variants in sequencing studies. Am J Hum Genet 89(3):354–367. https://doi.org/10.1016/j.ajhg.2011.07.015
71. Liu DJ, Leal SM (2010) A novel adaptive method for the analysis of next-generation sequencing data to detect complex trait associations with rare variants due to gene main effects and interactions. PLoS Genet 6(10): e1001156. https://doi.org/10.1371/journal.pgen.1001156
72. Price AL, Kryukov GV, de Bakker PI et al (2010) Pooled association tests for rare variants in exon-resequencing studies. Am J Hum Genet 86(6):832–838. https://doi.org/10.1016/j.ajhg.2010.04.005
73. Neale BM, Rivas MA, Voight BF et al (2011) Testing for an unusual distribution of rare variants. PLoS Genet 7(3):e1001322. https://doi.org/10.1371/journal.pgen.1001322
74. Basu S, Pan W (2011) Comparison of statistical tests for disease association with rare variants. Genet Epidemiol 35(7):606–619. https://doi.org/10.1002/gepi.20609
75. Lee S, Wu MC, Lin X (2012) Optimal tests for rare variant effects in sequencing association studies. Biostatistics 13(4):762–775. https://doi.org/10.1093/biostatistics/kxs014
76. Ladouceur M, Dastani Z, Aulchenko YS et al (2012) The empirical power of rare variant association methods: results from sanger sequencing in 1,998 individuals. PLoS Genet 8(2):e1002496. https://doi.org/10.1371/journal.pgen.1002496
77. Wu MC, Lee S, Cai T et al (2011) Rare-variant association testing for sequencing data with the sequence kernel association test. Am J Hum Genet 89(1):82–93. https://doi.org/10.1016/j.ajhg.2011.05.029
78. Pan W (2009) Asymptotic tests of association with multiple SNPs in linkage disequilibrium. Genet Epidemiol 33(6):497–507. https://doi.org/10.1002/gepi.20402
79. Ionita-Laza I, Lee S, Makarov V et al (2013) Sequence kernel association tests for the combined effect of rare and common variants. Am J Hum Genet 92(6):841–853. https://doi.org/10.1016/j.ajhg.2013.04.015
80. Hasegawa T, Kojima K, Kawai Y et al (2016) AP-SKAT: highly-efficient genome-wide rare variant association test. BMC Genomics 17 (1):745. https://doi.org/10.1186/s12864-016-3094-3
81. Lee S, Emond MJ, Bamshad MJ et al (2012) Optimal unified approach for rare-variant association testing with application to small-sample case-control whole-exome sequencing studies. Am J Hum Genet 91(2):224–237. https://doi.org/10.1016/j.ajhg.2012.06.007
82. Sun J, Zheng Y, Hsu L (2013) A unified mixed-effects model for rare-variant

association in sequencing studies. Genet Epidemiol 37(4):334–344. https://doi.org/10.1002/gepi.21717

83. Li H, Chen J (2016) Efficient unified rare variant association test by modeling the population genetic distribution in case-control studies. Genet Epidemiol 40(7):579–590. https://doi.org/10.1002/gepi.21995

84. Moutsianas L, Agarwala V, Fuchsberger C et al (2015) The power of gene-based rare variant methods to detect disease-associated variation and test hypotheses about complex disease. PLoS Genet 11(4):e1005165. https://doi.org/10.1371/journal.pgen.1005165

85. Greco B, Hainline A, Arbet J et al (2016) A general approach for combining diverse rare variant association tests provides improved robustness across a wider range of genetic architectures. Eur J Hum Genet 24(5):767–773. https://doi.org/10.1038/ejhg.2015.194

86. Dering C, Konig IR, Ramsey LB et al (2014) A comprehensive evaluation of collapsing methods using simulated and real data: excellent annotation of functionality and large sample sizes required. Front Genet 5:323. https://doi.org/10.3389/fgene.2014.00323

87. Yi N, Zhi D (2011) Bayesian analysis of rare variants in genetic association studies. Genet Epidemiol 35(1):57–69. https://doi.org/10.1002/gepi.20554

88. Quintana MA, Berstein JL, Thomas DC et al (2011) Incorporating model uncertainty in detecting rare variants: the Bayesian risk index. Genet Epidemiol 35(7):638–649. https://doi.org/10.1002/gepi.20613

89. Chen LS, Hsu L, Gamazon ER et al (2012) An exponential combination procedure for set-based association tests in sequencing studies. Am J Hum Genet 91(6):977–986. https://doi.org/10.1016/j.ajhg.2012.09.017

90. Logsdon BA, Dai JY, Auer PL et al (2014) A variational Bayes discrete mixture test for rare variant association. Genet Epidemiol 38(1):21–30

91. Fan R, Wang Y, Mills JL et al (2013) Functional linear models for association analysis of quantitative traits. Genet Epidemiol 37(7):726–742. https://doi.org/10.1002/gepi.21757

92. Luo L, Zhu Y, Xiong M (2012) Quantitative trait locus analysis for next-generation sequencing with the functional linear models. J Med Genet 49(8):513–524. https://doi.org/10.1136/jmedgenet-2012-100798

93. Luo L, Boerwinkle E, Xiong M (2011) Association studies for next-generation sequencing. Genome Res 21(7):1099–1108. https://doi.org/10.1101/gr.115998.110

94. Fan R, Wang Y, Mills JL et al (2014) Generalized functional linear models for gene-based case-control association studies. Genet Epidemiol 38(7):622–637. https://doi.org/10.1002/gepi.21840

95. Vsevolozhskaya OA, Zaykin DV, Greenwood MC et al (2014) Functional analysis of variance for association studies. PLoS One 9(9):e105074. https://doi.org/10.1371/journal.pone.0105074

96. Fan R, Wang Y, Boehnke M et al (2015) Gene level meta-analysis of quantitative traits by functional linear models. Genetics 200(4):1089–1104. https://doi.org/10.1534/genetics.115.178343

97. Wang Y, Liu A, Mills JL et al (2015) Pleiotropy analysis of quantitative traits at gene level by multivariate functional linear models. Genet Epidemiol 39(4):259–275. https://doi.org/10.1002/gepi.21895

98. Wijsman EM (2012) The role of large pedigrees in an era of high-throughput sequencing. Hum Genet 131(10):1555–1563. https://doi.org/10.1007/s00439-012-1190-2

99. De G, Yip WK, Ionita-Laza I et al (2013) Rare variant analysis for family-based design. PLoS One 8(1):e48495. https://doi.org/10.1371/journal.pone.0048495

100. Ionita-Laza I, Lee S, Makarov V et al (2013) Family-based association tests for sequence data, and comparisons with population-based association tests. Eur J Hum Genet 21(10):1158–1162. https://doi.org/10.1038/ejhg.2012.308

101. Chen H, Meigs JB, Dupuis J (2013) Sequence kernel association test for quantitative traits in family samples. Genet Epidemiol 37(2):196–204. https://doi.org/10.1002/gepi.21703

102. Schaid DJ, McDonnell SK, Sinnwell JP et al (2013) Multiple genetic variant association testing by collapsing and kernel methods with pedigree or population structured data. Genet Epidemiol 37(5):409–418. https://doi.org/10.1002/gepi.21727

103. Feng S, Pistis G, Zhang H et al (2015) Methods for association analysis and meta-analysis of rare variants in families. Genet Epidemiol 39(4):227–238. https://doi.org/10.1002/gepi.21892

104. Svishcheva GR, Belonogova NM, Axenovich TI (2014) FFBSKAT: fast family-based sequence kernel association test. PLoS One 9(6):e99407. https://doi.org/10.1371/journal.pone.0099407
105. Oualkacha K, Dastani Z, Li R et al (2013) Adjusted sequence kernel association test for rare variants controlling for cryptic and family relatedness. Genet Epidemiol 37 (4):366–376. https://doi.org/10.1002/gepi.21725
106. Jiang D, McPeek MS (2014) Robust rare variant association testing for quantitative traits in samples with related individuals. Genet Epidemiol 38(1):10–20. https://doi.org/10.1002/gepi.21775
107. Svishcheva GR, Belonogova NM, Axenovich TI (2015) Region-based association test for familial data under functional linear models. PLoS One 10(6):e0128999. https://doi.org/10.1371/journal.pone.0128999
108. Chen H, Lumley T, Brody J et al (2014) Sequence kernel association test for survival traits. Genet Epidemiol 38(3):191–197. https://doi.org/10.1002/gepi.21791
109. Cai T, Tonini G, Lin X (2011) Kernel machine approach to testing the significance of multiple genetic markers for risk prediction. Biometrics 67(3):975–986. https://doi.org/10.1111/j.1541-0420.2010.01544.x
110. Lin X, Cai T, Wu MC et al (2011) Kernel machine SNP-set analysis for censored survival outcomes in genome-wide association studies. Genet Epidemiol 35(7):620–631. https://doi.org/10.1002/gepi.20610
111. Fan R, Wang Y, Yan Q et al (2016) Gene-based association analysis for censored traits via fixed effect functional regressions. Genet Epidemiol 40(2):133–143. https://doi.org/10.1002/gepi.21947
112. Liu DJ, Leal SM (2015) Replicating sequencing-based association studies of rare variants. In: Zeggini E, Morris A (eds) Assessing rare variation in complex traits: design and analysis of genetic studies. Springer, New York, NY, pp 201–213. https://doi.org/10.1007/978-1-4939-2824-8_14

Chapter 6

Meta-Analysis of Common and Rare Variants

Kyriaki Michailidou

Abstract

Meta-analysis is a statistical technique that is widely used for improving the power to detect associations, by synthesizing data from independent studies, and is extensively used in the genomic analyses of complex traits. Estimates from different studies are combined and the results effectively provide the power of a much larger study. Meta-analysis also has the potential of discovering heterogeneity in the effects among the different studies. This chapter provides an overview of the methods used for meta-analysis of common and rare single variants and also for gene/region-based analyses; common variants are mainly identified via genome-wide association studies (GWAS) and rare variants through various types of sequencing experiments.

Key words Meta-analysis, Common variants, Rare variants, Aggregation analysis, Single variant analysis, GWAS, NGS

1 Introduction

Meta-analysis provides a powerful approach to combine data from different resources. It has been widely used in genomics in order to increase the power of single studies to detect associations with a specific trait or disease of interest [1, 2]. Sharing of genotype data between studies is not always possible, even within well-established collaborations, thus the need for alternative approaches for combining the effects from different studies has led to the wide use of meta-analyses in the field. The different meta-analysis techniques use summary statistics, are easy and quick to perform, are powerful, and practically provide the power of a much larger study.

Meta-analysis has been extensively used in order to assess Genome-wide association study (GWAS) data for millions of genotyped or imputed SNPs [2]. GWAS provide a cost-effective method for assessing the effect of common genetic variation across the genome [3, 4] and have been widely informed using imputation to publicly available genotype reference panels such as the HapMap [5], the 1000 Genomes Project Consortium [6], and the

Evangelos Evangelou (ed.), *Genetic Epidemiology: Methods and Protocols*, Methods in Molecular Biology, vol. 1793, https://doi.org/10.1007/978-1-4939-7868-7_6,

Haplotype Reference Consortium [7]. Over the last decade thousands of common variants, which are associated with complex diseases or traits, have been identified through imputation and meta-analyses of GWAS [8, 9]. More recently, custom arrays that focus on the replication of rare variants from sequencing experiments have been developed [10]. The identification of rare variants through genotyping arrays and imputation has been more problematic compared to common variants [11]. With the tremendous advances in next generation sequencing (NGS) technologies [12], it is now feasible to conduct large-scale whole-genome, whole-exome, and targeted sequencing experiments. Recently, novel statistical techniques have been developed for the analysis of the rare variants as single entities and also for their collective analysis in gene or regional tests. As in the common variant analysis, meta-analysis techniques will aid the increase of power to detect associations with rare variants. In the following sections, the different aspects of meta-analysis for common and rare variants are discussed.

1.1 Meta-Analysis Pre-Steps and Quality Control

Meta-analysis usually begins with the individual studies sharing summary statistics for each variant, including a regression estimate, standard error, *p*-value, sample size, imputation accuracy, and minor allele frequency (MAF). There are various steps that need to be taken into account before performing the meta-analysis in order to minimize bias. Studies need to harmonize their quality control measures and perform the analysis in the same/comparable way before being able to combine the results. Standardized quality control measures that need to be followed in each of the participating studies, for example in GWAS, include the removal of low call rate individuals and variants, removal of variants with genotype frequencies deviating from those expected under Hardy-Weinberg Equilibrium and variants with poor clusterplots [4]. Parameters for adjustments need to be set upfront so that the analyses are performed in a comparable way. Principal components should be calculated and adjusted for in the analyses [13] and appropriate genomic control can be applied to individual studies [14] in order to minimize bias due to population stratification. If the studies perform imputation they need to use the same reference panel and the same filters afterward (MAF and imputation accuracy) [15]. Different programs produce different quality metrics that need to be accounted for when performing the meta-analysis, for example "info score" from IMPUTE2 [16], "R^2" from MACH [17] and BEAGLE [18]. The individual study effect estimates need to be aligned to the same strand (usually more difficult for the ambiguous SNPs with A/T and C/G genotypes) and variants with large differences from the mean MAF need to be checked in more detail. Short insertion/deletions (INDEL) that are now being successfully imputed, using the 1000 Genomes Project data as reference, can have different annotations across the different imputation software that need to be carefully matched. For example some software keep the actual alleles from the reference panel whereas others provide the INDELs as D/I.

If the data come from sequencing experiments they need to be aligned on the same reference genome and low-quality variants need to be removed before the meta-analysis is performed, to avoid spurious associations due to sequencing errors. Furthermore, special care needs to be taken when combining the results of sequencing experiments that have been produced using different technologies. Different depth/coverage of the regions of interest or genotyping bias due to the differences in sequencing technologies can lead to the wrong conclusions. If the analyses are based on genes or regions with variable thresholds the classifications for SNPs/variants to be included in each gene/region need to be the same (for example minor allele frequency threshold). Before performing meta—analysis, a common statistical analysis plan needs to be adopted to ensure compatibility of the results and to aid a smooth execution [2].

2 Common Variants

Different analytical approaches have been proposed and have been extensively used for common variant meta-analyses [1, 2].

2.1 Fixed Effects

The most widely used technique for meta-analysis of common variants is the fixed-effects meta-analysis [1, 2]. The assumption behind the fixed-effect meta-analysis is that there is a single common underlying genetic effect in the different studies. This has been proven a powerful approach for discovery of common genetic variants and provides practically the same information as a pooled analysis of the raw data [19]. Different weights have been proposed with the most optimal weight being the inverse variance [20]; other weighting methods have also been used, such as the Mantel-Haesnzel method [21] or weights proportional to the sample size. The weighted effect and variance are calculated as:

$$\overline{\beta} = \frac{\sum_i^k w_i \beta_i}{\sum_i^k w_i}$$

$$\overline{v} = \frac{1}{\sum_i^k w_i}$$

where β_i is the effect estimate from each study, w_i is the weight assigned to each study and k is the number of studies. For the fixed-effects inverse variance meta-analysis, $w_i = \frac{1}{v_i}$, where v_i is the variance of each study [22]. The fixed-effect weighted test statistic follows a standard normal distribution:

$$\frac{\overline{\beta}}{\sqrt{\overline{v}}} \sim N(0,1)$$

2.2 Random Effects

When the underlying effects for each of the studies are assumed to be different but drawn from the same distribution with variance τ, random-effects meta-analysis should be used. When there is no presence of heterogeneity across the different studies, the random- and fixed-effects estimates will give approximately the same results. The most common methods for calculating the variance of the effect distribution are the method of moments [23] or likelihood-based methods [24]. Random-effects models have been used mainly for the determination of the generalizability of the results of the meta-analysis rather than for discovery purposes, as they are less powerful [2]. Most commonly researchers report both fixed- and random-effects meta-analysis results. The classic random-effects meta-analysis follows the inverse-variance scheme with the difference that the variance is now the sum of the within-study variance (v_i) plus the between-studies variance (τ^2) [22]:

$$w_i^* = \frac{1}{v_i^*}$$

$$v_i^* = v_i + \tau^2$$

$$\tau^2 = \frac{Q - (k-1)}{\sum_i^k w_i - \frac{\sum_i^k w_i^2}{\sum_i^k w_i}}$$

$$Q = \sum_i^k w_i \beta_i^2 - \frac{\left(\sum_i^k w_i \beta_i\right)^2}{\sum_i^k w_i}$$

where β_i is the effect estimate from each study, w_i is the weight assigned to each study, and k is the number of studies. The weighted effect and variance becomes

$$\overline{\beta}^* = \frac{\sum_i^k w_i^* \beta_i}{\sum_i^k w_i^*}$$

$$\overline{v}^* = \frac{1}{\sum_i^k w_i^*}$$

The test statistic then follows

$$\frac{\overline{\beta}^*}{\sqrt{\overline{v}^*}} \sim N(0,1)$$

Han and Eskin [25] observed that classical random effect models are underperforming even when there is heterogeneity present among the different studies. They proposed an alternative method for performing random effects meta-analysis whereby under the null hypothesis it is assumed that there is no heterogeneity. Han and Eskin [26] proposed the Binary Effects Assumption as another method for random effects meta-analysis. This method is based on two hypotheses; first that the effect is either present or absent in a study and second that if the studies have an effect then the effect is expected to be similar between the studies. A novel random effects model, based on a kernel machine framework, has been proposed by Shi et al. [27] for the meta-analysis of trans-ethnic studies. In the presence of substantial heterogeneity between the results in the different studies, further checking needs to be performed to explore the potential reasons behind this heterogeneity [25].

2.3 P-Value and Z Score Meta-Analyses

A more simplistic meta-analysis approach is the meta-analysis using the p-values of the individual studies [28], the test statistic takes the form:

$$X^2_{2k} = -2\sum\nolimits_i^k \log(p_i) \sim X^2_{2k}$$

where k is the number of studies and p_i the individual study p-value. Z score statistics-based meta-analysis [29] has also been used, the test statistic can be derived using the p-values together with the sample size information and direction of the effect. The Z-score can be calculated using the following equation:

$$Z = \frac{\sum_i^k Z_i w_i}{\sqrt{\sum_i^k w_i^2}} \sim N(0,1),$$

where

$$Z_i = \Phi^{-1}\left(1 - \frac{p_i}{2}\right) \times \text{direction of effect}$$

where w_i is the square root of the sample size and Φ is the standard normal cumulative distribution function. Although these methods are more straightforward to perform there is a substantial loss of power as no information regarding the direction of the effects in each study is used (for the p-value meta-analysis), a combined effect cannot be calculated and measures of heterogeneity cannot be obtained [2].

2.4 Bayesian Meta-Analysis

Although not as widely used as the other classical methods for meta-analysis, different Bayesian methods have been also adapted for different scenarios, with both fixed and random effects. Results obtained from Bayesian meta-analyses are directly comparable among/across different SNPs without the need for comparing power and adjusting for differences in the frequencies among different variants [30]. Choosing a suitable prior to be used for the meta-analysis is an important issue and certain assumptions need to be made. Results obtained via Bayesian meta-analysis include the Bayes Factor (BF). The conventional cutoff for a test to be significant ($BF > 10$) is not sufficient for GWAS, not due to issues of multiple testing as in frequentist testing but because the number of truly associated variants we expect to have is small [30]. Bayesian methods have also been developed for the meta-analysis of trans-ethnic GWAS data, where the studies are assigned into ethnic clusters and the effects are assumed to be the same in each ethnic group [31].

3 Rare Variants

The significant reduction in the cost of whole-exome and whole-genome sequencing in recent years has enabled large-scale sequencing experiments to be conducted [7, 32]. Chip-based rare variant experiments [10, 33] have also been performed for the assessment of rare variation.

Single variant tests for rare variants are more challenging to perform compared to common variants. The statistical tests need to be adapted for rare variants as there is usually only a small number of alternative allele counts and the current methods might not be as accurate [11]. Score type statistics have been shown to be more stable for rare variant association testing, especially for binary traits [34]; Wald statistics can be too conservative and likelihood type statistics too liberal.

3.1 Aggregation Tests

Rare variant experiments are underpowered to identify single variants associated with modest effects, even within a large sample size [11]. Different methods have been proposed to increase the power to detect associations by grouping variants into units of interest (regions). A large number of different aggregation tests have been developed to combine the effects of a subset of variants in order to obtain a region-level test statistic [11]. Aggregation testing increases the power to detect associations by combining the cumulative effects of rare variants and by reducing the number of tests performed [11, 34].

The various aggregation tests can be extended to include any subset of variants of interest and for convenience, for the rest of this chapter, these subsets will be referred to as a "region" of interest.

For example, in exome or whole-exome studies the region can be a specific exon of a single gene, all the exons of a single gene or all the exons of all the expressed genes in a genome. In the case of whole-genome studies the region can also be a genomic region (for example a sliding window of a pre-specified genomic length) or a subset of variants belonging to the same category (for example non-synonymous variants or variants that have a specific functional annotation according to functional classification software [35]). Some of the most widely used aggregation tests are discussed in more detail elsewhere in this book (*see* Chapter 5). These include the burden test or collapsing test, where a score is created for each set of variants in a region, for each study sample, and then this is compared to the disease/trait of interest. Collapsing tests can either calculate a binary value (0 rare alleles or at least one rare allele) such as CAST [36], or count the rare variants in each gene [37], or calculate a weighted sum of the rare alleles in the region [38]. Another form of collapsing test is the CMC test where the variants are grouped according to their MAF and then CAST is performed [39]. A different set of approaches are the variable threshold (VT) methods, where the decision of the MAF threshold for variants to be included in the region is obtained so that it gives the most significant result [34, 40]. Other methods developed are the variance-component (VC) tests that can detect associations in regions when variants are allowed to have opposite effects such as the C-alpha and SKAT [41, 42]. A combination of the burden and variance-component tests has also been developed such as the optimal unified SKAT-O, which takes the most significant linear combination of the burden and SKAT tests [43]. The majority of the different methods are applicable for quantitative measures, binary traits, and survival analysis data. Even when aggregating rare variants in regions of interest the power to detect associations is still small [11] and thus appropriate techniques for the meta-analysis of regional tests have been developed in order to increase the power to detect associations. Both fixed- and random-effects meta-analysis methods have been proposed for the regional tests. As estimates based on individual rare-variant regression are not stable the most optimal methods for meta-analysis of regional tests have been based on the meta-analysis of score statistics.

3.2 Meta-Analysis of Regional Tests

3.2.1 P Value and Z Score

Following a similar concept as the single variant meta-analysis the most straightforward method for regional meta-analysis is a *p*-value [28] or a *Z* score statistic [29] meta-analysis. A regional *p*-value or *Z* score is obtained from each study and then these are meta-analyzed. This is an attractive method when effect estimates cannot be calculated or shared between the different studies. However, these methods have been shown to suffer from substantial loss of information, especially when no information of sample size and direction of the effects is used, and thus these methods are not widely used [44]. Another simple method has been proposed by Lumley et al. [45] and is performed by the summation of the test statistics for each individual study, though it is not as powerful if variants are shared between studies.

More sophisticated methods that do not result in loss of information and provide results that are as powerful as a pooled analysis of individual level data have also been proposed. In the following sections a general framework for the meta-analysis of rare variant regional association tests will be described. These tests are based on the individual study score test summary statistics and the fact that the regional test statistic can be reconstructed using the individual variant score statistic from each study [44–48]. Fixed effects and random effects meta-analysis methods have been proposed for the most widely used regional tests. Individual studies share the summary score statistic for each variant and an average variance-covariance matrix for the region [44–48]. Others have also proposed meta-analysis methods for aggregation tests that are reconstructed using the effects and standard errors from the usual regression analyses together with the correlation matrix of the individual variants (which can also be obtained from public resources) [49]. This is an attractive method when score statistics cannot be obtained but there is a substantial loss of information since variants that do not produce valid effect estimates are not used [49]. In the next sections score-based meta-analysis tests will be described; these methods have been shown to be as powerful as the analysis of the pooled genotype data [44, 46, 47].

3.2.2 Fixed Effects

The main assumption behind fixed effect meta-analysis for regional tests is that there is a shared common genetic effect across the different k studies. If we assume that there are j variants in the region of interest, we can get the combined score (U_j) and combined variance (V_j) for each variant [44, 50]:

$$U_j = \sum_i^k U_{(j,i)} \text{ and } V_j = \sum_i^k V_{(jj,i)}$$

$$w = (w_1, w_2, \ldots, w_j)^T$$

where w is a vector of weights. If a variant is not present in a specific study then the corresponding score and variance are set equal to 0. The regional score (U) and variance/covariance matrix (V) are defined as

$$U = (U_1, U_2, \ldots, U_j)^T$$

$$V = \text{cov}(U)$$

The majority of the different methods use a normalized score statistic (for quantitative traits) for each variant [34, 46, 47] whereas Liu et al. [44] uses non-normalized scores.

Burden Tests

For the burden test, the assumption is that the combined score for the region is the same across the different studies $\beta_1 = \beta_2 = \ldots = \beta_k$. For testing the null hypothesis that $\beta_k = 0$, under the additive mode of inheritance, the meta-analysis test statistic takes the form [46]:

$$Q_{M-Burden} = \frac{U^{*2}}{V^*} \sim X_1^2$$

where $U^* = w^T U$ and $V^* = w^T V w$.

Equivalently form Liu et al. [44]:

$$Q_{M-Burden} = \frac{w^T U}{\sqrt{(w^T V w)}} \sim N(O, 1)$$

Weights are usually based on MAF threshold cutoff (for example MAF < 0.05 or MAF < 0.01) or the Madsen-Browning [38] weights, which up-weight rarer variants.

Variable Threshold (VT) Tests

A VT test can be constructed by calculating the burden test statistic at each MAF threshold (p):

$$Q_{M-VT} = \max_p Q_{M-\text{Burden}}(p)$$

The p-value can then be calculated by comparing the test statistic to a multivariate normal distribution of U [34].

Variance Components (VC) Test, SKAT, and SKAT-O

For the VC tests, the mean of the genetic effect of the variants in the region is assumed to be the same across studies. The mean μ of the effect of the variants in the region is assumed to follow a multivariate normal distribution with mean 0 and covariance matrix $\tau_w W$. For testing the null hypothesis that the mean of the variant level effects $\mu = 0$, the meta-analysis test statistic takes the form [44, 46]:

$$Q_{M-\text{SKAT}} = U^T W U$$

where W is an jxj diagonal matrix of rare variant-specific weights, usually a function of the MAF, for example if W is a diagonal Beta (MAF_i, a_1, a_2) this is equal to the SKAT statistic [41] and if W is an identity matrix then it produces the meta-analysis statistic for the C-alpha test [42]. The p-value of the test statistic can then be obtained by comparing the test statistic to a mixture of χ_1^2 distributions, $\sum_i^j \lambda_i \chi_{1,i}^2$ where λ_i is the ith eigenvalue of $V^{1/2} W V^{1/2}$ [44, 46, 47].

An optimal unified test, SKAT-O [43], has been proposed; for this test the most optimal linear combination of SKAT and burden test is selected. The meta-analysis formula for SKAT-O takes the form [34, 43]

$$Q_{\text{hom-SKAT-O}} = \rho Q_{M\text{-Burden}} + (1 - \rho) Q_{M\text{-SKAT}}$$

Intuitively if $\rho = 1$ the test correspond to the meta-analysis of burden test and if $\rho = 0$, to the meta-analysis of the SKAT statistic. ρ is calculated so that it produces the most significant result, the p-value of the test can be obtained using a one-dimensional numerical integration [43].

3.2.3 Random-Effects

Random-effects meta-analysis for regional tests assumes that the genetic effects of the different studies are not the same but are derived from the same distribution [51]. Heterogeneity between and across studies is expected to be a bigger issue for rare variants compared to common variants, as they are population specific [51]. Random-effects models for aggregation tests have been based on the Han and Eskin [25] single variant meta-analysis method that has been shown to be more powerful compared to other classical methods.

Burden Test

Under the random effects model for the burden test, the combined effects of the different studies are drawn from:

$$\beta_i = \mu + \xi_i, \quad i = 1, \ldots, k$$

where μ represents the average combined genetic effect among studies and ξ_i represents the deviation of the effect of study k from the mean μ, and is assumed to follow a multivariate normal distribution with mean 0 and variance σ. The test for $\mu = 0$ and $\sigma = 0$ takes the form [51]:

$$Q_{RM\text{-Burden}} = Q_{M\text{-Burden}} + \frac{\left(\sum_i^k U_i^2 - \sum_i^k V_i\right)^2}{2\sum_i^k V_i^2}$$

For the VT test we test:

$$Q_{RM-VT} = \max_p Q_{RM\text{-Burden}}(p),$$

which is the maximum of the random-effects burden tests obtained with a MAF threshold p [51].

SKAT and SKAT-O

In order to obtain the test statistic for the SKAT meta-analysis we assume that the mean of the genetic effects of the variants in each region, for each study, is drawn from the distribution:

$$\beta_i = \mu + \xi_i, \quad i = 1, \ldots, k$$

where μ is the mean of the effects of the j variants across the k studies and ξ_i is the deviation of the effects of the kth study from the mean effect [34, 51]. Random effects models have been proposed for the SKAT and SKAT-O tests, by Lee et al. [47], the Het-SKAT and Het-SKAT-O and by Tang et al. [51], the RE-SKAT and RE-SKAT-O. RE-SKAT aims to detect mean effects and heterogeneity and HET-SKAT aims to detect heterogeneity in the absence of mean effects [46].

Tang and Lin [46] performed extensive simulation testing to compare the power of the different statistical models. They compared three different genetic structure models: rare variant model (for this model it is assumed that 50% of the variants with MAF < 0.5% are causal), low-frequency-variant model (where 50% of all variants are assumed to be causal), and opposite effects model (where 50% of the variants are assumed to be causal, 80% of the causal variants are risk, and 20% of the causal variants are protective) [46]. Under these genetic models they evaluated the different meta-analysis methods for the fixed- and random-effects burden, VT, SKAT, and SKAT-O models using normalized score statistics [46]. The tests were performed assuming that the effect of each study is a random variable with mean μ and variance τ. Two different mean effect values, $\mu = 0$ and $\mu = 0.25$, were tested and the variance τ was allowed to vary between 0 and 0.25. For $\mu = 0.25$ and when genetic heterogeneity was small the fixed-effects burden and VT models were more powerful than their equivalent random-effects models and the fixed-effect SKAT and SKAT-O had similar power to their corresponding random-effects models [46]. In the presence of strong heterogeneity the random-effect models were more powerful to the equivalent fixed-effects. The simulations showed that under the rare variant model VT tests were the most powerful whereas for the opposite effects model SKAT and SKAT-O were more powerful than burden and VT models [46]. Under the opposite effects structure model, the random effects models for SKAT and SKAT-O (HET-SKAT and HET-SKAT-O) proposed by Lee et al. [47] were less powerful compared to random effects models proposed by Tang et al. [51] (RE-SKAT and RE-SKAT-O) when the heterogeneity was low, and slightly more powerful when the heterogeneity was large [46]. Under the assumption that $\mu = 0$, the random effects models were more powerful in the presence of strong heterogeneity. For the rare and low-frequency variant models RE-SKAT-O was the most powerful whereas for the opposite effects model HET-SKAT and HET-SKAT-O were more powerful [46]. Tang and Lin [46] further compared the different methods using normalized and non-normalized score statistics and illustrated that the use of non-normalized score-type statistics can result in power loss. It is obvious that no single test is more powerful under all different genetic models and since the underlying genetic model is not known upfront, it is important that the different methods are explored in each different case.

4 Heterogeneity

There can be numerous reasons underlying between-study heterogeneity in genomic studies, including differences due to different populations being studied and environmental or lifestyle factors. Other potential sources of heterogeneity include genotyping errors, differences in genotyping platforms, variants being imputed or genotyped in the different studies, or differences in the definitions of the phenotype or trait [2]. Different measures of heterogeneity have been proposed and used in the literature for assessing the between-study differences in underlying models for the common variants in GWAS. The Cochran's Q-statistic [20] and the I^2 metric [52] have been widely used in common variant meta-analyses. Q statistic is used for testing the hypothesis of no heterogeneity between studies and I^2 is a measure of the proportion of the total variability that is due to heterogeneity and takes values between 0 and 100%. Usually, a Q statistic p-value of <0.1 is regarded as significant heterogeneity, $I^2 > 50\%$ is considered moderate heterogeneity and $I^2 > 75\%$ is considered as high heterogeneity [52].

Heterogeneity is expected to play a more significant role in the meta-analyses of rare variant studies as rare variants are population specific [53] and can be more sensitive to sequencing technologies errors, quality control measures, and differences in regional annotations [51].

5 Meta-Analysis Software

The majority of the software developed for the common variant meta-analysis perform both fixed- and random–effects meta-analysis for binary and quantitative traits and also allow for genotyped and imputed variants. For the common variant single variant meta-analysis, METAL [54], META [55], GWAMA [56], PLINK [57] and different R packages [58] like MetABEL [59] have been most widely used. MANTRA [31] and TransMeta [27] have been used for the meta-analysis of results from multiethnic studies and METASOFT for the new random effects model proposed by Han and Eskin [25] and the binary effects assumption [26]. The different software require input of individual study summary statistics including p-values, sample size, estimate of the regression coefficient, standard errors, and imputation quality metrics. GWAMA, META, and METASOFT perform both fixed-

and random effects meta-analysis whereas METAL, PLINK, and MetABEL perform only fixed effects meta-analysis. META and METAL also perform *z*-score-based meta-analysis and META-SOFT implements two additional random-effects meta-analysis tests; a test that is optimal for detecting associations in the presence of heterogeneity and a test that is optimal when some studies have an effect and others do not. All software allow for genomic control adjustments and also produce measures of heterogeneity across the different studies (Cochran's Q *p*-value and I^2).

Different software have been developed for the meta-analysis of the regional rare variant test statistics including meta-analysis of score statistics (MASS) [50], RAREMETAL [60], MAGA and different R packages like MetaSKAT [47] and seqMeta [48]. Each package has their own function or complementary software for the calculation of the score statistics and covariance matrices of each individual study to be used subsequently for the meta-analysis. MASS, MetaSKAT, and seqMeta can be used to obtain summary statistics for both quantitative and binary traits whereas RAREMETAL can currently only be used for quantitative traits. seqMETA can also be used for survival analysis data and allows for different selection weights for the Burden and SKAT part of the SKAT-O. RAREMETAL and seqMeta also support the analysis of family data and conditional analyses. Furthermore, Tang and Lin developed a software to convert the summary statistics of the different rare variant meta-analysis software (PreMeta) as they are not always compatible [46]. This allows for the easier exchange of summary level statistics across the different studies without the need for each analyst to perform the analysis using the same software. Tang and Lin [46] have also proposed different transformation methods that are implemented in PreMeta which aim to achieve normality and reduce the type I error; the inverse-normal transformation (INT) and rescaled INT (R-INT). MAGA allows for the reconstruction of the regional test statistic using the single variant results from each study (effect estimates and standard errors) and uses correlation matrices from one of the component studies or publicly available resources [49]. The method implemented in MAGA is attractive when each of the component studies cannot obtain the score statistics and information matrices, but has limitation due to the fact that rare variants for which the effect cannot be estimated are not used in the analysis [49].

6 Discussion

Meta-analysis provides a powerful tool for the combination of the results of different studies in order to identify associations that would have not been found through a single study. This has proven an extremely successful method in GWAS and aided the identification of thousands of robustly associated common variants with complex traits. Although different meta-analysis techniques have been proposed, the fixed-effects meta-analysis has been most widely used in GWAS. The field of genetics is currently being driven by rare variant studies and a large number of sequencing experiments are currently being performed. Larger power will need to be achieved in order to identify rare variant associations and aggregation methods and meta-analysis will clearly play an important role in this identification. As the underlying genetic effects of rarevariants are not known upfront and currently there is not a universally more powerful rare variant meta-analysis method and a collection of approaches need to be explored. Further validation will need to be performed to regions identified through meta-analyses of aggregation tests.

References

1. Zeggini E, Ioannidis JP (2009) Meta-analysis in genome-wide association studies. Pharmacogenomics 10(2):191–201. https://doi.org/10.2217/14622416.10.2.191
2. Evangelou E, Ioannidis JP (2013) Meta-analysis methods for genome-wide association studies and beyond. Nat Rev Genet 14(6):379–389. https://doi.org/10.1038/nrg3472
3. Manolio TA (2010) Genomewide association studies and assessment of the risk of disease. N Engl J Med 363(2):166–176. https://doi.org/10.1056/NEJMra0905980
4. Pearson TA, Manolio TA (2008) How to interpret a genome-wide association study. JAMA 299(11):1335–1344. https://doi.org/10.1001/jama.299.11.1335
5. International HapMap Consortium (2005) A haplotype map of the human genome. Nature 437(7063):1299–1320. https://doi.org/10.1038/nature04226
6. 1000 Genomes Project Concortium, Auton A, Brooks LD et al (2016) A reference panel of 64,976 haplotypes for genotype imputation. Nat Genet 48(10):1279–1283. https://doi.org/10.1038/ng.3643
7. Haplotype Reference, C (2016) A reference panel of 64,976 haplotypes for genotype imputation. Nat Genet 48:1279
8. Visscher PM, Brown MA, McCarthy MI, Yang J (2012) Five years of GWAS discovery. Am J Hum Genet 90(1):7–24. https://doi.org/10.1016/j.ajhg.2011.11.029
9. Welter D, MacArthur J, Morales J et al (2014) The NHGRI GWAS catalog, a curated resource of SNP-trait associations. Nucleic Acids Res 42 (Database issue):D1001–D1006. https://doi.org/10.1093/nar/gkt1229
10. Do R, Kathiresan S, Abecasis GR (2012) Exome sequencing and complex disease: practical aspects of rare variant association studies. Hum Mol Genet 21(R1):R1–R9. https://doi.org/10.1093/hmg/dds387
11. Lee S, Abecasis GR, Boehnke M et al (2014) Rare-variant association analysis: study designs and statistical tests. Am J Hum Genet 95 (1):5–23. https://doi.org/10.1016/j.ajhg.2014.06.009
12. Ansorge WJ (2009) Next-generation DNA sequencing techniques. New Biotechnol 25 (4):195–203. https://doi.org/10.1016/j.nbt.2008.12.009
13. Price AL, Patterson NJ, Plenge RM et al (2006) Principal components analysis corrects for stratification in genome-wide association studies. Nat Genet 38(8):904–909. https://doi.org/10.1038/ng1847
14. Devlin B, Roeder K (1999) Genomic control for association studies. Biometrics 55 (4):997–1004
15. de Bakker PI, Ferreira MA, Jia X et al (2008) Practical aspects of imputation-driven meta-analysis of genome-wide association studies. Hum Mol Genet 17(R2):R122–R128. https://doi.org/10.1093/hmg/ddn288
16. Howie BN, Donnelly P, Marchini J (2009) A flexible and accurate genotype imputation method for the next generation of genome-wide association studies. PLoS Genet 5(6): e1000529. https://doi.org/10.1371/journal.pgen.1000529

17. Howie B, Fuchsberger C, Stephens M et al (2012) Fast and accurate genotype imputation in genome-wide association studies through pre-phasing. Nat Genet 44(8):955–959. https://doi.org/10.1038/ng.2354
18. Browning BL, Browning SR (2009) A unified approach to genotype imputation and haplotype-phase inference for large data sets of trios and unrelated individuals. Am J Hum Genet 84(2):210–223. https://doi.org/10.1016/j.ajhg.2009.01.005
19. Lin DY, Zeng D (2010) Meta-analysis of genome-wide association studies: no efficiency gain in using individual participant data. Genet Epidemiol 34(1):60–66. https://doi.org/10.1002/gepi.20435
20. Cochran WG (1954) The combination of estimates from different experiments. Biometrics 10:101–129
21. Mantel N, Haenszel W (1959) Statistical aspects of the analysis of data from retrospective studies of disease. J Natl Cancer Inst 22 (4):719–748
22. Borenstein M, Hedges LV, Higgins JP et al (2010) A basic introduction to fixed-effect and random-effects models for meta-analysis. Res Synth Methods 1(2):97–111. https://doi.org/10.1002/jrsm.12
23. DerSimonian R, Laird N (1986) Meta-analysis in clinical trials. Control Clin Trials 7 (3):177–188
24. Hardy RJ, Thompson SG (1996) A likelihood approach to meta-analysis with random effects. Stat Med 15:619–629
25. Han B, Eskin E (2011) Random-effects model aimed at discovering associations in meta-analysis of genome-wide association studies. Am J Hum Genet 88(5):586–598. https://doi.org/10.1016/j.ajhg.2011.04.014
26. Han B, Eskin E (2012) Interpreting meta-analyses of genome-wide association studies. PLoS Genet 8(3):e1002555. https://doi.org/10.1371/journal.pgen.1002555
27. Shi J, Lee S (2016) A novel random effect model for GWAS meta-analysis and its application to trans-ethnic meta-analysis. Biometrics 72(3):945–954. https://doi.org/10.1111/biom.12481
28. Fisher RA (1925) Statistical methods for research workers. Oliver and Boyd, Edinburgh
29. Stouffer SA (1949) Adjustment during army life. Princeton University Press, Princeton, NJ
30. Stephens M, Balding DJ (2009) Bayesian statistical methods for genetic association studies. Nat Rev Genet 10(10):681–690. https://doi.org/10.1038/nrg2615
31. Morris AP (2011) Transethnic meta-analysis of genomewide association studies. Genet Epidemiol 35(8):809–822. https://doi.org/10.1002/gepi.20630
32. Lek M, Karczewski KJ, Minikel EV et al (2016) The OncoArray consortium: a network for understanding the genetic architecture of common cancers. Cancer Epidemiol Biomark Prev 26:126. https://doi.org/10.1158/1055-9965.EPI-16-0106
33. Amos CI, Dennis J et al (2017) The OncoArray Consortium: A Network for Understanding the Genetic Architecture of Common Cancers. Cancer Epidemiol Biomark Prev 26(1): 126–135
34. Lin DY, Tang ZZ (2011) A general framework for detecting disease associations with rare variants in sequencing studies. Am J Hum Genet 89(3):354–367. https://doi.org/10.1016/j.ajhg.2011.07.015
35. Wang K, Li M, Hakonarson H (2010) ANNOVAR: functional annotation of genetic variants from high-throughput sequencing data. Nucleic Acids Res 38(16):e164. https://doi.org/10.1093/nar/gkq603
36. Morgenthaler S, Thilly WG (2007) A strategy to discover genes that carry multi-allelic or mono-allelic risk for common diseases: a cohort allelic sums test (CAST). Mutat Res 615(1–2):28–56. https://doi.org/10.1016/j.mrfmmm.2006.09.003
37. Morris AP, Zeggini E (2010) An evaluation of statistical approaches to rare variant analysis in genetic association studies. Genet Epidemiol 34(2):188–193. https://doi.org/10.1002/gepi.20450
38. Madsen BE, Browning SR (2009) A groupwise association test for rare mutations using a weighted sum statistic. PLoS Genet 5(2): e1000384. https://doi.org/10.1371/journal.pgen.1000384
39. Li B, Leal SM (2008) Methods for detecting associations with rare variants for common diseases: application to analysis of sequence data. Am J Hum Genet 83(3):311–321. https://doi.org/10.1016/j.ajhg.2008.06.024
40. Price AL, Kryukov GV, de Bakker PI et al (2010) Pooled association tests for rare variants in exon-resequencing studies. Am J Hum Genet 86(6):832–838. https://doi.org/10.1016/j.ajhg.2010.04.005
41. Wu MC, Lee S, Cai T et al (2011) Rare-variant association testing for sequencing data with the sequence kernel association test. Am J Hum Genet 89(1):82–93. https://doi.org/10.1016/j.ajhg.2011.05.029

42. Neale BM, Rivas MA, Voight BF et al (2011) Testing for an unusual distribution of rare variants. PLoS Genet 7(3):e1001322. https://doi.org/10.1371/journal.pgen.1001322
43. Lee S, Wu MC, Lin X (2012) Optimal tests for rare variant effects in sequencing association studies. Biostatistics 13(4):762–775. https://doi.org/10.1093/biostatistics/kxs014
44. Liu DJ, Peloso GM, Zhan X et al (2014) Meta-analysis of gene-level tests for rare variant association. Nat Genet 46(2):200–204. https://doi.org/10.1038/ng.2852
45. Lumley T, Brody J, Dupuis J, Cupples A (2013) Meta-analysis of a rare variant association test. http://stattech.wordpress.fos.auckland.ac.nz/files/2012/11/skat-meta-paper.pdf
46. Tang ZZ, Lin DY (2015) Meta-analysis for discovering rare-variant associations: statistical methods and software programs. Am J Hum Genet 97(1):35–53. https://doi.org/10.1016/j.ajhg.2015.05.001
47. Lee S, Teslovich TM, Boehnke M et al (2013) General framework for meta-analysis of rare variants in sequencing association studies. Am J Hum Genet 93(1):42–53. https://doi.org/10.1016/j.ajhg.2013.05.010
48. Voorman A, Brody J, Chen H, Lumley T, Davis B (2017) seqMeta: Meta-analysis of region-based tests of rare DNA variants. R package version 1.6.7. https://CRAN.R-project.org/package=seqMeta
49. Hu YJ, Berndt SI, Gustafsson S et al (2013) Meta-analysis of gene-level associations for rare variants based on single-variant statistics. Am J Hum Genet 93(2):236–248. https://doi.org/10.1016/j.ajhg.2013.06.011
50. Tang ZZ, Lin DY (2013) MASS: meta-analysis of score statistics for sequencing studies. Bioinformatics 29(14):1803–1805. https://doi.org/10.1093/bioinformatics/btt280
51. Tang ZZ, Lin DY (2014) Meta-analysis of sequencing studies with heterogeneous genetic associations. Genet Epidemiol 38(5):389–401. https://doi.org/10.1002/gepi.21798
52. Higgins JP, Thompson SG (2002) Quantifying heterogeneity in a meta-analysis. Stat Med 21 (11):1539–1558. https://doi.org/10.1002/sim.1186
53. Nelson MR, Wegmann D, Ehm MG et al (2012) An abundance of rare functional variants in 202 drug target genes sequenced in 14,002 people. Science 337(6090):100–104. https://doi.org/10.1126/science.1217876
54. Willer CJ, Li Y, Abecasis GR (2010) METAL: fast and efficient meta-analysis of genomewide association scans. Bioinformatics 26 (17):2190–2191. https://doi.org/10.1093/bioinformatics/btq340
55. Liu JZ, Tozzi F, Waterworth DM et al (2010) Meta-analysis and imputation refines the association of 15q25 with smoking quantity. Nat Genet 42(5):436–440. https://doi.org/10.1038/ng.572
56. Magi R, Morris AP (2010) GWAMA: software for genome-wide association meta-analysis. BMC Bioinformatics 11:288. https://doi.org/10.1186/1471-2105-11-288
57. Purcell S, Neale B, Todd-Brown K et al (2007) PLINK: a tool set for whole-genome association and population-based linkage analyses. Am J Hum Genet 81(3):559–575. https://doi.org/10.1086/519795
58. R Core Team (2015) R: a language and environment for statistical computing. R Foundation for Statistical Computing, Vienna
59. Aulchenko YS, Ripke S, Isaacs A et al (2007) GenABEL: an R library for genome-wide association analysis. Bioinformatics 23 (10):1294–1296. https://doi.org/10.1093/bioinformatics/btm108
60. Feng S, Liu D, Zhan X et al (2014) RAREMETAL: fast and powerful meta-analysis for rare variants. Bioinformatics 30(19):2828–2829. https://doi.org/10.1093/bioinformatics/btu367

Chapter 7

Gene-Gene and Gene-Environment Interactions

Andrew T. DeWan

Abstract

Identifying gene–gene and gene–environment interactions may help us to better describe the genetic architecture for complex traits. While advances have been made in identifying genetic variants associated with complex traits through more dense panels of genetic variants and larger sample sizes, genome-wide interaction analyses are still limited in power to detect interactions with small effect sizes, rare frequencies, and higher order interactions. This chapter outlines methods for detecting both gene-gene and gene-environment interactions both through explicit tests for interactions (i.e., ones in which the interaction is tested directly) and non-explicit tests (i.e., ones in which an interaction is allowed for in the test, but does not test for the interaction directly) as well as approaches for increasing power by reducing the search space. Issues relating to multiple test correction, replication, and the reporting of interaction results in publications.

Key words Interaction, Epistasis, Environment, GWAS, Power, Replication

1 Introduction

An interaction results when the effect of one factor is only evident in the presence of another. These factors could be genetic markers and/or environmental exposures. Much has been written on the topic of gene-gene (also known as epistasis) and gene-environment interactions with several comprehensive reviews of study designs and methods for analyzing both gene-gene [1–3] and gene-environment interactions [4, 5]. But why are we interested in studying interactions? Both gene-gene and gene-environment and potentially gene-gene-environment interactions allow us to better describe the underlying genetic architecture of a particular trait and as such we can begin to fill in the missing heritability [6] for a particular phenotype.

Biological interactions were originally defined as the situation when the phenotypic effect of one gene was only evident in the presence of a second gene [7]. In contrast, a statistical interaction is defined as a departure from a linear model combining two or more genetic factors (or a genetic factor and environmental factor) [8].

Evangelos Evangelou (ed.), *Genetic Epidemiology: Methods and Protocols*, Methods in Molecular Biology, vol. 1793, https://doi.org/10.1007/978-1-4939-7868-7_7, © Springer Science+Business Media, LLC, part of Springer Nature 2018

Another way to think about this is that biological interactions are observed at the individual level and statistical interactions at the population level, but this does not imply that observing evidence of one will lead to observing evidence of another [9]. The traditional method to test for statistical interactions is to use a regression-based model that includes main effect variables representing each genetic factor and an interaction term (the product of the main effect variables), and then testing for the significance of the interaction term after adjusting for the main effects. However, several other methods exist to test for statistical interactions and these will be discussed as well.

We now have the ability to conduct very dense genome-wide association studies with up to five million genetic markers genotyped at one time and millions more imputed using large reference panels from population-based sequencing projects. The combinatorial problem can be immense if you attempt to look at all possible marker combinations with little power to detect significant interactions after accounting for all interactions tested. Given the exponential improvements in computational power and the relative ease of parallel computing, the computational hurdles of examining all pairwise gene-gene interactions are not insurmountable, and exhaustive searches of higher order interactions will follow. However, the immense power constraints on currently available sample sizes, while improving with studies routinely examining 10,000 to more than 500,000 subjects, are still underpowered to detect interactions with modest effect sizes ($OR < 1.2$) and low frequency variants (minor allele frequency [MAF] < 0.01). Though marker pruning using linkage disequilibrium can reduce this problem somewhat, there are several other data reduction approaches that will be discussed based on prior biological knowledge or statistical evidence for association. These can mitigate the multiple testing burden but depend heavily on the quality of this prior information.

Similar to gene-gene interactions, gene-environment interactions arise when the effect of a genetic factor on a phenotype is dependent on the presence or absence of an environmental factor. Statistically, this can be tested in a similar fashion as for gene-gene interactions traditionally done using a regression-based model with main effects for the genetic factor and environmental factor and an interaction term and testing for the significance of the interaction term. This environmental factor may be one traditionally thought of as an environmental exposure such as smoking, indoor NO_2 levels, or sun exposure, but these could also be other potentially genetically influenced phenotypes such as obesity, blood glucose levels, or birthweight that may be influencing the effect of the genetic factor depending on the value of these secondary phenotypes.

As outlined below, direct assessment of interactions (termed as "explicit" test) is often less powerful than joint tests that include either an interaction term or allow for interaction but do not test for the significance of the interaction directly (termed as "non-explicit" test). This classification of tests for interactions will be used throughout this chapter as different approaches and tests are discussed.

2 Materials

2.1 Data

2.1.1 Genotype Data

The core of both gene-gene and gene-environment interaction analyses is obtaining high-quality genotype data. One may use data generated specifically for a particular project, but there are also many outstanding datasets available for analysis from a number of online repositories.

If samples are being genotyped for the specific project there are many options available. There are whole genome microarray panels of markers based on relatively even coverage across the genome, panels of markers that maximize the coverage for specific race/ ethnic groups, and panels that allow custom markers to be added-on to existing panels to increase coverage of specific genes of interest or previously associated markers. There are also panels of markers that target specific regions of the genome such as the exonic regions, cancer-associated genes, and metabolic genes. The selection of the right microarray will depend on your specific study hypotheses, type of study, and budget. Lower throughput genotyping can be done for single variants to hundreds of variants simultaneously depending again on the hypotheses and goals of the project.

Genotyping known panels of markers is not the only choice for interaction studies. One could choose to utilize sequencing-based approaches to genotype unknown variants and/or low frequency and rare variants. Whole genome or whole exome sequencing could be utilized for hypothesis-free analyses or targeted sequencing if specific genes or pathways are hypothesized to be involved in the interaction(s).

If secondary data analysis is an option, there are a plethora of datasets with genome-wide data available as well as extensive phenotype data. Two such repositories are the database of genotype and phenotype (dbGaP) maintained by NCBI primarily of studies conducted in the United States (https://www.ncbi.nlm.nih.gov/gap) and the European Genome-phenome Archive (EGA) maintained by EBI primarily of studies conducted in Europe (https://www.ebi.ac.uk/ega/home). These databases contain hundreds of datasets accessible through an application to the respective data access committees.

2.1.2 Environmental Data

The environmental factors that could be considered in a study of gene-environment interactions are extremely broad. These include chemical (e.g., polychlorinated biphenyl (PCB)), physical (e.g., airborne particulate matter), biological (e.g., viral infections), and lifestyle (e.g., physical activity). The measurement of each of these individual environmental factors is going to vary widely depending on the environmental factor of interest. This could range from measuring NO_2 levels in the air via chemiluminescence, measuring radiation exposure via a dosimeter, conducting a daily food diary to estimate saturated fat intake, or reviewing charts to collect data on BMI history. The discussion in this chapter will focus on environmental exposures at one time point, but there is some evidence that longitudinal environmental data may increase the power to detect gene-environment interactions for common diseases [10].

2.1.3 Biological/Functional Data

For analyses that are pursuing a hypothesis-driven approach and/or filtering based on biological information, one may want to utilize prior biological or functional data. There are a variety of databases and programs that can be accessed to provide this type of information. One could simply curate information from publications in the scientific literature through systemic reviews of publications in databases such as PubMed. Data on functionality of variants can be obtained more systematically from databases such as ENCODE (Encyclopedia of DNA Elements) [11] that contains a comprehensive list of functional elements at both the RNA and protein levels and is available for viewing or downloading from the UCSC Genome Browser (www.genome.ucsc.edu/ENCODE). Direct annotation of variants could be conducted using a program such as Annovar [12] to annotate variants as to their respective genes, coding vs. noncoding, and predicted functional consequence. An alternative annotation program more directly related to filtering variants for interaction analyses is Biofilter which allows for the annotation of variants based on previous association studies and biological knowledge, filtering variants based on specific biological hypotheses, and building sets of testable variant interactions based on implication indices compiled from available data [13].

2.1.4 Previous Statistical Data

For analyses that filter variants based on prior statistical knowledge, data from one's own GWAS or single-variant association study could be used, results mined from previous publications or, alternatively, association results obtained from databases such as the GWAS Catalog (http://www.ebi.ac.uk/gwas/). While results from previous publications or the GWAS Catalog are a convenient and useful resource, they have the disadvantage of being biased toward reporting only genome-wide significant results and other nominally significant results will likely not be available and should be kept in mind when planning this type of analysis approach.

2.2 Software

Below are a listing of programs that can be used to conduct gene-gene and/or gene-environment interaction analyses with other programs mentioned and described throughout the chapter. This is not an exhaustive list and is only an example of programs that are commonly used to assess interactions in genetic epidemiological studies. Additional programs not directly related to the interaction analysis such as for computing eigenvalues from principal components analyses (e.g., EIGENSTRAT [14]) and imputation of variants (e.g., IMPUTE2 [15]) are not listed.

2.2.1 PLINK

This is a suite of tools designed to conduct genome association analyses, including both gene-gene and gene-environment interactions [16]. The primary interaction analyses are based on logistic and linear regression. They can accommodate both gene-gene and gene-environment interactions on the genome-wide scale or on a smaller number of variants by creating subsets of genetic variants to test again each other or the environmental factor. The program has the flexibility to conduct both explicit tests for interaction by testing for the significance of the interaction term directly in the regression model or a non-explicit joint test by testing the main and interactions effects. There is also a faster option for conducting genome-wide gene-gene interactions (*fast-epistasis*) based on the Z-score for the differences in OR for SNP-SNP combinations between cases and controls or for cases alone (case-only test).

2.2.2 CASSI

This is a software package that is specifically designed to conduct genome-wide gene-gene interaction analyses in a computationally efficient manner ([17]; https://www.staff.ncl.ac.uk/richard.howey/cassi/index.html). This package corrects a minor error in the Wu et al. statistic [18] in the calculation of the variance for estimated rather than observed haplotypes and in the *fast-epistasis* variance originally implemented in PLINK.

2.2.3 BOOST

The Boolean Operation-based Screening and Testing (BOOST) program was designed to efficiently screen and then explicitly test for genome-wide gene-gene interactions [19]. The screening phase involves a non-iterative procedure to approximate the likelihood ratio and then all variant pairs that survive this screening are subjected to a classical likelihood ratio test in the testing phase.

2.2.4 MDR

The Multifactor Dimensionality Reduction (MDR) software package [20] is designed to conduct data mining on discrete variables and can be used to detect both gene-gene and gene-environment interactions for dichotomous outcomes [21]. The traditional MDR approach is a non-explicit test for interaction as it is a nonparametric test that combines factors that may be interacting in order to best discriminate the subjects among the dichotomous outcome. An extension of the MDR has been developed that incorporates a permutation-based approach that can explicitly test for interactions [22]. A recent extension to the MDR has implemented a t-test approach that allows for quantitative outcomes [23]. The MDR method, however, is designed primarily for smaller sets of markers, but parallel computing could be utilized to conduct a genome-wide analysis.

3 Methods

3.1 Quality Control (QC)

No analysis can be successful without high-quality data. The specific steps of the genotype QA/QC will depend on the type of assay used to generate the genotypes. These range from single-variant assays based on PCR, whole genome microarray genotyping, and whole-exome and whole-genome sequencing. A brief outline of the QC steps for each is outlined below.

3.1.1 Single-Variant QC

The primary steps are to assess the overall performance of the individual genotyping assays through examination of the variant call rate (variant call rate = total number of genotype calls/total number of individuals genotyped) and Hardy-Weinberg Equilibrium (HWE). While the thresholds chosen to include variants can be arbitrary, typically one would look for variant call rates >98% (which should be examined in cases and controls separately if conducting a case-control analysis to ensure no bias due to differences in call rates between cases and controls) and HWE p-values $>10^{-4}$ which if conducting a case-control study are assessed only in controls. Without the benefit of genome-wide genotype data it is impossible to assess the data for population stratification, but adjustments can be made in the analysis (if using regression-based methods) for relevant covariates that may capture potential stratification such as self-reported race/ethnicity.

3.1.2 Microarray QC

As with single-variant QC, one will examine both the individual variant call rates and HWE to ensure that each variant probe is generating high-quality genotype data with similar thresholds applied as mentioned above. However, additional steps can and should be taken into account. The individual subject call rates should be examined first to determine if there were general problems with the individual array and/or DNA. These call rate thresholds may range from 93% to 98% and are often suggested by the array manufacturer-based past performance of the array (subject call rate = total number of genotype calls for an individual subject/total number of variants attempted to be genotyped). Poorly performing subjects should be removed prior to any downstream QC steps. Population stratification should be assessed using a genome-wide procedure such as principal components analysis to determine if there are slight variations in the genotype frequencies between subpopulations within your dataset. This procedure can detect any systematic differences that may be due to differences in allele frequencies arising ancestry differences, but also due to experimental/processing differences (e.g., plate effects). If significant principal components (PCs) are detected it is suggested that these PCs be adjusted for in the analysis. If the analysis assumes unrelated subjects it is suggested that the dataset be examined for cryptic relatedness using a procedure such as estimate pairwise identity-by-decent (IBD). This pairwise measure that is often used is $\widehat{p}_i$. Again, the threshold for identifying cryptically related subjects is arbitrary one often chooses a threshold ranging from 0.125 to 0.2 and then eliminates one of the two subjects in this cryptically related pair. This can be done randomly, or one may want to eliminate the subjects based on the subject call rate (eliminating the subject with a fewer genotype calls) or if it is a case-control study and a cryptically related pair is comprised of a case subject and a control subject it may be beneficial to eliminate the control if cases are in short supply.

To assess whether or not the QC steps that have been taken are successful prior to conducting an interaction analysis, it would be beneficial to conduct a genome-wide single-variant analysis and examine QQ plots and/or estimate λ from the data after adjusting for PCs and other covariates. QQ plots can be generated using an R script such as qqman.r (https://CRAN.R-project.org/package=qqman) and λ estimated using PLINK. Deviations from the expected line on the QQ plot are not expected except at the tail (i.e., the true positives) and with deviations along much of the expected line being an indication of residual population stratification. λ estimates greater than 1.05 are routinely seen as indicators of population stratification and additional PCs should be adjusted for until the lambda value falls below this threshold. This assessment is typically done in single-variant analyses prior to any interaction analyses.

3.1.3 Sequencing QC

Specific workflows for alignment, variant calling, and variant QA/QC and filtering are described in detail elsewhere (*see* Ref. 24 for a detailed step-by-step pipeline covering the major sequencing analysis tools). Briefly, a standard analysis pipeline would start by aligning the FASTQ raw sequence reads to a reference genome using the Burrows-Wheeler Aligner (BWA, [25]).Then converting to BAM format, sorting, indexing, marking PCR duplicates and merging into one BAM file using SAMtools [26]. Finally, locally realigning the BAM file around insertion/deletions, recalibrating and calling variants using HaplotypeCaller in the Genome Analysis Toolkit (GATK, [27, 28]).

Variant QC can utilize a variety of different metrics, but an example of one approach is how we conducted our QC in our whole-exome sequence analysis of a family segregating asthma [29]. Variants were flagged (and not considered further in our analysis) if they met any of the following criteria: three or more variants detected within 10 bp; four or more alignments map to different locations equally well; coverage of less than five reads; quality score <50; low quality for a particular sequence depth (variant confidence/unfiltered depth <1.5); and strand bias (Phred-scaled *p*-values using Fisher's Exact Test >200). There are many variations that can be employed in your QC pipeline, but the most important aspect is achieving the highest quality set of variants to retain in your analysis.

3.1.4 Linkage Disequilibrium Pruning

Reducing the number of variants considered in the analysis, regardless of genotyping method, can be accomplished by linkage disequilibrium (LD) pruning. LD is an indication of the correlation, or non-independence, between variants and can be measured using r^2 or D'. A typical r^2 threshold used to prune variants is 0.8, but a lower threshold can be used to eliminate more variants at the risk of excluding some that are independently informative. This procedure is particularly important when conducting a case-only gene-gene interaction analysis (discussed in Subheading 3.2.12) as the variants must not be correlated with each other.

3.2 Gene-Gene Interaction Analysis

The basic analysis is straightforward, the assessment of a deviation from an additive or multiplicative model containing two or more variants. This is traditionally assessed through regression-based modeling but many different methods are available and several methods will be discussed below. One could divide these approaches into explicit vs. non-explicit tests for interactions, with explicit tests determining if the null hypothesis of the sum on the additive/linear scale or the product on the multiplicative scale of the joint effects of the two variants is contributing to the outcome with the alternative hypothesis being that the joint effect of the two variants is greater or less than the expected. Non-explicit tests are able to determine if the grouping of variants is associated with the outcome, but not necessarily that the variants together deviate from an additive or multiplicative model. Different inheritance models can be imposed on the genetic variants in the interaction models (*see* **Note 1**) and the issue of outcome scale is also an important consideration when interpreting interactions (*see* **Note 2**).

Regression-based approaches are attractive not only for their ability to explicitly detect interactions in the data, but because of the ability to adjust for multiple covariates. In a genome-wide setting this is important so that significant principal components can be adjusted to remove population stratification, but other potential confounders can be adjusted as well, including age, sex, etc. depending on the outcome of interest.

3.2.1 Logistic Regression

For dichotomous outcomes, a logistic regression model is one of the most straightforward approaches for testing an interaction, either explicitly or non-explicitly. In the following logistic regression model we are modeling the probability of our dichotomous outcome (p) using an intercept (β_0), two genetic variants (SNP1 and SNP2, for example) and their respective main effects (β_1 and β_2) and their interaction effect (β_3):

$$\log\left(\frac{p}{1-p}\right) = \beta_0 + \beta_1\text{SNP1} + \beta_2\text{SNP2} + \beta_3\text{SNP1} \times \text{SNP2}$$

In this model, we can test for the significance of the interaction effect of the two variants by testing the null hypothesis that $\beta_3 = 0$. This is an explicit test for interaction in that we are testing for an interaction after adjusting for the main effects (i.e., independent effects) of the two genetic variants. This model will produce an effect estimate (β_3) which can easily be converted to an OR by $\exp\beta_3$. It should be noted that the main effects should not be interpreted as the main effect of the variants (or the variant and the environmental factor) since they are adjusted for the interaction term in the model.

Alternatively, we can test for the significance of the joint effects of the two variants by using a 2 degree of freedom likelihood ratio test of the full model against a model in which there is neither an interaction term nor main effect term for one of the SNPs:

$$\log\left(\frac{p}{1-p}\right) = \beta_0 + \beta_1\text{SNP1}$$

While this model contains an interaction term, this is a non-explicit test for interaction as we are testing the significance of the main effect of one of the SNPs and interaction term combined. This may be seen as a less desirable test but this can be more powerful for detecting significant signals [30]. However, this joint test can be significant if either of the main effects is strong enough or if both main effects are strong enough without a significant interaction term (β_3). As will be discussed later, one may want to screen combinations of variants for joint effects and then follow up for explicit tests of an interaction only on the limited set of variants demonstrating significant joint effects.

When reporting the results of regression-based analyses, it is important to report not only the significance of the interaction (p-value), but also the parameter estimate of the interaction as well as those of the main effects (*see* **Note 3**).

3.2.2 Linear Regression

For continuous outcomes, linear regression can be used to test for interactions in much the same way as logistic regression for dichotomous outcomes. βs are not converted to ORs, but are rather interpreted directly with the sign of β_3, an indication of the direction of the interaction, and the p-value for the likelihood ratio test of the full model versus one without the interaction term an indication of the significance of the interaction term. A two degree of freedom joint test can also be constructed.

3.2.3 Nonparametric Analyses

The most popular nonparametric method for interaction analysis are the multidimensional reduction methods. These are based on the idea that across a contingency table of two or more genetic variant genotype combinations or genotype and discrete environmental factor combinations, each square in the contingency table can be divided into increasing risk and decreasing risk in the context of the phenotype. These collapsed contingency tables can then be tested for association with the phenotype. This is typically done by splitting the data into a training set (to build the collapsed contingency table) and a testing set to determine the classification error. The data are split multiple times and the model is assessed by the classification error and prediction error estimated from these multiple cross-validations [21]. Due to the fact that this is a nonparametric method, a p-value is obtained for the set of factors included in the model, but an effect estimate is not. The significance of the model is interpreted as the significance of the group of factors (genetic variants or genetic variant(s) and environmental factors) but cannot be interpreted as direct evidence of an interaction.

The model-based MDR (MB-MDR) methodology is an extension of the classic MDR framework that allows for the direct testing of interactions through the use of the Wald statistic on high and low-risk genotype categories [22, 31]. The significance of the interaction is then tested using permutation testing of the maximum Wald statistic and can be considered an explicit test of an interaction.

3.2.4 Multiple Test Correction

One of the biggest challenges in conducting genome-wide analysis in general, and more specifically interaction analysis, particularly gene-gene interactions, is the multiple testing problem. Given that hundreds of thousands or millions of variants are considered in most genome-wide studies, the chance of detecting a false positive is immense. This is even more apparent when multiple environmental factors are considered and most problematic when all pairwise variant interactions are considered in an exhaustive gene-gene interaction search. Traditionally, genome-wide studies have adopted a Bonferroni correction to adjust for the number of variants analyzed, but this can be overly conservative, especially for dense maps of markers in high LD. However, other procedures such as the False Discovery Rate (FDR; [32]), LD-based variant counting to account only for the number of independent tests [33] and permutation testing [34, 35] have been adopted. Permutation testing, while attractive because it accounts for the number of independent tests by maintaining the LD structure in the permuted data, is computationally intensive, even more so when all pairwise variant combinations need to be considered in thousands of permuted datasets. Therefore, the FDR or LD-based methods are more attractive alternatives.

3.2.5 Genome-Wide (Exhaustive) Approaches

A typical genome-wide association study will genotype between 100,000 and 1,000,000 singe-nucleotide polymorphisms. While exponential advances in computational power mean that the computing power to run the analysis on the pairwise tests required for a panel of 500,000 SNPs (2.5×10^{11} tests) is not insurmountable and with parallel computing relatively quick, the major hurdle is power. While large multi-center consortium studies mean that the number of subjects for many subjects has greatly increased, with studies reaching 50,000 or more subjects depending on the frequency of the disease or phenotype, these may still not be powerful enough to detect significant interactions on the genome-wide scale. In a study of genome-wide data obtained from the Resource for Genetic Epidemiology Research on Adult Health and Aging (GERA), using 45,171 subjects for ten phenotypes and conducting an exhaustive search for interactions, we failed to identify any genome-wide significant interactions, suggesting that we were underpowered to detect interactions with apparently weak effect sizes [36].

As demonstrated in Table 1, for a genome-wide gene-gene interaction study of 200,000 markers using an exhaustive approach, requires more than 30,000 cases and 30,000 controls to achieve genome-wide significance for two loci each with an MAF of 0.2 and an interaction OR of 1.2. All power calculations presented in this chapter were performed in Quanto [37]. The power calculations assumed a population risk of the disease of 0.1 and a log-additive mode of inheritance and a main effect of each variant of 1.2. For a case-control study with 5000 cases and 5000 controls, a reasonably sized case-control GWAS, and 200,000 markers genotyped, the minimal detectable OR is just over 1.6 (Table 2). For an interaction OR of 1.5, the number of markers considered would need to be reduced to around 2000 to detect a significant interaction among all pairs of interactions (4,000,000) and at an interaction OR of 1.2, only one interaction can be considered as only a nominally associated interaction is detectable (Table 3).

This lack of power can be daunting, but as detailed in the following sections there are several ways to increase power by reducing the number of tests through filtering or using biologically informed combinations of variants.

Table 1
Power of interaction analysis

	Number of cases and controls					
Interaction type	5000	10,000	20,000	30,000	40,000	50,000
G-G	0.000	0.003	0.164	0.654	0.940	0.995
G-E	0.024	0.032	0.317	0.717	0.928	0.988

Table 2
Power of case-control and case-only gene-gene interaction analyses

intOR	Case-control	Case-only
1.1	0.000	0.000
1.2	0.000	0.013
1.3	0.004	0.547
1.4	0.076	0.992
1.5	0.388	1.000
1.6	0.782	1.000
1.7	0.961	1.000
1.8	0.996	1.000
1.9	1.000	1.000
2.0	1.000	1.000

3.2.6 Data Reduction Approaches

In order to overcome the multiple testing burden of a genome-wide screen for all gene-gene interactions, it may be advantageous to focus on a subset of SNPs that may have a one or more properties that may make the interaction analysis more likely to detect a significant interaction. If we reduce our set of 200,000 SNPs down to 2000 we can now detect an interaction OR of 1.5 using a set of 5000 cases and 5000 controls (Table 3). Below I outline a series of methods to reduce the set of SNPs considered.

Filtering by Allele Frequency

The simplest method to increase power to detect interactions is to impose a filter by minor allele frequency (MAF). Depending on the sample size and subsequent power estimates, it may be advantageous to filter out all SNPs with MAFs less than the power to detect a reasonable interaction effect size (e.g., all SNPs with an MAF <0.2).

Table 3
Power of gene-gene interaction analysis by interaction OR and number of markers

# Markers	intOR = 1.2	intOR = 1.4	intOR = 1.5
200,000	0.000	0.076	0.388
100,000	0.000	0.107	0.465
20,000	0.000	0.221	0.649
10,000	0.001	0.289	0.724
2000	0.004	0.488	0.869
1000	0.008	0.584	0.914
200	0.037	0.793	0.975
100	0.066	0.864	0.988
20	0.219	0.966	0.999
10	0.337	0.986	1.000
5	0.488	0.995	1.000
2	0.713	0.999	1.000
1	0.865	1.000	1.000

Filtering by Marginal Effects

While a significant marginal and/or main effect is not required to detect a significant interaction, there are few reports of significant interactions without also having detectable main effects. Therefore, it may be advantageous to filter based on marginal effects (i.e., single-variant effect) and only include those variants that have, for example, a single-variant association *p*-value of <0.05 (nominal significance threshold). This should reduce the number of SNPs to approximately 5% of the starting number (for our 500,000 SNPs this would result in 6.25×10^8 tests). This approach may be too stringent, as it requires both variants be nominally significant. An alternative approach would be to select a set of SNPs reaching a predefined significance threshold (e.g., $p < 10^{-4}$) and testing this set of SNPs against all other SNPs. In our example with 500,000 SNPs we would select ~50 SNPs with $p < 10^{-4}$ and test for an interaction with the remaining 499,450 for a total of 2.5×10^{-7} SNPs. This balances the requirement that there be some marginal effect of one of the SNPs with being able to detect interactions with SNPs showing no marginal effects but having a significance effect on disease only in the presence of a second SNP.

Candidate Gene Approaches

Filtering based on prior evidence of a gene's involvement in a particular disease is another approach to reducing the search space for interactions. Candidate genes could be selected by systematically reviewing the literature or for some diseases databases of candidate genes exist based on association studies, linkage analyses, and/or expression studies. For example, there are databases for preterm birth [38], preeclampsia [39], and non-syndromic hearing loss [40] for which one can obtain lists of candidate genes. By annotating variants to their respective genes using programs such as Annovar [12] only those SNPs annotated to the set of candidate genes can be selected for inclusion in the interaction analysis. As for the marginal effects, it may be advantageous to consider those SNPs within candidate genes against all other SNPs genotyped. In this way, it is possible to detect interactions with SNPs in novel genes not previously identified to be associated with the disease of interest.

Filtering by Function

Filtering by the effects of specific variants is another approach to reducing the search space. Again, variants can be annotated, but now the selection may be made based on being a coding variant or a splicing variant that is more likely to be functional. Other biological information could also be utilized such as examining interactions between SNPs in genes known to be involved in protein-protein interactions with the rationale being that SNPs in these biologically interacting genes are more likely to also show evidence of a statistical interaction. Similarly, one could examine interactions between variants within transcription factors and those within their binding sites.

3.2.7 Multistage Approaches

In order to maintain a genome-wide approach but overcome the hurdle of the immense multiple testing problem, it may be beneficial to employ a multistage approach. This is possible in situations in which a study has a large sample size, but still not adequately powered to detect significant interactions genome-wide. In a study of asthma, we first screened all pairwise interactions (9.1×10^{10}) in a small subset of the data and then carried through all interaction with a suggestive significance ($p < 10^{-5}$) to a follow-up stage of independent subjects and then attempted to replicate the top SNPs in a third set of independent subjects [41]. While this approach did not identify any genome-wide significant interactions, it did identify a candidate interaction between SNPs in two regions of the genome. The major advantage of this type of approach is that it allows for an unbiased examination of the SNPs without relying on previously reported biological and/or association data.

3.2.8 Gene-Based Interaction Tests

Another approach to reduce the multiple testing burden and combine information across multiple variants is to conduct a gene-based test of interaction. By considering each gene as a unit in the interaction rather than each individual variant, the total number of interactions considered is significantly reduced, thus increasing power. One such approach combines interaction p-values across all combinations of genetic variants in two genes into a single gene-gene interaction *p*-value that also accounts for linkage disequilibrium [42].

It should be appreciated that these gene-based tests can be applied to the setting of rare variant which are increasingly being studied. Extensions to rare variant tests to incorporate gene-gene and gene-environment interactions have been developed and include SKAT [43] which can handle gene-gene interactions and iSKAT [44] and rareGE [45] for gene-environment interactions.

3.2.9 Replication

Regardless of the analysis approach taken to identify gene-gene interactions, the gold standard is to conduct a replication analysis using an independent dataset. While fairly common for single-variant association studies, this is less routinely followed for gene-gene interaction analyses, as demonstrated in our systematic review of asthma gene-gene interactions where only 15.2% of interactions were attempted to be replicated [46]. The challenge is often identifying an appropriate replication dataset in which both variants were genotyped. Through the use of imputation the variant to be replicated could be imputed if they were not directly in the independent dataset.

A challenge for any replication of a genetic effect is the directionality of the effect. Differences due to the populations selected that can alter the minor allele frequencies and linkage disequilibrium structure can result in differences in both the magnitude and direction of effect [47]. This is amplified when looking at two or more loci as the probability of subtle differences can result in differences in the direction of effect when looking at interactions.

3.2.10 Meta-Analysis

This data analysis technique is commonly used to pool data across multiple studies and increase evidence for an association with a genetic variant. Meta-analysis is an attractive analytical technique because it can be used to increase power by substantially increasing the total sample size. While relatively straightforward for single-variant analyses using either fixed or random effects models [48] or by combining *p*-values [49], this is not always the case for gene-gene and gene-environment interactions. Differences in the analytical strategy and the way in which the results are presented may make meta-analyses more challenging. The *p*-value approach does not take into account the effect estimates, but this may be a better first approach as it can be used on a much broader set of analytical strategies such as MDR, regression-based approaches, and Random Forrest methods, for example. Meta-analysis methods that account for the effect estimate are more attractive because they can account for heterogeneity in both the effect estimates and between populations.

3.2.11 Case-Only Approach

The case-only study design to detect interactions was first described for gene-environment interactions [50, 51]. This design is premised on the idea that the variant is independent of the environmental exposure in the population. In the presence of a gene-environment interaction, there would be an association between the variant and the environmental exposure among cases only and this can be most easily tested using the regression-based approaches described above (linear or logistic depending on the environmental exposure being investigated); however, it should be noted that when using the case-only design the main effects of the variant and the environmental exposure cannot be determined as this is only possible using a case-control design.

The case-only design is more powerful than the case-control design (Table 4; 5000 cases and 5000 controls for case-control and 5000 cases for case-only, main effects ORs of 1.2 for both the environmental factor and genetic variant, a frequency of the environmental exposure of 0.25 in the population and MAF of 0.2, population risk of disease of 0.1 and 200,000 genetic markers). The major caveat is that there is an assumption that there is independence between the genetic variant and the environmental factor, i.e., that there is no association between these factors among the source population. Violation of this assumption can lead to biased estimates of the OR and there is a recommendation that a case-only gene-environmental interaction analysis only proceed for environmental factors with population-specific data [52]. This independence may be difficult to establish in population-based data, so independence could be tested for among controls (e.g., when a

Table 4
Power of case-control and case-only gene-environment interaction analyses

intOR	Case-control	Case-only
1.1	0.000	0.001
1.2	0.002	0.063
1.3	0.038	0.564
1.4	0.211	0.962
1.5	0.541	1.000
1.6	0.829	1.000
1.7	0.959	1.000
1.8	0.994	1.000
1.9	0.999	1.000
2.0	1.000	1.000

case-only analysis is being conducted among a case-control study) or replication of the finding among an independent case-control study. This is of particular importance when the environmental factor could be under genetic influence such as BMI. The substantial power gain of the case-only study makes this analysis strategy relatively attractive, but this is somewhat diminished by the strong independence assumption and the need to test this assumption in a set of population-based samples.

The case-only approach can also be utilized to detect gene-gene interactions [53]. In the presence of an interaction between two genetic variants there will be an association between these genetic variants among cases. This is most easily tested using a logistic regression model using one of the genetic markers as the dependent variable. As with case-only gene-environment interaction analyses, only the interaction can be examined and not the main effects of the genetic variants. Independence of the genetic variants in the source population is assumed, but this is much easier to achieve given the large amounts of genome-wide genotype data available for many diverse populations (e.g., HapMap [54]) or the use of LD pruning among controls, if available (*see* Subheading 3.1.4).

3.2.12 Three or More Variants

Gene-gene interactions are not limited to pairwise interactions. Higher order interactions involving three or more variants have been reported (e.g., renin-angiotensin system SNPs and hypertension [55]) and can be modeled in the regression framework. The problem is that as higher order interactions are considered the data become more and more sparse and the power to detect a significant interaction decreases. One approach to detecting higher order interactions would be to use a nonparametric, non-explicit method such as MDR to screen for potential higher order combinations of variants and then subsequently explicitly test for the interaction on a subset of the best performing combinations using a regression-based method.

3.3 Gene-Environment Interaction Analysis

At the core, the analysis of gene-environment interactions does not fundamentally differ from gene-gene interactions. The analysis can be conducted using the regression-based or nonparametric approaches described above with the same caveats for testing for explicit vs. non-explicit interactions in the dataset. Joint, or non--explicit, tests may be used to screen the data to detect potential interactions, followed by explicit tests to determine if an interaction exists between the identified variant and the environmental factor. In the logistic regression framework, one of the genetic variant variables is replaced by the environmental exposure of interest and the significance of the interaction β is tested in the model. Using the non-explicit MDR approach, the environmental variable is entered into the algorithm with the caveat that the environmental factor must be categorical in order for the reduction algorithm to work.

The power to detect gene-environment interactions suffers from the same lack of power on the genome-wide scale as gene-gene interactions. More than 30,000 cases and controls are required to detect an interaction OR of 1.2 (Table 1) under similar parameters as the gene-gene interactions analysis (main effects of OR = 1.2 for gene and environmental factors, MAF of 0.2, environmental prevalence of 0.25, population risk of disease of 0.1 and 200,000 genetic markers tested). Using 5000 cases and 5000 controls, the smallest detectable OR is just under 1.6 (Table 4). The same approaches to increase power by reducing the search space can be applied to the search for gene-environment interaction analyses, through all of the data reduction techniques described for gene-gene interactions.

It cannot be stressed enough that replication is the key to describing true positive gene-environment interactions, as was discussed for gene-gene interactions. As mentioned previously for gene-gene interaction replication, if the exact genetic variants are not directly genotyped in the independent dataset, imputation can be used to estimate the genotypes to be replicated. While this will work for the genetic variants in gene-environment interactions to be replicated, this is not the case if there is not comparable environmental data in the independent dataset. This can make the identification and selection of an appropriate dataset for replication more challenging for gene-environment interactions, but makes the replication of the findings no less important.

3.3.1 Modifiable Environmental Factors

One attractive aspect of identifying and describing gene-environment interactions for a complex disease is that this gives us the possibility of potentially modifying one contributing factor to a disease. At this point in time, inherited genetic variants are not modifiable, but if, for example, a significant gene-environment interaction were identified for obesity with a genetic variant and high saturated fat diet, individuals carrying the risk variant could be more strongly encouraged to reduce their saturated fat intake. Despite the general benefit we could all gain from reducing our saturated fat intake, this may be more effective if it were targeted to individuals based on their genetic profile and increased risk for obesity when both factors are present (beyond the additive main effects).

3.3.2 Gene-Gene-Environment Interactions

We should not think of gene-gene and gene-environment interactions as being mutually exclusive. As with higher order gene-gene interactions, interactions involving multiple genetic variants and an environmental factor are possible to model. The same issues with power due to sparsity of data and the number of unique combinations of factors apply, but given sufficient sample size these types of interaction models can be tested. It may be more important in this setting to attempt a screening step using a non-explicit approach and then apply an explicit test only to the set of interactions that surpass an initial significance threshold.

3.4 Conclusions

I have outlined several methods for conducting interaction analysis to detect both gene-gene and gene-environment interactions. However, it should be clear that there is no optimal method to detect either type of interaction. The method(s) chosen are often dictated based on the type of data you have available (e.g., case-control, case-only), the number of markers you have genotyped, and the number of subjects you have included. I strongly recommend reporting the results of explicit tests for interaction as this will greatly improve ability of other groups to attempt to replicate your results and meta-analyze where appropriate, but the use of non-explicit tests for interaction can be extremely useful to initially screen large numbers of interactions and when sample sizes are limited. We must continue to invest time and resources into identifying interactions in genome-wide data as this will help us to fill in the missing heritability gap and better understand the genetic architecture of complex traits.

4 Notes

1. Inheritance models: It should be noted that as with single-variant approaches, inheritance models can be imposed on the variants that include additive, multiplicative, dominant, recessive, and overdominant. These inheritance models can be imposed on the variants in the interaction model independently and can be considered in a combinatorial fashion for variant 1 and variant 2 (e.g., additive × additive, additive × multiplicative, additive × dominant, etc.). However, if this is done, care must be taken to account for this additional multiple testing. These models can be problematic when they are misspecified as they can reduce power which makes nonparametric approaches attractive.
2. Scale: The scale on which the outcome is measured or evaluated can influence whether or not an interaction exists between two variants or between a variant and an environmental factor. It needs to be kept in mind that there may be a monotone transformation of the outcome that could remove the interaction. For example, on the odds ratio scale, an interaction may exist between two SNPs (coded dichotomously as in a dominant model) in which the OR for having dominant alleles at both SNPs is greater than the sum of the ORs for having one dominant allele at each SNP. However, on the log(OR) scale this interaction is removed and termed a removable interaction. If there is no monotone transformation that can remove this interaction it is termed essential. The method to detect these types of interactions is described in a paper by Wu et al. [56].

3. Reporting of interaction results: As was previously outlined in our paper [46], there are several recommendations for how results of interaction analyses are reported in order to increase the interpretability and replicability of the interaction. Effect estimates should be provided so that both the strength and direction of the interaction can be assessed. If a regression-based approach is used, parameter estimates of the main effects and the interaction term should be provided. If a nonparametric approach is used, such as MDR, effect estimates are not produced, however, counts of cases and controls for the contingency table of genotype combinations should be provided. This will allow for a better assessment of the interaction and the possibility to incorporate the data into a meta-analysis.

References

1. Niel C, Sinoquet C, Dina C et al (2015) A survey about methods dedicated to epistasis detection. Front Genet 6:285
2. Ritchie MD (2015) Finding the epistasis needles in the genome-wide haystack. Methods Mol Biol 1253:19–33
3. Gusareva ES, Van Steen K (2014) Practical aspects of genome-wide association interaction analysis. Hum Genet 133(11):1343–1358
4. Tiret L (2002) Gene-environment interaction: a central concept in multifactorial diseases. Proc Nutr Soc 61(4):457–463
5. Ottman R (1990) An epidemiologic approach to gene-environment interaction. Genet Epidemiol 7(3):177–185
6. Manolio TA, Collins FS, Cox NJ et al (2009) Finding the missing heritability of complex diseases. Nature 461(7265):747–753
7. Bateson W (1909) Mendel's principles of heredity. Cambridge University Press, Cambridge
8. Cordell HJ (2002) Epistasis: what it means, what it doesn't mean, and statistical methods to detect it in humans. Hum Mol Genet 11 (20):2463–2468
9. Moore JH (2005) A global view of epistasis. Nat Genet 37(1):13–14
10. Ma J, Thabane L, Beyene J et al (2016) Power analysis for population-based longitudinal studies investigating gene-environment interactions in chronic diseases: a simulation study. PLoS One 11(2):e0149940
11. Dunham I, Kundaje A, Aldred SF et al (2012) An integrated encyclopedia of DNA elements in the human genome. Nature 489 (7414):57–74
12. Wang K, Li M, Hakonarson H (2010) ANNOVAR: functional annotation of genetic variants from high-throughput sequencing data. Nucleic Acids Res 38(16):e164
13. Bush WS, Dudek SM, Ritchie MD (2009) Biofilter: a knowledge-integration system for the multi-locus analysis of genome-wide association studies. Pac Symp Biocomput:368–379
14. Price AL, Patterson NJ, Plenge RM et al (2006) Principal components analysis corrects for stratification in genome-wide association studies. Nat Genet 38(8):904–909
15. Howie BN, Donnelly P, Marchini J (2009) A flexible and accurate genotype imputation method for the next generation of genome-wide association studies. PLoS Genet 5(6): e1000529
16. Purcell S, Neale B, Todd-Brown K et al (2007) PLINK: a tool set for whole-genome association and population-based linkage analyses. Am J Hum Genet 81(3):559–575
17. Ueki M, Cordell HJ (2012) Improved statistics for genome-wide interaction analysis. PLoS Genet 8(4):e1002625
18. Wu X, Dong H, Luo L et al (2010) A novel statistic for genome-wide interaction analysis. PLoS Genet 6(9):e1001131
19. Wan X, Yang C, Yang Q et al (2010) BOOST: a fast approach to detecting gene-gene interactions in genome-wide case-control studies. Am J Hum Genet 87(3):325–340
20. Hahn LW, Ritchie MD, Moore JH (2003) Multifactor dimensionality reduction software for detecting gene-gene and gene-environment interactions. Bioinformatics 19(3):376–382
21. Ritchie MD, Hahn LW, Roodi N et al (2001) Multifactor-dimensionality reduction reveals high-order interactions among estrogen-metabolism genes in sporadic breast cancer. Am J Hum Genet 69(1):138–147

22. Calle ML, Urrea V, Malats N et al (2010) mbmdr: an R package for exploring gene-gene interactions associated with binary or quantitative traits. Bioinformatics 26 (17):2198–2199
23. Gui J, Moore JH, Williams SM et al (2013) A simple and computationally efficient approach to multifactor dimensionality reduction analysis of gene-gene interactions for quantitative traits. PLoS One 8(6):e66545
24. Van der Auwera GA, Carneiro MO, Hartl C et al (2013) From FASTQ data to high confidence variant calls: the genome analysis toolkit best practices pipeline. Curr Protoc Bioinformatics 43:11.10 1–11.1033
25. Li H, Durbin R (2010) Fast and accurate long-read alignment with Burrows-Wheeler transform. Bioinformatics 26(5):589–595
26. Li H, Handsaker B, Wysoker A et al (2009) The sequence alignment/map format and SAMtools. Bioinformatics 25(16):2078–2079
27. McKenna A, Hanna M, Banks E et al (2010) The genome analysis toolkit: a MapReduce framework for analyzing next-generation DNA sequencing data. Genome Res 20 (9):1297–1303
28. DePristo MA, Banks E, Poplin R et al (2011) A framework for variation discovery and genotyping using next-generation DNA sequencing data. Nat Genet 43(5):491–498
29. Dewan AT, Egan KB, Hellenbrand K et al (2012) Whole-exome sequencing of a pedigree segregating asthma. BMC Med Genet 13 (1):95
30. Marchini J, Donnelly P, Cardon LR (2005) Genome-wide strategies for detecting multiple loci that influence complex diseases. Nat Genet 37(4):413–417
31. Calle ML, Urrea V, Vellalta G, Malats N, Steen KV (2008) Improving strategies for detecting genetic patterns of disease susceptibility in association studies. Stat Med 27 (30):6532–6546
32. Benjamini Y, Hochberg Y (1995) Controlling the false discovery rate: a practical and powerful approach to multiple testing. J R Stat Soc B 57 (1):289–300
33. Nyholt DR (2004) A simple correction for multiple testing for single-nucleotide polymorphisms in linkage disequilibrium with each other. Am J Hum Genet 74(4):765–769
34. North BV, Curtis D, Sham PC (2002) A note on the calculation of empirical P values from Monte Carlo procedures. Am J Hum Genet 71 (2):439–441
35. North BV, Curtis D, Sham PC (2003) A note on calculation of empirical P values from Monte Carlo procedure. Am J Hum Genet 72 (2):498–499
36. Murk W, DeWan AT (2016) Exhaustive genome-wide search for SNP-SNP interactions across 10 human diseases. G3 (Bethesda) 6 (7):2043–2050
37. Gauderma WJ, Morrison JM, QUANTO 1.1: A computer program for power and sample size calculations for genetic-epidemiology studies. http://hydra.usc.edu/gxe2006
38. Uzun A, Sharma S, Padbury J (2012) A bioinformatics approach to preterm birth. Am J Reprod Immunol 67(4):273–277
39. Uzun A, Triche EW, Schuster J et al (2016) dbPEC: a comprehensive literature-based database for preeclampsia related genes and phenotypes. Database (Oxford). https://doi.org/10.1093/database/baw006. pii:baw006
40. Shearer AE, Eppsteiner RW, Booth KT et al (2014) Utilizing ethnic-specific differences in minor allele frequency to recategorize reported pathogenic deafness variants. Am J Hum Genet 95(4):445–453
41. Murk W, DeWan AT (2016) Genome-wide search identifies a gene-gene interaction between 20p13 and 2q14 in asthma. BMC Genet 17(1):102
42. Ma L, Clark AG, Keinan A (2013) Gene-based testing of interactions in association studies of quantitative traits. PLoS Genet 9(2):e1003321
43. Wu MC, Lee S, Cai T et al (2011) Rare-variant association testing for sequencing data with the sequence kernel association test. Am J Hum Genet 89(1):82–93
44. Lin X, Lee S, Wu MC et al (2016) Test for rare variants by environment interactions in sequencing association studies. Biometrics 72 (1):156–164
45. Chen H, Meigs JB, Dupuis J (2014) Incorporating gene-environment interaction in testing for association with rare genetic variants. Hum Hered 78(2):81–90
46. Murk W, Bracken MB, DeWan AT (2015) Confronting the missing epistasis problem: on the reproducibility of gene-gene interactions. Hum Genet 134(8):837–849
47. Greene CS, Penrod NM, Williams SM et al (2009) Failure to replicate a genetic association may provide important clues about genetic architecture. PLoS One 4(6):e5639
48. Fleiss JL (1993) The statistical basis of meta-analysis. Stat Methods Med Res 2(2):121–145
49. Fisher RA (1948) Combining independent tests of significance. Am Stat 2:30
50. Piegorsch WW, Weinberg CR, Taylor JA (1994) Non-hierarchical logistic models and

case-only designs for assessing susceptibility in population-based case-control studies. Stat Med 13(2):153–162

51. Begg CB, Zhang ZF (1994) Statistical analysis of molecular epidemiology studies employing case-series. Cancer Epidemiol Biomark Prev 3 (2):173–175
52. Hodgson ME, Olshan AF, North KE et al (2012) The case-only independence assumption: associations between genetic polymorphisms and smoking among controls in two population-based studies. Int J Mol Epidemiol Genet 3(4):333–360
53. Yang Q, Khoury MJ, Sun F et al (1999) Case-only design to measure gene-gene interaction. Epidemiology 10(2):167–170
54. The International HapMap Consortium (2003) The international HapMap project. Nature 426:789–796
55. Yang CH, Lin YD, Wu SJ et al (2015) High order gene-gene interactions in eight single nucleotide polymorphisms of renin-angiotensin system genes for hypertension association study. Biomed Res Int 2015:454091
56. Wu C, Zhang H, Liu X et al (2009) Detecting essential and removable interactions in genome-wide association studies. Stat Interface 2(2):161–170

Chapter 8

Genetic Association in the HLA Region

Loukas Moutsianas and Javier Gutierrez-Achury

Abstract

The MHC/HLA region has been consistently associated with a large number of complex traits, including but not limited to, most immune-mediated ones. Efforts to pinpoint drivers of this commonly encountered association peak at the short arm of chromosome 6, however, have been challenging, owing to the high density of genes and the long and extended linkage disequilibrium that are characteristic of this region.

The development of methods to impute classical HLA alleles and amino acids from SNP genotyping data has offered an important additional layer of information to the investigators seeking to fine map the signal in the region. As a result, imputation-aided association analyses are now typically employed to shed light on the relationship of this locus with disease susceptibility and response to drugs.

In this chapter we discuss how the signal in the HLA region can be interrogated in practice, from performing the imputation to understanding its output and to incorporating it into downstream analysis. In addition, we recount some of the analytical approaches that are commonly used and suggest ways in which the findings from such imputation-aided analyses can be interpreted.

Key words HLA, MHC, Imputation, Association studies, Immune-mediated diseases, Autoimmunity, HLA*IMP:02, SNP2HLA, HIBAG

1 Introduction

The Major Histocompatibility Complex (MHC), located on the short arm of chromosome 6, is the most gene-rich region of the human genome and it contains the most polymorphic genes known to date [1]. The MHC complex first attracted attention when it was realized that genes in the region were the main reason behind graft rejection between unrelated individuals of the same species. Nowadays, the complex is recognized as the cornerstone of self-nonself discrimination and it has been associated with hundreds of diseases, including virtually all immune-mediated ones, as well as with adverse effects of various drugs [2–4]. The first MHC molecules in humans were discovered in the surface of white blood cells and the respective genes were accordingly named human leukocyte antigens (HLA) genes. The terms MHC region and HLA region have been used interchangeably in this chapter.

Evangelos Evangelou (ed.), *Genetic Epidemiology: Methods and Protocols*, Methods in Molecular Biology, vol. 1793, https://doi.org/10.1007/978-1-4939-7868-7_8, © Springer Science+Business Media, LLC, part of Springer Nature 2018

The MHC-HLA complex is divided into three main regions named class I, class III, and class II. The HLA classical genes are located in class I and II regions (Fig. 1) and are primarily involved in the presentation of peptide antigens to T-cells. Classical class I molecules are ordered by physical position, HLA-A, HLA-C, and HLA-B. They are heterodimers consisting of four domains. Three of them are coded by the respective HLA genes, forming the transmembrane region and the peptide-binding groove (the position in the protein where the peptide antigen is being presented). The fourth domain, a β_2 microglobulin molecule coded elsewhere in the genome (in chromosome 15), brings stability to the structure. Classical class II molecules are HLA-DR, HLA-DQ, and HLA-DP. They are also heterodimers, but both genes forming the protein are encoded in the MHC region (e.g., HLA-DQ is encoded by HLA-DQA1 and HLA-DQB1 genes) and they both participate in the formation of the peptide-binding groove. Apart from their structure, the two classes of molecules differ in the cell types they are expressed in, the type of immune cells they primarily interact with, the length of the peptides they typically present, and the sites from which they typically derive the peptides they present (cytosol for class I versus endosomes for class II proteins).

The experimental determination of HLA types, commonly referred to as HLA typing, was historically performed using serological tests. The methodology was based on the binding specificity of antigen presenting cells to specific antibodies, helping to determine a group of alleles based on serological recognition. Due to their inability to offer further discrimination between alleles of the same serotype, these methods are called low resolution. Molecular typing methods, such as sequence-specific primers (PCR-SSP) or sequencing-based typing (SBT), offer higher resolution. Initially, such methods typically only focused on genomic regions which code for the peptide-binding groove of the HLA molecules. These include exons 2 and 3 of class I HLA genes and the typing of exon 2 for class II HLA genes. However, more recent SBT methods, often using high-throughput sequencing data, offer gene polymorphism determination across the whole coding region or even the full-length gene (e.g., [5–7]).

1.1 HLA Imputation Algorithms

The availability of classical HLA types for the individuals included in an association study could be crucial for understanding their role in disease susceptibility; however, experimental determination of the allelic subtypes has been relatively costly and as such, it has generally been prohibitive for large datasets. A cost-effective alternative that was considered, as data from SNP genotyping platforms became more widely available, was to use dense genotyping data to try and pinpoint single SNPs that would provide good tags for specific HLA alleles. In a landmark study, it was found that while a subset of the classical HLA alleles could be tagged by such SNPs,

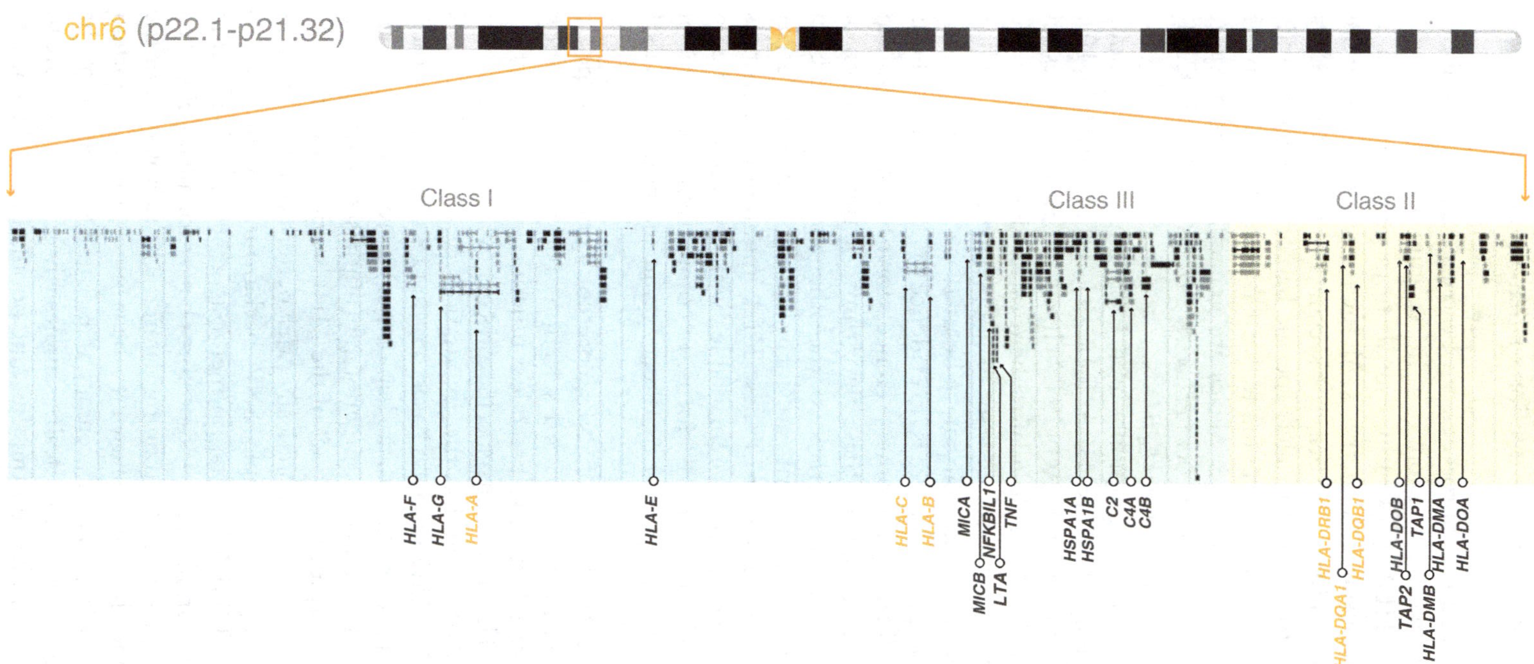

Fig. 1 Schematic representation of the HLA region. The MHC region is located in the short arm of chromosome 6 and expands for approximately 5 Mb. The three sub-regions, Class I (blue), Class III (green), and Class II (yellow), harbor hundreds of genes, many of which are involved in the immune response (a small subset of them in each region are tagged by name). The HLA classical genes are located in Class I and Class II regions. The genes highlighted (yellow) at the bottom correspond to the HLA genes that are typically imputed by the different imputation algorithms

these were likely to differ by population and tagging accuracy using a single SNP was generally inferior to that using multiple SNPs instead [8].

HLA imputation approaches can be considered probabilistic, more sophisticated extensions of the tagging methods. These methods infer HLA types of individuals from genotyping data in the region using statistical methods. All such approaches utilize the linkage disequilibrium (LD) between specific HLA alleles and SNPs in the region to model the allele-specific haplotypic backgrounds and generally require a set of samples with available SNP genotypes and HLA data, as reference. Alleles are generally imputed for at least the six classical HLA loci (*HLA-A*, *HLA-C*, *HLA-B*, *HLA-DRB1*, *HLA-DQA1*, *HLA-DQB1*).

Four of the most commonly used HLA imputation methods from genotyping data are HLA*IMP [9], HLA*IMP:02 [10], SNP2HLA [11], and HIBAG [12]. While this section focuses on HLA*IMP/IMP:02, all four aforementioned algorithms require similar input (e.g., all require a set of samples with available HLA allelic and genotype data as input, to be used as a reference), return comparable output, and there is no evidence of one of the methods clearly outperforming the others. Hence, downstream analysis can be conducted using any of these algorithms for the imputation of HLA alleles. Some characteristics of the other algorithms and brief notes on their relative merits are included in Subheading 4 (*see* **Note 1**). The performance of these HLA imputation algorithms on European individuals is remarkable, with the accuracy being over 90% for all but the DRB1 locus. In comparison, accuracies of 96–99% have been reported by direct typing methods for class I HLA alleles [13].

In HLA*IMP, the sets of SNPs representing each haplotype are selected via an iterative forward selection- backward elimination process, where a likelihood-based loss function is applied to different subsets. This is a locus-specific process, leading to different subsets of SNPs used for the imputation of each HLA locus [14]. The HLA*IMP model is based on the Li & Stephens method [15], and requires phased data (haplotypes) as reference. In contrast, HLA*IMP:02 works on genotype (unphased) data, is based on a graphical haplotype model of the MHC region, uses all available SNPs, and should theoretically offer better accuracy for HLA alleles appearing in multiple SNP backgrounds compared to HLA*IMP [9]. HLA imputation methods generally benefit from larger training sample sizes, and perform better for alleles observed with high frequency in the training dataset. The sample size of the reference panel has been shown to be a much more important determinant of imputation accuracy than the SNP density of the genotyping platform [11]. Ideally, samples whose HLA types are to be imputed should come from the same population as the samples in the reference panel, or at least the latter should contain samples from the same population as the ones to be imputed. Population-specific reference panels are thus crucial for the accurate imputation of HLA alleles across all methods, as it has been demonstrated across imputation algorithms. This realization has more recently led to the construction of multiple Asian HLA imputation reference panels (e.g., with Japanese [16], Chinese [17], and Korean [18] individuals) which show marked improvements in the imputation accuracy for individuals from these populations. For instance, HLA imputation accuracy in Japanese individuals increased from ~75% to over 90% when a Japanese reference panel was used instead of a European one, even though the latter contained over five times more samples [16].

1.2 HLA Nomenclature

All HLA alleles are coded by the gene name, followed by an asterisk and a number of numerical fields separated by colons. The first field (digits between the asterisk and the first colon) contains the type of the allele (allele family) [19]. Alleles that differ in the first field are said to be different at a 2-digit resolution. The second field separates alleles that differ in nucleotide positions that determine the amino acid (AA) sequences they code for. Alleles that code for identical AA sequences thus have the same digits in the second field and are said to be the same at a 4-digit resolution. The third field splits alleles that differ at the coding sequence but by synonymous substitutions only; these are said to be different at a six-digit resolution. Alleles that only differ in intronic or flanking regions differ at their fourth field and are said to be different at an eight-digit resolution. More information on the nomenclature for the HLA genes can be found at http://hla.alleles.org/nomenclature/naming.html [20]. The vast majority of association analyses on the MHC region to-date that include HLA alleles (typed or imputed) are conducted at a resolution of not more than four digits.

2 Methods

2.1 Data Input and Filtering

SNPs within the extended MHC region (xMHC) on chromosome 6 (29.9 –33.6 Mb for Hg19/GRCh37) are used for imputation. The filtering steps on the genotypes that are to be used for the HLA imputation are similar to the ones used for genome-wide association studies [21] and are also discussed elsewhere in this book (*see* Chapter 3). Missing data and issues with strand alignment are particularly important for the imputation process. For this reason, all HLA imputation algorithms mentioned here have in-built strand alignment routines and filters for missing data (although the threshold for missingness varies between the algorithms). Sites with differential missingness between cases and controls could lead to differences in imputation quality for specific alleles and should therefore also be removed. In our recent study [22], we used a p-value cutoff of 10^{-3} for differential missingness.

```
IndividualID Chromosome HLAC Q Q2 P
Sample35009 1 0702 0.990230537924458 0.990230537924458 NA
Sample35009 2 0701 0.944803282749089 0.935573062909424 NA
Sample00388 1 1203 0.99999998514765 0.99999998514765 NA
Sample00388 2 0303 0.995772040088735 0.995772025299167 NA
Sample15115 1 0701 0.999842442893582 0.999842442893582 NA
Sample15115 2 0303 0.751617678487644 0.751499255781089 NA
Sample35032 1 0701 0.992018490537126 0.992018490537126 NA
Sample35032 2 0702 0.989392763517362 0.981495915812849 NA
Sample13414 1 0303 0.999984114937413 0.999984114937413 NA
Sample13414 2 0701 0.999927697111961 0.99991181319791 NA
Sample16561 1 0702 0.990231180897962 0.990231180897962 NA
Sample16561 2 0303 0.987972993878332 0.978335664423436 NA
Sample09801 1 0501 0.999999999984806 0.999999999984806 NA
Sample09801 2 0501 0.999988330130418 0.999988330115224 NA
```

Fig. 2 Sample output from HLA*IMP:02, for the "best guess" file. Imputations shown here are at the 4-digit level, for HLA-C. There are two rows per sample, containing the imputed HLA allele with the higher posterior probability for each of the haplotypes (chromosomes). However, in HLA*IMP:02 the two rows are interchangeable (they are simply ranked in the order each allele was called) and thus contain no information about the phasing of the alleles. The first column contains the SampleID, the third column contains the imputed HLA alleles (without the colon between the first two fields), and columns 4, 5 contain confidence measures on the imputations. Specifically, for the first called allele columns Q and Q2 are identical and contain the marginal probability of the specified allele. For the second allele, Q is the conditional probability of the second allele given the first, and Q2 is the joint probability for the two alleles. This (Q2 of the second called allele) is the posterior probability typically used in uncertainty-aware analyses

2.2 Imputation Output

There are two main output files per HLA locus produced by HLA*IMP:02:

1. A "best guess" file, where the two most likely alleles for each individual are reported (*see* Fig. 2), together with the corresponding imputation quality values (Q and Q2 in the case of HLA*IMP:02) that reflect the confidence in the imputed alleles for that individual, and
2. A "full posteriors" file containing posterior probabilities across all possible combinations of HLA alleles for that locus, for each individual.

There will typically be two sets of the above files, one at a 4- and one at a 2-digit resolution. Analogous files are produced by the other imputation software, while SNP2HLA also returns amino acid sequences for the HLA genes by default (*see* **Note 1**). The joint posterior probability for the pair of alleles of each locus will be typically used in downstream analyses. For sample 15115 in Fig. 2, the allelic pair with the highest joint posterior at locus *HLA-C* is 07:01-03:03. The "full posteriors" file provides additional information on alternative allelic pairs for each individual. For Sample 15115, as seen in Table 1, the other likely pair is 07:01-03:04, with a posterior probability of 0.25. Hence, the two most likely

Table 1
HLA-C allele combinations with joint posterior of 10^{-5} or higher as returned by HLA*IMP:02 for Sample15115 (*see* also Fig. 2)

HLA-C alleles for Sample15115	Q2
07:01–03:03	0.751499
07:01–03:04	0.24834
07:04–03:03	1.00E−04
07:04–03:04	3.00E−05
03:03–03:03	2.00E−05
03:03–03:04	1.00E−05

combinations both consist of an HLA-C*07 and an HLA-C*03 alleles, so the algorithm's confidence in the results at a low resolution is much higher. Indeed, in the respective entry at the 2-digit resolution output file, the highest joint posterior probability is over 0.999 for the HLA-C*07, HLA-C*03 pair (alleles at a 2-digit resolution are coded with a set of zeros at field 2 in HLA*IMP:02, so the entries for the two alleles would be 0700, 0300). This is quite common in practice and can be useful in the analysis (*see* **Note 2**).

2.3 Validation

The availability of typed HLA alleles for a subset of the samples for which the imputation is conducted could increase confidence in the imputations, especially if the individuals come from a population that is not well represented in the reference panel used for the imputation. This is worth considering during study design, if resources are available. In general, and in the absence of such information, accuracy can be expected to be better for higher-frequency HLA alleles, and at a two-digit resolution (*see* **Note 2**).

In addition to the imputed HLA alleles, HLA*IMP:02 returns results from a so-called 2/3–1/3 cross-validation experiment with every imputed dataset. In this context, the term validation is used with respect to the adequacy of the specific subset of the SNPs used for the imputation:

1. The reference set, for which known (typed) HLA data are available for all samples, is split into 2/3 (to be used as training) and 1/3 (to be used for testing),
2. The *same* set of SNPs used for the imputation of the user's dataset is used to impute HLA types in the testing set (1/3 of the samples) that was kept out of the training set, and a series of detailed imputation quality measures are offered.

Specifically, allele-specific sensitivity, specificity, and positive predictive values are reported for different calling thresholds (T) on posteriors (typically $T = 0$, $T = 0.50$, and $T = 0.70$). In addition, complete lists of all mis-imputed alleles per locus are provided, so that the user can identify specific (systematic) patterns that will need to be considered in the association analysis (*see* Table 2).

Table 2
Output from a 2/3–1/3 cross validation returned from HLA*IMP:02 as part of an imputation of European samples using the Immunochip genotyping array

Locus	RealAllele	ImputedAllele	*N*
A	101	201	0.5
A	101	301	0.5
A	101	2402	0.5
A	202	205	2
A	205	1101	1
A	206	201	2
A	2301	201	0.5
A	2301	2402	0.5
A	2403	2402	1
A	2601	2501	2
A	2608	2601	2
A	2901	2902	2
A	3301	3300	1
A	3303	3101	2
A	6601	2601	4
A	6801	301	0.5
A	6824	6801	1
A	7406	3201	1
A	7410	3201	1

The threshold used for these calls was $T = 0.5$. This is the output for *HLA-A* alleles. The file reveals mis-imputation patterns for specific alleles. For instance, from rows 1, 6, 7 we see that the algorithm erroneously imputes allele HLA-A*02:01 in some cases where the real allele is HLA-A*01:01, HLA-A*02:06, or HLA-A*23:01. The fourth column is an indicator of the frequency of each mis-imputation. In this example, a total of 74 individuals with at least a copy of HLA-A*02:01 were included in the validation set (this number is included in a separate output file), so the imputation quality is actually high for this allele. Notice that no alleles were mis-imputed as being HLA-A*02:01, so the allele was imputed with 100% sensitivity in the testing set

Good performance in this validation experiment means that the subset of SNPs that were available for the imputation can be considered sufficient to yield high-quality imputations. This is a very useful diagnostic when the genotyping chip is non-standard. However, these metrics should *not* be interpreted as a measure of the imputation quality, unless reference and imputation panels are both derived from the same population. In that case, the actual imputation quality is likely to be better, because the whole reference set will be used as reference instead of just 2/3 of it.

2.4 Association Analysis Using Imputed HLA Alleles Only

The "best guess" file, such as the one produced by HLA*IMP:02 or HIBAG, can be easily transformed to a format that is accepted as input by programs which are used for association analyses, such as SNPTEST2 [23, 24] or PLINK [25]. Table 3 shows how the example output from Fig. 2 can be converted into a suitable file format for input into SNPTEST2. SNP2HLA outputs a file containing allele dosage data which can be directly used for downstream analysis in PLINK. It is recommended that the posterior probabilities returned by the algorithms are used for downstream analyses, instead of hard calls. This is because the posterior probabilities account for the uncertainty from the imputation process. Alternatively, a hard threshold on the posteriors can be used (e.g., a call threshold of $T = 0.7$ is commonly used for comparative analyses in the HLA*IMP:02 manuscript [10]). Either way, each HLA allele is commonly treated as a bi-allelic variant, with values in the range [0, 2] for dosage data or 0, 1, or 2 for discrete data, indicating the copies of the specific HLA allele for an individual.

Table 3
Example of how the output from the imputation shown in Fig. 2 can be transformed into a format for downstream analysis

HLAC1	C0303	31346171	A	C	1	0	0	0	1	0	0	1	0	1	0	0	0	1	0	0	1	0	1	0	0
HLAC2	C0501	31346171	A	C	1	0	0	1	0	0	1	0	0	1	0	0	1	0	0	1	0	0	0	0	1
HLAC3	C0701	31346171	A	C	0	1	0	1	0	0	0	1	0	0	1	0	0	1	0	1	0	0	1	0	0
HLAC4	C0702	31346171	A	C	0	1	0	1	0	0	1	0	0	0	1	0	1	0	0	0	1	0	1	0	0
HLAC5	C0703	31346171	A	C	1	0	0	1	0	0	1	0	0	1	0	0	1	0	0	1	0	0	1	0	0
HLAC6	C1203	31346171	A	C	1	0	0	0	1	0	1	0	0	1	0	0	1	0	0	1	0	0	1	0	0

In this case, it is transformed into a genotype file format that can be used in SNPTEST2 [24]. *See* http://www.stats.ox.ac.uk/~marchini/software/gwas/file_format.html for details on the format. Hard calls are used here instead of probabilities, for visual clarity. Instead of a SNP per row, here each row represents a specific HLA-C allele at 4-digit resolution. Hence, alleles A, C in columns 4, 5 are arbitrarily chosen to preserve the required format. Triplet 1 0 0 means the individual contains no copies of that allele, triplet 0 1 0 means the individual contains one copy of the allele, and triplet 0 0 1 means that the individual contains two copies of the allele. For instance, from columns 6–8 it can be seen that the first individual contains a copy each of HLA-C*07:01 and HLA-C*07:02

In a single-variant (univariate) model, each HLA allele will be commonly tested for association with the trait of interest in the same way that a SNP would be, i.e., by employing the same covariates in the model to correct for age or population stratification. In a multi-variate setting, multiple HLA alleles from the same locus may be included in the same model. This can theoretically lead to combinations of HLA alleles that cannot occur in reality and hence to an altered probability space, if they are treated as independent variants. Hereafter, we treat the variants as if being independent (but *see* **Note 3**).

A typical genome-wide association study using SNPs will assume a multiplicative model (additive on the log-scale) for the effect of each SNP. However, the effects of some HLA alleles in complex traits have been shown to deviate from this model. For instance, such is the case with HLA-B*27 in Ankylosing Spondylitis (AS) [26], HLA-C*06:02 in Psoriasis [27], or HLA-DRB1*15:01, HLA-DRB1*03:01 in Multiple Sclerosis (MS) [22] which seem to exhibit deviations from the multiplicative model. Therefore, in a stepwise model, we would recommend looking for such deviations from additivity before adding each additional term to the model. A simple forward selection approach to construct a general model of the HLA-allele risk in a binary complex trait (similar to one of the analyses we employed in [22]) is as follows:

1. Start with a baseline model including all covariates and perform logistic regression on the trait using each HLA allele in turn and assuming a general model (i.e., two separate terms for each allele, with different effects assumed for heterozygotes and homozygotes).
2. Focusing on the HLA allele which led to the model with the highest likelihood from the previous step, compare models where the allele's effect is assumed to be additive, dominant, recessive, over-dominant, or general and choose the effect that yields the best fit to the data. Model comparison can be conducted using Bayesian Information Criterion (BIC) or Akaike Information Criterion (AIC).
3. Add the HLA allele with the chosen effect back in the model and continue the process until there is no further increase in the BIC/AIC score or until there are no HLA alleles for which the p-value falls below a set significant threshold (e.g., alpha $= 5 \times 10^{-8}$).

A backward elimination step could be added in the process above. In that case, each allele could be removed in turn from the model at each iteration and the resulting model compared to the one with all alleles in, to ensure that the full model still yields the best fit to the data. Moreover, all models of how the allele affects the trait (dominant, recessive, etc.) could be separately included in the parameter space at the beginning of the algorithm, removing **step 2**.

The above process attempts to dissect the association signal in the MHC region by building a model that *only* includes effects of specific HLA alleles. Using imputed data, however, analysis of the extended MHC region can be conducted using SNPs, imputed HLA alleles at various loci at 4- or 2-digit resolution (*see* **Note 2**), imputed amino-acids, or combinations of these data in a variety of models. The interpretation of the results from such analyses is rarely straightforward and the analytical approach generally depends on the specific question being asked (*see* **Note 4**).

2.5 Interrogation of Imputed Amino Acid Polymorphisms within HLA Genes

Amino acid residues at specific positions in the coding sequence have been long known to affect susceptibility to a trait, such as *HLA-DQB1* position 57 for Type 1 diabetes (T1D) [28]. Hence, the inclusion of imputed AA polymorphisms in the analysis of the MHC region could provide further insights on disease pathogenesis. With this in mind, imputation of polymorphic amino acids in the HLA genes is provided by default by the SNP2HLA software [11]. Figure 3 shows a sample output from an imputed allele dosage file from SNP2HLA, focusing on AA polymorphisms. This file can be directly used for downstream analysis. Such functionality is not provided by default by the HLA*IMP/IMP:02 or HIBAG software, but imputed AA residues are straightforward to obtain by using the classical HLA imputations (*see* **Note 5**).

The association analysis for AA polymorphisms is typically done in two ways. In one of them, every polymorphic position is treated in a "binary," residue-specific fashion, in the same way we treated each allele at each HLA locus (or SNPs in a usual GWAS analysis).

```
AA_DQB1_70_32740627_G   P    A    1.918   2.000   0.002   0.104   2.000
AA_DQB1_70_32740627_R   P    A    0.103   0.000   1.999   1.903   0.000
AA_DQB1_70_32740627_E   P    A    0.021   0.000   0.001   0.007   0.000
AA_DQB1_67_32740636     I    V    0.046   0.000   0.006   1.131   0.000
AA_DQB1_66_32740639     D    E    0.046   0.000   0.006   1.131   0.000
AA_DQB1_57_32740666_V   P    A    0.061   0.000   0.001   0.024   0.000
AA_DQB1_57_32740666_D   P    A    1.932   2.000   1.985   0.208   2.000
AA_DQB1_57_32740666_A   P    A    0.048   0.000   0.013   1.773   0.000
AA_DQB1_57_32740666_S   P    A    0.022   0.000   0.001   0.015   0.000
AA_DQB1_57_32740666_VD  P    A    1.972   2.000   1.987   0.227   2.000
AA_DQB1_57_32740666_VA  P    A    0.088   0.000   0.014   1.788   0.000
AA_DQB1_57_32740666_VS  P    A    0.062   0.000   0.001   0.032   0.000
```

Fig. 3 Sample output from imputed allele dosage file (.dosage) from SNP2HLA, focusing on AA polymorphisms. In AA positions 66, 67, there are only two amino acids available in the reference panel (D, E and I, V, respectively) and can be seen in columns 2, 3 of the respective rows. In position 70, there are three different AAs in the reference, G, R, and E, and the presence (dosage) of each is coded in separate rows. Note that now the specific amino acid is mentioned as part of the variant's name (AA_DQB1_70_32740627_G, etc.) and columns 2 and 3 have entries P, A. In position 57 there are four different AAs, V, D, A and S. In this case, the program outputs each in a separate line as before, but also adds lines with pairwise combinations of the two (VD, VA, VS) so they can also be readily tested for association. Naming conventions are the same as for the case of three AA residues

In the case of the amino acids at position 57 of HLA-DQB1, for instance, which could be Valine (V), Aspartic Acid (D), Alanine (A), and Serine (S), each of the four residues would be separately included in the model with its dosage data values in the range [0, 2], to look for associations between the specific AA residue at that position and the trait of interest.

To look for the association of *all* residues at a specific AA position with the trait, an omnibus test could be employed, where for an AA position with *m* different residues, *m-1* of them would be simultaneously included in the model, each with their respective effect (commonly the most frequent would be left out as the reference one). The omnibus p-value could then be obtained by comparing the above model to a model without any AA effects, using a log-likelihood ratio test that follows a χ^2 distribution with *m-1* degrees of freedom [29, 30].

2.6 Interpretation of Results

HLA imputation will be commonly conducted after the discovery of an association between a trait and variants in the MHC region. Imputation-aided analysis is expected to pinpoint one or more specific alleles that may explain the observed association. In some cases, such an allele does exist; in our study on Psoriasis allele HLA-C*06:02 was found to have a stronger signal than the top hit SNP and also led to a model which fitted the case-control data significantly better than the model with the top SNP [27]. While this was a known association, these results convincingly supported the argument that the main signal in the region is indeed driven by the HLA allele. Similarly, in our analysis of the HLA region in celiac disease (CeD), imputation-aided analysis allowed us to confirm the known association at the HLA-DQ locus and to determine five new variants across the region that appear to act independently of the known association. This also highlighted the possible role of class I genes in the pathogenesis of CeD [29].

However, there are studies where the signal at a SNP is much stronger than that at the HLA allele (e.g., [31, 32]). The association of HLA-DPB1*03:01 with multiple sclerosis is a characteristic example (*see* **Note 6**). In such cases, it is difficult to pinpoint the driver of the observed association, and simply drawing attention to the most associated HLA allele while ignoring the SNP can be misleading. The SNP could be tagging variation(s) outside the classical HLA alleles (e.g., variation in the class III region, *see* **Note** 7) or contribution from one or more HLA alleles in partial linkage disequilibrium (LD) with it. It may also be due to the fact that the allele(s) tagged by the SNP has not been imputed very well. This is more likely for alleles that have low frequency in the reference panel or for samples for which there was no reference data from the same population to be used by the imputation algorithm.

If the goal of the MHC analysis is to identify specific HLA alleles which are convincingly associated with a complex trait of interest, a more conservative (and robust) approach would only include in the model those HLA alleles whose signals are *stronger* than these of the SNPs in LD with them. As an example, Goyette et al. [33] analyzed the MHC association with inflammatory bowel disease (IBD) and focused on HLA alleles, but built models that also considered SNPs in the region, as well as AA residues. While for Crohn's disease they found the strongest signal to be coming from an HLA allele, DRB1*01:03, for ulcerative colitis (UC) they found tens of SNPs and AA variants with stronger association signals than the top HLA allele. However, all of them seemed to be acting independently of the top HLA allele and were correlated with the most associated SNP instead, thus supporting the hypothesis that DRB1*01:03 is likely a driver of one of the associations between the MHC region and UC.

Due to the extended linkage disequilibrium structure in the region, it is not uncommon for HLA alleles in different loci to show comparable evidence for association with a trait. This is characteristic in the case of MS and narcolepsy, where a haplotype containing DRB1*15:01 and DQB1*06:02 alleles showed strong evidence for association in studies on European populations. Due to the LD between the two alleles in these populations, the further refinement of the signal was more challenging. Given that such extended haplotypes are often population-specific, association studies in populations where the LD between the specific HLA alleles is less (*e.g.,* [34, 35]) can help to identify the driver of the observed association. Alternatively, studies specifically focusing on individuals who do not have one of the candidate HLA alleles (*e.g.,* [36]) can be helpful. Such studies helped to determine that the MHC association in MS is DRB1*15:01, but in narcolepsy DQB1*06:02. Large imputation-based studies on European populations may also provide an insight of the potential driver of an association in such cases, e.g., through comparison of models containing each of the alleles in turn, or by checking whether the signal of one of the alleles is fully explained by the other. However, care should be taken as small differences in such analyses could also be the result of differential imputation quality between the two alleles.

AA residues can also be included in the algorithm of Subheading 2.4, either from the start (during model selection, e.g., with each residue at each polymorphic AA position coded in a binary fashion and being included in the parameter space) or in the end, to further interrogate whether the signal seen at an HLA locus is likely driven by specific amino acid residues at that locus (*see* **Note 4** for some additional examples of models being applied in practice).

3 Conclusive Remarks

The fine-mapping of the association between the MHC region and complex traits has been greatly facilitated by the availability of accurate, efficient methods for the imputation of classical HLA alleles and amino acids. Imputation-aided HLA analysis can help to pinpoint specific HLA alleles or amino acid residues that may be the drivers of the observed associations, allow for more accurate analyses for secondary associations signals, or even highlight new associations to traits where the signals may not be explained by variation in the classical HLA genes in class I or class II regions.

As in the case of the genome-wide association studies using SNPs, a regression framework is commonly used for the association of the MHC region with the disease. However, the parameter space, the models used, and the overall analytical approach can vary widely across traits and analyses. Accordingly, the interpretation of the outcomes from such analyses depends on the specific questions being asked.

The availability of large, population-specific reference panels can lead to further advances in fine-mapping of the signal in the MHC region, exploiting the differential LD structure across populations. This will be further aided by the inclusion of non-classical HLA loci to the reference datasets. Moreover, the inclusion of HLA data typed at higher resolution will allow us to look into the role of synonymous and intronic variation, or variation in the UTR regions of the HLA genes.

Most of the analysis performed to date on the HLA region has been on European and more recently Asian samples. The construction of HLA imputation reference panels from other underrepresented populations (e.g., African, South-American) could be invaluable in further dissecting the signal in the HLA region, as well as in discovering novel population-specific effects.

Sequence-based HLA imputation/determination methods (*e.g.*, [37–39] or methods using even RNA-seq data (*e.g.*, [40]) have been developed, but are not commonly used in practice yet. However, as whole-genome and whole-exome data become increasingly available for association analyses of complex traits, such methods are bound to become commonplace. With them, new analytical approaches will likely be required.

4 Notes

1. HIBAG is an ensemble classifier which is based on a bootstrap aggregation technique known as "bagging." Subsets of the individuals in the reference panel are sampled with replacement to create several bootstrap samples. A classifier is subsequently

built for each of the bootstrap samples, each based on a different subset of the SNPs in the region. The SNP selection process is conducted in an iterative, computationally tractable way, where subsets of SNPs are randomly picked from the full set and tested one by one for improvement in the prediction of HLA types, with the best one being added to the classifier each time until no further improvement is noted. Each classifier will return a prediction probability for each HLA allele, and the algorithm's output is a vector of genotype probabilities averaged over the results of all classifiers [12]. The algorithm is implemented in an R package and it comes with pre-calculated classifiers for a range of different ancestries. This is very useful in practice, as it can be used for imputation without the need for providing access to a reference panel. As such, it has a comparative advantage over SNP2HLA, which requires a reference panel that has to be obtained externally for the imputation of samples of European ancestry. In addition, the HIBAG implementation allows the building of new classifiers from user-provided reference data, something that adds flexibility to the method compared to HLA*IMP, HLA*IMP:02. When using the pre-calculated classifiers, the HLA loci imputed by HIBAG are *HLA-A*, *HLA-C*, *HLA-B*, *HLA-DRB1*, *HLA-DQA1*, *HLA-DQB1*, and *HLA-DPB1*.

SNP2HLA uses Beagle [41] for the imputation of HLA alleles and amino acid (AA) sequences. It is the only HLA imputation software among the commonly used ones that presently outputs AA sequences by default. *See* **Note 5** for how to get imputed AA sequences from other HLA imputation software. In contrast to HIBAG and HLA*IMP:02, SNP2HLA outputs the phased HLA/AA data. This feature could be useful, e.g., in the construction and analysis of extended haplotypes across multiple HLA loci. When using the T1DGC reference panel for imputation (a European ancestry reference panel of over 5000 individuals with typed HLA alleles put together by the T1 Diabetes Genetics Consortium), the HLA loci that are imputed are *HLA-A*, *HLA-C*, *HLA-B*, *HLA-DRA1*, *HLA-DRB1*, *HLA-DQA1*, *HLA-DQB1*, and *HLA-DPB1*. *HLA-DRA1* is not imputed by HLA*IMP, HLA*IMP:02, or HIBAG with the pre-calculated classifiers. However, HLA*IMP:02 imputes alleles at loci HLA-DRB3, HLA-DRB4, and HLA-DRB5, but at a 2-digit resolution only.

A very useful characteristic of HLA*IMP:02 that is not shared by the other software is the provision of imputation quality metrics from a 2/3–1/3 cross-validation study on the reference panel, using the identical set of SNPs as these used for the user's imputation (*see* Subheading 2.3 for more details).

Scripts for running SNP2HLA are freely available online, as is the software that SNP2HLA uses for imputation (Beagle) and filtering (PLINK). Hence, in line with HIBAG, it can be directly downloaded and used, in contrast to HLA*IMP:02, which is now exclusively licensed to Affymetrix and requires registration via the company's website.

In terms of imputation quality, all software discussed in this chapter have demonstrated high prediction accuracy for individuals of European ancestry and there is no study to suggest that one clearly outperforms the others. Studies comparing imputations conducted via SNP2HLA vs HLA*IMP, HLA*IMP:02, either across all imputed alleles [42] or across alleles that appear more associated in the particular study or are more relevant to the study's research questions, found the results to be comparable [31, 42, 43]. There are few specific alleles in [42] for which SNP2HLA appears to be doing much better than HLA*IMP or vice versa (e.g., DQA1*05:01 and DRB1*14:01, respectively), but this is most likely an outcome of the specific reference panels used, rather than the imputation method per se.

We also compared the imputations from HLA*IMP:02 and HIBAG (using pre-calculated classifiers) on a European cohort of ~2800 individuals without known HLA types and found the concordance between the two software to be over 80% across all loci (*see* Fig. 4). When only high confidence calls were taken into account, the agreement increased to over 95%. In the vast majority of the cases where results were discordant even when posterior probabilities indicated high confidence, the allele that HIBAG called was not present in the HLA*IMP:02 reference panel. The remainder of the high confidence discordant calls was for a very small number of

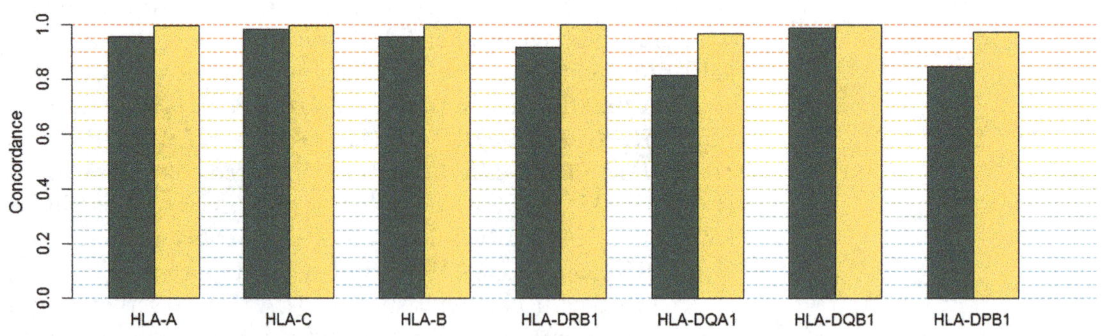

Fig. 4 Concordance between imputations. Concordance between imputations obtained via HLA*IMP:02 and HIBAG for a European (Swedish) cohort of 2872 individuals. Bars in green represent concordance across all calls (i.e., without applying a call threshold) while bars in yellow represent concordance across calls for which both imputation programs report posterior probabilities of 0.9 or more. Concordance is calculated as the fraction of individuals for which imputations for both alleles agree at a 4-digit resolution

specific alleles. In the case of *HLA-C*, for instance, in all but two cases where a disagreement was observed, HLA*IMP:02 called HLA-C*05:01 while HIBAG called HLA-C*07:01.

To conclude, the imputation of the alleles of interest using more than one imputation algorithm may be a worthwhile effort to increase confidence in an association.

2. Most commonly used HLA imputation algorithms presently offer HLA imputations at both a 2- and a 4-digit resolution. Typically, the analysis will either be conducted with the higher resolution available, or alleles at both resolutions will be included in the model selection process. However, there are cases where a 2-digit resolution may be preferable. This is particularly true when the individuals to be imputed come from a population which is not well represented in the reference panel; in such cases, the accuracy of imputation has been found to be higher at a 2-digit resolution [10]. Likewise, most HLA alleles that are not imputed well at a 4-digit imputation will typically be correctly imputed at 2-digit resolution. This is also reported for imputations by SNP2HLA [11]. The 2/3–1/3 validation results returned by HLA*IMP:02 will often contain such examples (alleles mis-imputed at 4d-resolution but correctly imputed at 2d). Moreover, in the example shown in Subheading 2.2, we saw that the 2-digit allele was imputed with very high confidence, but the algorithm was less certain about the specific 4-digit HLA allele. Finally, when we compared results between HIBAG and HLA*IMP:02 (*see* **Note 1**), most of the high confidence discordant calls the two algorithms made where both HLA alleles were included in the reference panels agreed at a 2-digit level.
3. For two alleles at the same HLA locus (a two-variant model) there are three impossible combinations (hom - hom, hom - het, het - hom). For instance, an individual cannot have two copies of allele HLA-A*02:01 and a copy of allele HLA-A*03:01, and the respective probability should be set to zero. In practice, in an analysis conducted using HLA*IMP, we found the difference between the actual probabilities and these assuming independence between the two alleles to generally be low, and not affecting the model's outcome. Specifically, using imputed HLA data from a European cohort, we calculated the sum of the probabilities of the three impossible combinations across all pairs of HLA alleles, for all classical loci, and found that even in the worst case scenario the sum only exceeded 0.1 in less than 3% of the individuals with that specific pair of HLA alleles. Even in that worst case, the difference in the model's outcome (estimated effect size and p-value) when using the two sets of probabilities was negligible [unpublished results]. This suggests that the impact of treating each HLA

allele independently of another on the same locus in a multivariate setting may be minimal. However, the confirmation of results from such multivariate models using the correct probability space (the information required is contained in the "full posteriors" file mentioned in the previous section) can increase confidence in the results.

4. Some analyses focus on a specific HLA gene, in order to identify all alleles associated with the trait at that locus (*e.g.*, [30, 33]). This may happen after the locus has been initially identified as associated with the trait, either through a SNP, a specific HLA allele, or via an omnibus test, such as the one described for amino acids in Subheading 2.5. The intuition behind this "locus-centric" approach is that, since an HLA locus has already been associated with a trait, it is likely to harbor multiple disease-modifying alleles. Hence, the hypothesis being asked is how many alleles at that particular locus are associated with the trait. However, given the extended LD in the region, alleles at each locus may also be tagging variation from neighboring loci. In the study on UC [33], for instance, HLA-DQA1*03:01 seems to be tagging an effect also explained by three different *HLA-DRB1* alleles. However, the association p-value for the DQA1 allele is over ten orders of magnitude more significant than that of the strongest of the three HLA-DRB1 alleles. In such cases, model comparison can be applied to assess whether the data is better explained by a locus-centric model (e.g., one where alleles from a specific locus are preferentially added to the model, then other loci are investigated sequentially), or under a more general model built like the one in Subheading 2.4. In addition, the associated alleles from the same locus can be further interrogated for shared patterns that may explain the observed effect, such as shared AA residues at specific positions. Finally, *see* **Note 3** for analyses including alleles at the same locus.

   An extension of the locus-centric model mentioned above is the interrogation of a subset of the HLA loci, before including the rest. This approach could be followed due to prior statistical or biological knowledge implicating these particular loci with the trait in question. Hu et al. [44] follow this approach in the context of T1D, focusing on allelic and AA effects for loci HLA-DRB1, HLA-DQA1, HLA-DQB1 before including other loci. In the same paper, Hu et al. looked for interactions between common haplotypes and T1D, by building a model that included the effects of all common DRB1-DQA1-DQB1 haplotypes as additive terms, as well as all possible pair-wise interactions between these haplotypes [44]. If m is the number of common haplotypes included in the model, this full interaction model has an additional $m^*(m-1)/2$ degrees of freedom. Lenz et al. [45] follow a similar analytical approach to look for interactions in five immune-mediated diseases. They work with either single- or multi-locus haplotypes, depending on the trait in question, and build a global model with all common haplotypes in, but also including an additional term per haplotype, to capture deviations from additivity. This model has an additional m degrees of freedom. They then compare this model to the one containing all pairwise interactions that was also used by Hu et al., to assess which of the models is a better fit to the data, by conducting a log-likelihood ratio test between the two, which follows a χ^2 distribution with $m^*(m-1)/2 - m$ degrees of freedom. Using variations of these models, they found that for many of the alleles showing deviations from additivity, the effect was better explained using a pairwise haplotypic interaction term instead. Interestingly, we observed the opposite effect in MS, where deviations from additivity in the effect of the main associated alleles gave rise to apparent interaction effects between these alleles and SNPs outside the MHC region. The effect disappeared once a general model was assumed for each of the alleles [22].

The analysis of multi-locus HLA haplotypes requires phased data. HLA*IMP and SNP2HLA return phased HLA imputation data, but not HLA*IMP:02 and HIBAG. Using genotype data for an analogous analysis, it can only be assessed whether an individual carries copies of all the alleles on the extended haplotype. While such analysis can be informative, it will not fully capture potential interaction effects between the alleles on the same haplotype [22].

5. HLA*IMP/IMP:02 and HIBAG do not return imputed AA polymorphisms as part of their imputation output. However, the imputed HLA alleles can be used to probabilistically infer the residues at each position, using the alignments provided online by IMGT/HLA (https://www.ebi.ac.uk/ipd/imgt/hla/align.html). This can be done as follows:
   (a) For a classical HLA locus (say DQB1), make a list of all alleles that are present in the dataset after imputation,
   (b) Use the sequence alignment tool of IMGT/HLA to align the amino acid sequences of all the alleles in the list. To do this, select the locus to align and pick "Protein – Full Length Protein" in the features. Next, add your list of HLA alleles to the required sequences at STEP 2.
   (c) The option "Show mismatches between sequences" when selecting alignment display options in STEP3 can be helpful to visually identify polymorphic positions. Select this and the numbering in blocks and proceed to align the sequences.

```
AA Pos.            -31        -21        -11         -1        10         20         30         40         50      57 60
DQB1*05:01:01:01   MS WKKSLRIPGD LRVATVTLML AILSSSLAEG RDSPEDFVYQ FKGLCYFTNG TERVRGVTRH IYNREEYVRF DSDVGVYRAV TPQGRPVAEY
DQB1*05:05:01      ** ********** ********** ********** *****----- ---------- ---------- -------A-- ---------- ------S---
DQB1*02:01:01      -- ---A-----G --A------- SM--TPV--- ---------- ---M------ -----L-S-S ------I--- -----EF--- -LL-L-A---
DQB1*03:01:01:01   -- ---A-----G --A------- -M--TPV--- ---------- --AM------ -----Y---Y -------A-- ----E----- --L-P-D---
DQB1*03:01:01:02   -- ---A-----G --A------- -M--TPV--- ---------- --AM------ -----Y---Y -------A-- ----E----- --L-P-D---
DQB1*03:01:01:03   -- ---A-----G --A------- -M--TPV--- ---------- --AM------ -----Y---Y -------A-- ----E----- --L-P-D---
DQB1*03:01:01:04   -- ---A-----G --A------- -M--TPV--- ---------- --AM------ -----Y---Y -------A-- ----E----- --L-P-D---
DQB1*03:01:01:05   -- ---A-----G --A------- -M--TPV--- ---------- --AM------ -----Y---Y -------A-- ----E----- --L-P-D---
DQB1*04:01:01      -- ---A-----G ---------- -M--TPV--- --------F- ---M------ --L------Y -------A-- ---------- --L--LD---
```

Fig. 5 Sample output from the sequence alignment tool of IMGT/HLA for some AA sequences of HLA-DQB1 alleles. The first sequence (in this case DQB1*05:01) is used as the reference. For every other sequence, positions where the AA residue is the same as in the reference are represented by dashes. The AA position is shown in the top row. Note that DQB1*03:01:01:01 -- DQB1*03:01:01:05 all have the same AA sequence since they are the same at a 4-digit resolution. There are four different amino acids in position 57 (highlighted in red), as we saw in the output file from SNP2HLA in Fig. 3

(d) The output will look like the one shown in Fig. 5. Note that the AA residues are only shown when they are different from the reference (the sequence on the top) and are otherwise replaced by dashes. All positions where there are entries other than dashed lines in the columns after the first are polymorphic.

(e) For each polymorphic position, the expected posterior probability can be calculated by summing for each individual the posterior probabilities of each of the HLA alleles which share the particular AA at that position. For instance, the posterior probability that an individual has AA Y at position 30 of the protein sequence in the example shown in Fig. 5 is equal to the sum of probabilities that the respective individual has of having HLA-DQB1*03:01 or HLA-DQB1*04:01.

Once the posterior probabilities for each individual are calculated across all polymorphic AAs of all imputed HLA alleles, they can be easily transformed for downstream analysis in the same way it was done for imputed HLA alleles (*see* Subheading 2.4).

Note that in theory there is a slight difference between using SNP2HLA–derived imputed amino acid polymorphisms, and polymorphisms estimated from classical HLA alleles. The former have been directly imputed and may have different posterior probabilities associated with them (i.e., they do not have to be equal to the sum of the posteriors of the HLA alleles carrying the particular AA at that position). In practice, we found the difference between the two sets of probabilities to be negligible (unpublished data). This is hardly surprising, since a substantial difference between the two could lead to inconsistencies between the imputed HLA alleles and the HLA alleles that would result from the imputation of AA polymorphisms.

6. As a case example, a signal in the HLA-DPB1 region was first reported for multiple sclerosis (MS) at genome-wide significance in 2010 [46]. The lead SNP was reported as being moderately correlated with a specific HLA-DPB1 allele, HLA-DPB1*03:01. Subsequent studies using much larger sample sizes and imputed HLA alleles have replicated this association. In these studies, the association of HLA-DPB1*03:01 with MS was genome-wide significant. However, despite the fact that different imputation algorithms (HLA*IMP in [9], HLA*IMP:02 in [10], SNP2HLA in [30]) were used for the imputation, and two different reference panels were employed, the signal of the most associated SNP was found to be consistently stronger than that of HLA-DPB1*03:01. While this could still be due to mis-imputation of HLA-DPB1*03:01, an independent study reports good accuracy in the imputation of this allele [42]. It is therefore unclear whether HLA-DPB1*03:01 and the lead SNP tag the same signal or not. Alternatively, they could be tagging an AA polymorphism, as suggested in [42], though still the signal at the SNP is stronger. In any case, in the light of the statistical evidence so far, it is potentially misleading to just refer to the association signal in the HLA-DPB1 region for MS as simply coming from HLA-DPB1*03:01.
7. While the focus of this is on the imputation of classical HLA alleles and their amino acid sequences, and their association with complex traits, the MHC region contains various other genes with known or putative immune functions. These include, but are not limited to [1]:
    (a) *MICA* and *MICB* in class I region,
    (b) the *TNF* gene, lymphotoxin-alpha (*LTA*) and lymphotoxin-beta (*LTB*), *NFKBIL1*, genes involved in stress response such as *HSPA1A* and *HSPA1B*, as well as components of the complement cascade such as *C2*, *C4A*, and *C4B* in class III region, and
    (c) *TAP1*, *TAP2* in class II region.
    (d) Several non-classical HLA genes such as *HLA-F*, *HLA-G*, *HLA-E* in class I and *HLA-DOA*, *HLA-DOB*, *HLA-DMA*, *HLA-DMB* in class II region.

Any association signal in the MHC region could be tagging an effect in one of the above genes. Hence, while the imputation of classical HLA alleles offers an invaluable additional layer of interrogation of the variation in the MHC region, the classical HLA alleles alone should by no means be expected to fully explain an observed association.

A recent paper on schizophrenia offers an example where an association of the MHC region with the trait, previously attributed to classical HLA alleles such as B*08:01, is likely tagging variation in the *C4A*, *C4B* genes which affects expression of C4 [47]. Three HLA alleles have genome-wide significant p-values in this study, but they are all several orders of magnitude weaker than the effect at the lead SNP. The authors found a relationship between *C4A* and *C4B* expression and their structural variation, and then used SNPs to statistically impute different *C4A*/*C4B* alleles. The imputed *C4A* expression was most strongly associated with Schizophrenia than any of the classical HLA alleles or AA residues (but not the main SNP) and seemed to be tagging most of the association with the classical HLA alleles.

References

1. Trowsdale J, Knight JC (2013) Major histocompatibility complex genomics and human disease. Annu Rev Genomics Hum Genet 14:301–323. https://doi.org/10.1146/annurev-genom-091212-153455
2. Moon J, Kim TJ, Lim JA et al (2016) HLA-B*40:02 and DRB1*04:03 are risk factors for oxcarbazepine-induced maculopapular eruption. Epilepsia 57:1879. https://doi.org/10.1111/epi.13566
3. Sousa-Pinto B, Correia C, Gomes L et al (2016) HLA and delayed drug-induced hypersensitivity. Int Arch Allergy Immunol 170 (3):163–179. https://doi.org/10.1159/000448217
4. Stamp LK, Day RO, Yun J (2016) Allopurinol hypersensitivity: investigating the cause and minimizing the risk. Nat Rev Rheumatol 12 (4):235–242. https://doi.org/10.1038/nrrheum.2015.132
5. Voorter CE, Palusci F, Tilanus MG (2014) Sequence-based typing of HLA: an improved group-specific full-length gene sequencing approach. Methods Mol Biol 1109:101–114. https://doi.org/10.1007/978-1-4614-9437-9_7
6. Ehrenberg PK, Geretz A, Baldwin KM et al (2014) High-throughput multiplex HLA genotyping by next-generation sequencing using multi-locus individual tagging. BMC Genomics 15:864. https://doi.org/10.1186/1471-2164-15-864
7. Hosomichi K, Jinam TA, Mitsunaga S et al (2013) Phase-defined complete sequencing of the HLA genes by next-generation sequencing. BMC Genomics 14:355. https://doi.org/10.1186/1471-2164-14-355
8. de Bakker PI, McVean G, Sabeti PC et al (2006) A high-resolution HLA and SNP haplotype map for disease association studies in the extended human MHC. Nat Genet 38 (10):1166–1172. https://doi.org/10.1038/ng1885
9. Dilthey AT, Moutsianas L, Leslie S et al (2011) HLA*IMP – an integrated framework for imputing classical HLA alleles from SNP genotypes. Bioinformatics 27(7):968–972. https://doi.org/10.1093/bioinformatics/btr061
10. Dilthey A, Leslie S, Moutsianas L et al (2013) Multi-population classical HLA type imputation. PLoS Comput Biol 9(2):e1002877. https://doi.org/10.1371/journal.pcbi.1002877
11. Jia X, Han B, Onengut-Gumuscu S et al (2013) Imputing amino acid polymorphisms in human leukocyte antigens. PLoS One 8(6): e64683. https://doi.org/10.1371/journal.pone.0064683
12. Zheng X, Shen J, Cox C et al (2014) HIBAG – HLA genotype imputation with attribute bagging. Pharmacogenomics J 14(2):192–200. https://doi.org/10.1038/tpj.2013.18
13. Erlich RL, Jia X, Anderson S et al (2011) Next-generation sequencing for HLA typing of class I loci. BMC Genomics 12:42. https://doi.org/10.1186/1471-2164-12-42
14. Leslie S, Donnelly P, McVean G (2008) A statistical method for predicting classical HLA alleles from SNP data. Am J Hum Genet 82 (1):48–56. https://doi.org/10.1016/j.ajhg.2007.09.001
15. Li N, Stephens M (2003) Modeling linkage disequilibrium and identifying recombination hotspots using single-nucleotide polymorphism data. Genetics 165(4):2213–2233
16. Okada Y, Momozawa Y, Ashikawa K et al (2015) Construction of a population-specific HLA imputation reference panel and its

application to Graves' disease risk in Japanese. Nat Genet 47(7):798–802. https://doi.org/10.1038/ng.3310

17. Zhou F, Cao H, Zuo X et al (2016) Deep sequencing of the MHC region in the Chinese population contributes to studies of complex disease. Nat Genet 48(7):740–746. https://doi.org/10.1038/ng.3576
18. Kim K, Bang SY, Lee HS et al (2014) Construction and application of a Korean reference panel for imputing classical alleles and amino acids of human leukocyte antigen genes. PLoS One 9(11):e112546. https://doi.org/10.1371/journal.pone.0112546
19. Marsh SG, Albert ED, Bodmer WF et al (2010) Nomenclature for factors of the HLA system, 2010. Tissue Antigens 75(4):291–455. https://doi.org/10.1111/j.1399-0039.2010.01466.x
20. Robinson J, Soormally AR, Hayhurst JD et al (2016) The IPD-IMGT/HLA database - new developments in reporting HLA variation. Hum Immunol 77(3):233–237. https://doi.org/10.1016/j.humimm.2016.01.020
21. Anderson CA, Pettersson FH, Clarke GM et al (2010) Data quality control in genetic case-control association studies. Nat Protoc 5 (9):1564–1573. https://doi.org/10.1038/nprot.2010.116
22. Moutsianas L, Jostins L, Beecham AH et al (2015) Class II HLA interactions modulate genetic risk for multiple sclerosis. Nat Genet 47(10):1107–1113. https://doi.org/10.1038/ng.3395
23. Marchini J, Howie B (2010) Genotype imputation for genome-wide association studies. Nat Rev Genet 11(7):499–511. https://doi.org/10.1038/nrg2796
24. Wellcome Trust Case Control Consortium (2007) Genome-wide association study of 14,000 cases of seven common diseases and 3,000 shared controls. Nature 447 (7145):661–678. https://doi.org/10.1038/nature05911
25. Chang CC, Chow CC, Tellier LC et al (2015) Second-generation PLINK: rising to the challenge of larger and richer datasets. Gigascience 4:7. https://doi.org/10.1186/s13742-015-0047-8
26. Evans DM, Spencer CC, Pointon JJ et al (2011) Interaction between ERAP1 and HLA-B27 in ankylosing spondylitis implicates peptide handling in the mechanism for HLA-B27 in disease susceptibility. Nat Genet 43(8):761–767. https://doi.org/10.1038/ng.873
27. Genetic Analysis of Psoriasis Consortium and the Wellcome Trust Case Control Consortium, Strange A, Capon F et al (2010) A genome-wide association study identifies new psoriasis susceptibility loci and an interaction between HLA-C and ERAP1. Nat Genet 42 (11):985–990. https://doi.org/10.1038/ng.694
28. Todd JA, Bell JI, McDevitt HO (1987) HLA-DQ beta gene contributes to susceptibility and resistance to insulin-dependent diabetes mellitus. Nature 329(6140):599–604. https://doi.org/10.1038/329599a0
29. Gutierrez-Achury J, Zhernakova A, Pulit SL et al (2015) Fine mapping in the MHC region accounts for 18% additional genetic risk for celiac disease. Nat Genet 47(6):577–578. https://doi.org/10.1038/ng.3268
30. Patsopoulos NA, Barcellos LF, Hintzen RQ et al (2013) Fine-mapping the genetic association of the major histocompatibility complex in multiple sclerosis: HLA and non-HLA effects. PLoS Genet 9(11):e1003926. https://doi.org/10.1371/journal.pgen.1003926
31. McMahon G, Ring SM, Davey-Smith G et al (2015) Genome-wide association study identifies SNPs in the MHC class II loci that are associated with self-reported history of whooping cough. Hum Mol Genet 24 (20):5930–5939. https://doi.org/10.1093/hmg/ddv293
32. Moutsianas L, Enciso-Mora V, Ma YP et al (2011) Multiple Hodgkin lymphoma-associated loci within the HLA region at chromosome 6p21.3. Blood 118(3):670–674. https://doi.org/10.1182/blood-2011-03-339630
33. Goyette P, Boucher G, Mallon D et al (2015) High-density mapping of the MHC identifies a shared role for HLA-DRB1*01:03 in inflammatory bowel diseases and heterozygous advantage in ulcerative colitis. Nat Genet 47 (2):172–179. https://doi.org/10.1038/ng.3176
34. Oksenberg JR, Barcellos LF, Cree BA et al (2004) Mapping multiple sclerosis susceptibility to the HLA-DR locus in African Americans. Am J Hum Genet 74(1):160–167. https://doi.org/10.1086/380997
35. Han F, Lin L, Li J et al (2012) HLA-DQ association and allele competition in Chinese narcolepsy. Tissue Antigens 80(4):328–335. https://doi.org/10.1111/j.1399-0039.2012.01948.x
36. Mignot E, Kimura A, Lattermann A et al (1997) Extensive HLA class II studies in 58

non-DRB1*15 (DR2) narcoleptic patients with cataplexy. Tissue Antigens 49(4):329–341

37. Liu C, Yang X, Duffy B et al (2013) ATHLATES: accurate typing of human leukocyte antigen through exome sequencing. Nucleic Acids Res 41(14):e142. https://doi.org/10.1093/nar/gkt481
38. Szolek A, Schubert B, Mohr C et al (2014) OptiType: precision HLA typing from next-generation sequencing data. Bioinformatics 30(23):3310–3316. https://doi.org/10.1093/bioinformatics/btu548
39. Dilthey AT, Gourraud PA, Mentzer AJ et al (2016) High-accuracy HLA type inference from whole-genome sequencing data using population reference graphs. PLoS Comput Biol 12(10):e1005151. https://doi.org/10.1371/journal.pcbi.1005151
40. Boegel S, Scholtalbers J, Lower M et al (2015) In silico HLA typing using standard RNA-Seq sequence reads. Methods Mol Biol 1310:247–258. https://doi.org/10.1007/978-1-4939-2690-9_20
41. Browning BL, Browning SR (2009) A unified approach to genotype imputation and haplotype-phase inference for large data sets of trios and unrelated individuals. Am J Hum Genet 84(2):210–223. https://doi.org/10.1016/j.ajhg.2009.01.005
42. Wissemann WT, Hill-Burns EM, Zabetian CP et al (2013) Association of Parkinson disease with structural and regulatory variants in the HLA region. Am J Hum Genet 93(5):984–993. https://doi.org/10.1016/j.ajhg.2013.10.009
43. Chen D, Gaborieau V, Zhao Y et al (2015) A systematic investigation of the contribution of genetic variation within the MHC region to HPV seropositivity. Hum Mol Genet 24(9):2681–2688. https://doi.org/10.1093/hmg/ddv015
44. Hu X, Deutsch AJ, Lenz TL et al (2015) Additive and interaction effects at three amino acid positions in HLA-DQ and HLA-DR molecules drive type 1 diabetes risk. Nat Genet 47(8):898–905. https://doi.org/10.1038/ng.3353
45. Lenz TL, Deutsch AJ, Han B et al (2015) Widespread non-additive and interaction effects within HLA loci modulate the risk of autoimmune diseases. Nat Genet 47(9):1085–1090. https://doi.org/10.1038/ng.3379
46. Field J, Browning SR, Johnson LJ et al (2010) A polymorphism in the HLA-DPB1 gene is associated with susceptibility to multiple sclerosis. PLoS One 5(10):e13454. https://doi.org/10.1371/journal.pone.0013454
47. Sekar A, Bialas AR, de Rivera H et al (2016) Schizophrenia risk from complex variation of complement component 4. Nature 530(7589):177–183. https://doi.org/10.1038/nature16549

Chapter 9

Novel Methods for Family-Based Genetic Studies

Qi Yan

Abstract

The recent development of microarray and sequencing technology allows identification of disease susceptibility genes. Although the genome-wide association studies (GWAS) have successfully identified many genetic markers related to human diseases, the traditional statistical methods are not powerful to detect rare genetic markers. The rare genetic markers are usually grouped together and tested at the set level. One of such methods is the sequence kernel association test (SKAT), which has been commonly used in the rare genetic marker analysis. In recent publications, SKAT has been extended to be applicable for family-based rare variant analysis. Here, I present three published statistical approaches for family-based rare variant analysis for: 1. continuous traits, 2. binary traits, and 3. multiple correlated traits.

Key words Statistical analysis, Sequence kernel association test, Mixed model, Rare genetic markers, Gene-based analysis

1 Introduction

With the advances in high-throughput microarray and sequencing technology, significant progress has been made in identifying disease susceptibility genes [1, 2]. Such progress requires the use of appropriate statistical methods. Genome-wide association studies (GWAS) have been widely used for identifying common genetic markers (i.e., single nucleotide polymorphisms [SNPs]) associated with human diseases [3–7]. In a typical GWAS, a large number of genetic markers are genotyped on hundreds or even thousands of subjects, and every genetic marker is subsequently tested, one by one, through single-marker tests (e.g., linear regression for continuous traits and logistic regression for binary traits). However, the single-marker association test is not powerful to detect rare genetic markers (i.e., low minor allele frequency [MAF], such as MAF $<$ 0.05 or 0.01) that confer susceptibility to complex human diseases [8, 9].

As a complement to the single-marker test, set-based tests become more and more attractive [10–12]. If multiple real

Evangelos Evangelou (ed.), *Genetic Epidemiology: Methods and Protocols*, Methods in Molecular Biology, vol. 1793, https://doi.org/10.1007/978-1-4939-7868-7_9,

causative genetic markers have small individual effects, single-marker test may not identify these weak signals. On the other hand, set-based tests have higher power because they combine the individual effects and thus may be able to detect the small effects. In addition, set-based tests could be more biologically meaningful. For example, genetic markers from the same gene can be grouped in a set. And finally, set-based approaches greatly reduce the burden of multiple testing in genome-wide studies. In recent years, many set-based statistical methods have been developed to evaluate the joint effect of a group of rare genetic markers in a predefined region [9–11, 13–23]. One such test that is commonly used is the sequence kernel association test (SKAT) [11, 22, 23], a flexible, computationally efficient, and regression-based approach. In SKAT, predefined weights can be assigned to each genetic marker in the set. This increases the power when prior information shows that certain types of markers may be associated with a trait. Furthermore, SKAT's test statistic follows a mixture of chi-square distributions. Thus, p-values can be computed analytically without performing resampling.

Family-based designs have been widely used in association studies of complex human diseases [24–27]. The GWAS with unrelated samples often employ general linear models, but the general linear models may result in an inflated Type I error rate when the familial correlation is ignored. Thus, in family-based studies, a linear mixed model including a random effect is usually used to account for the familial correlations. The covariance of random polygenic effects between all subjects is proportional to their kinship coefficients and linear mixed models with a kinship matrix have been commonly used in family-based genetic studies [28–32].

2 Methods

2.1 SKAT for Continuous Traits in Family Samples

The SKAT has been extended to be applicable for continuous traits in family samples [33–35] using the framework of linear mixed models. We assume that the $n \times 1$ vector of the trait $\mathbf{y}$ follows a linear mixed model. The trait is assumed to follow a normal distribution, shown as

$$\mathbf{y} = \mathbf{X}\boldsymbol{\beta} + \mathbf{G}\boldsymbol{\gamma} + \boldsymbol{\delta} + \boldsymbol{\varepsilon},$$

where $\mathbf{X}$ is an $n \times p$ covariate matrix, $\boldsymbol{\beta}$ is a $p \times 1$ vector for fixed effects parameters (an intercept and $p - 1$ covariates), $\mathbf{G}$ is an $n \times q$ genotype matrix for q genetic markers of interest, $\boldsymbol{\gamma}$ is a $q \times 1$ vector for the random effects of genetic markers, $\boldsymbol{\delta}$ is an $n \times 1$ vector to account for the familial correlations, and $\boldsymbol{\varepsilon}$ is an $n \times 1$ vector for the random error. The random effects $\boldsymbol{\gamma}$ are assumed to follow a normal distribution with mean 0 and variance $\tau\mathbf{W}$, so the null hypothesis

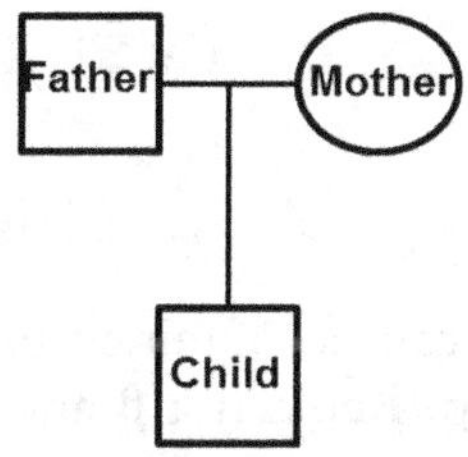

$$\Phi = \begin{bmatrix} 1 & 0 & 0.5 \\ 0 & 1 & 0.5 \\ 0.5 & 0.5 & 1 \end{bmatrix} \begin{matrix} \text{Father} \\ \text{Mother} \\ \text{Child} \end{matrix}$$

(columns: Father, Mother, Child)

Fig. 1 $n \times n$ twice kinship matrix

being tested is H_0: $\boldsymbol{\gamma} = 0$ that is equivalent to testing H_0: $\tau = 0$. A variance component score test known as the locally most powerful test can be used to test this H_0 [22] under the framework of mixed models. In addition, $\boldsymbol{\delta}$ follows a normal distribution with mean 0 and variance $\sigma_\delta^2\boldsymbol{\Phi}$, where $\boldsymbol{\Phi}$ is twice the $n \times n$ kinship matrix (Fig. 1). Also it is assumed that error $\boldsymbol{\varepsilon}$ is normally distributed and uncorrelated with $\boldsymbol{\gamma}$, as in:

$$\boldsymbol{\gamma} \sim N(0, \quad \tau\mathbf{W})$$

$$\boldsymbol{\delta} \sim N\left(0, \quad \sigma_\delta^2\boldsymbol{\Phi}\right),$$

$$\boldsymbol{\varepsilon} \sim N\left(0, \quad \sigma_E^2\mathbf{I}\right),$$

where $\mathbf{W}$ is a predefined $q \times q$ diagonal weight matrix for each of the genetic markers and may use $\sqrt{w_i} = Beta(MAF_i, 1, 25)$ as recommended in SKAT [22], and σ_E^2 is the error variance.

For a linear mixed model, we use the log-likelihood

$$l = -\frac{1}{2}\log|\boldsymbol{\Sigma}| - \frac{1}{2}(\mathbf{y} - \mathbf{X}\boldsymbol{\beta})'\boldsymbol{\Sigma}^{-1}(\mathbf{y} - \mathbf{X}\boldsymbol{\beta}),$$

where $\boldsymbol{\Sigma} = \text{var}(\mathbf{y}) = \tau\mathbf{GWG}' + \sigma_\delta^2\boldsymbol{\Phi} + \sigma_E^2\mathbf{I}$. In the log-likelihood, the first term $-\frac{1}{2}\log|\boldsymbol{\Sigma}|$ is fixed and independent of trait $\mathbf{y}$ when replacing $\boldsymbol{\Sigma}$ with its estimator.

To derive the score test for H_0: $\tau = 0$, we take the first derivative of the log-likelihood with respect to τ

$$\frac{\mathrm{d}l}{\mathrm{d}\tau} = -\frac{1}{2}\text{tr}\left(\boldsymbol{\Sigma}^{-1}\mathbf{GWG}'\right) + \frac{1}{2}(\mathbf{y} - \mathbf{X}\boldsymbol{\beta})'\boldsymbol{\Sigma}^{-1}\mathbf{GWG}'\boldsymbol{\Sigma}^{-1}(\mathbf{y} - \mathbf{X}\boldsymbol{\beta}),$$

where $\frac{\mathrm{d}l}{\mathrm{d}\tau}$ is the score function of τ. The first term is fixed and independent of $\mathbf{y}$. We take twice the second term to be derived as our test statistic Q.

Under the null hypothesis (i.e., H_0: $\boldsymbol{\gamma} = 0$), the linear mixed model is $\mathbf{y} = \mathbf{X}\boldsymbol{\beta} + \boldsymbol{\delta} + \boldsymbol{\varepsilon}$, where $\boldsymbol{\delta} \sim N\left(0, \sigma_\delta^2\boldsymbol{\Phi}\right)$ and $\boldsymbol{\varepsilon} \sim N\left(0, \sigma_E^2\mathbf{I}\right)$. Therefore, $\boldsymbol{\Sigma} = \sigma_\delta^2\boldsymbol{\Phi} + \sigma_E^2\mathbf{I}$. After replacing with their maximum likelihood estimators (MLE),

$$\widehat{\boldsymbol{\beta}} = \left(\mathbf{X}'\widehat{\boldsymbol{\Sigma}}^{-1}\mathbf{X}\right)^{-1}\mathbf{X}'\widehat{\boldsymbol{\Sigma}}^{-1}\mathbf{y},$$

$$\widehat{\boldsymbol{\Sigma}} = \widehat{\sigma}_{\delta}^{2}\boldsymbol{\Phi}+\widehat{\sigma}_{E}^{2}\mathbf{I}.$$

The MLE can be obtained using the function lmekin from R package kinship. Replacing $\widehat{\boldsymbol{\beta}}$ and $\widehat{\boldsymbol{\Sigma}}$ with their MLE, we have test statistics.

$$\mathrm{Q} = \left(\mathbf{y}-\mathbf{X}\widehat{\boldsymbol{\beta}}\right)'\widehat{\boldsymbol{\Sigma}}^{-1}\mathbf{GWG}'\widehat{\boldsymbol{\Sigma}}^{-1}\left(\mathbf{y}-\mathbf{X}\widehat{\boldsymbol{\beta}}\right).$$

Under null hypothesis, the variance of residual is

$$\begin{aligned}\mathrm{var}\left(\mathbf{y}-\mathbf{X}\widehat{\boldsymbol{\beta}}\right) &= \mathrm{var}\left(\mathbf{y}-\mathbf{X}\left(\mathbf{X}'\widehat{\boldsymbol{\Sigma}}^{-1}\mathbf{X}\right)^{-1}\mathbf{X}'\widehat{\boldsymbol{\Sigma}}^{-1}\mathbf{y}\right)\\ &= \widehat{\boldsymbol{\Sigma}}-\mathbf{X}\left(\mathbf{X}'\widehat{\boldsymbol{\Sigma}}^{-1}\mathbf{X}\right)^{-1}\mathbf{X}' = \mathbf{P}_0.\end{aligned}$$

The statistic Q is a quadratic form of $\left(\mathbf{y}-\mathbf{X}\widehat{\boldsymbol{\beta}}\right)$ and follows a mixture of chi-square distributions [36] under H_0. Thus,

$$\mathrm{Q} \sim \sum_{i=1}^{q}\lambda_i\chi_{1,i}^{2},$$

where λ_i is the eigenvalues of the matrix $\mathbf{W}^{\frac{1}{2}}\mathbf{G}'\widehat{\boldsymbol{\Sigma}}^{-1}\mathbf{P}_0\widehat{\boldsymbol{\Sigma}}^{-1}\mathbf{G}\mathbf{W}^{\frac{1}{2}}$ [33], which can be proved by the Theorem of the Distribution of Quadratic Forms and the Theorem of Equal Eigenvalues. The p-values can be calculated by different algorithms, such as Davies' method [37] using the function davies from R package CompQuadForm. The algorithm has been implemented in R and the software is available in Chen et al. [33].

2.2 SKAT for Binary Traits in Family Samples

The SKAT has been extended to handle binary traits in family samples. The method is based on a generalized linear mixed model framework that is general and can be applied to a large range of studies with different types of traits. The model setup is presented in a manner very similar to the previous section. We assume that the $n \times 1$ vector of the binary trait $\mathbf{y}$ is shown as

$$\mathrm{logit}(P(\mathbf{y}=1)) = \mathrm{logit}(\boldsymbol{\mu}) = \eta = \mathbf{X}\boldsymbol{\beta}+\mathbf{G}\boldsymbol{\gamma}+\boldsymbol{\delta},$$

where $\mathbf{X}\boldsymbol{\beta}$, $\mathbf{G}\boldsymbol{\gamma}$, and $\boldsymbol{\delta}$ are the same as described in the previous section, and $\boldsymbol{\mu}$ is the mean of $\mathbf{y}$. We still assume that the random effects $\boldsymbol{\gamma}$ are normally distributed with mean 0 and variance $\tau\mathbf{W}$, so the null hypothesis being tested is H_0: $\boldsymbol{\gamma} = 0$ that is equivalent to testing H_0: $\tau = 0$. We have

$$\boldsymbol{\gamma} \sim N(0,\ \ \tau\mathbf{W})$$

$$\boldsymbol{\delta} \sim N\left(0, \quad \sigma_\delta^2 \boldsymbol{\Phi}\right),$$

where $\mathbf{W}$ is a predefined $q \times q$ diagonal weight matrix for each variant. For a generalized linear mixed model, we use the quasi-likelihood [38].

$$ql = -\frac{1}{2}\log|\boldsymbol{\Sigma}| - \frac{1}{2}(\mathbf{y}^* - \mathbf{X}\boldsymbol{\beta})'\boldsymbol{\Sigma}^{-1}(\mathbf{y}^* - \mathbf{X}\boldsymbol{\beta}),$$

where $\mathbf{y}^*$ is the working trait vector that is equal to $\mathbf{H}^{-1}(\mathbf{y} - \boldsymbol{\mu}) + \eta$, $\boldsymbol{\Sigma} = \mathbf{R}^{-1} + \tau\mathbf{GWG}' + \sigma_\delta^2\boldsymbol{\Phi}$, $\mathbf{H}$ is a diagonal matrix with diagonal elements equal to $\frac{\partial\mu_i}{\partial\eta_i} = \partial\frac{e^{\eta_i}}{1+e^{\eta_i}}\Big/\partial\eta_i = \frac{e^{\eta_i}}{1+e^{\eta_i}}\left(1 - \frac{e^{\eta_i}}{1+e^{\eta_i}}\right) = \mu_i(1 - \mu_i)$, and $\mathbf{R}$ is also a diagonal matrix with diagonal elements equal to $\left\{\mathrm{var}\left(y_i|\gamma_i, \delta_i\right)/\left(\frac{\partial\mu_i}{\partial\eta_i}\right)^2\right\}^{-1} = \mu_i(1 - \mu_i)$ [38]. In the quasi-likelihood, the first term $-\frac{1}{2}\log|\boldsymbol{\Sigma}|$ is fixed and independent of phenotype $\mathbf{y}$ when replacing $\boldsymbol{\Sigma}$ with its estimator.

We take the first derivative of the quasi-likelihood with respect to τ to derive the score test for H_0: $\tau = 0$,

$$\frac{dql}{d\tau} = -\frac{1}{2}\mathrm{tr}\left(\boldsymbol{\Sigma}^{-1}\mathbf{GWG}'\right) + \frac{1}{2}(\mathbf{y}^* - \mathbf{X}\boldsymbol{\beta})'\boldsymbol{\Sigma}^{-1}\mathbf{GWG}'\boldsymbol{\Sigma}^{-1}(\mathbf{y}^* - \mathbf{X}\boldsymbol{\beta}),$$

where $\frac{dql}{d\tau}$ is the score function. Following the same rationale as described in the above section, we take twice the second term to be derived as our test statistic Q.

Under the null hypothesis, the generalized linear mixed model is $\mathrm{logit}(P(\mathbf{y} = 1)) = \mathbf{X}\boldsymbol{\beta} + \boldsymbol{\delta}$. When solving an iterated weighted least squares (IWLS) problem, it can be also written as

$$\mathbf{y}^* = \mathbf{X}\boldsymbol{\beta} + \boldsymbol{\delta} + \boldsymbol{\varepsilon}^*,$$

where $\mathbf{y}^*$ is the working trait vector, $\boldsymbol{\varepsilon}^* \sim N(0, \quad \mathbf{R}^{-1})$, and $\boldsymbol{\delta} \sim N\left(0, \quad \sigma_\delta^2\boldsymbol{\Phi}\right)$. Therefore, $\boldsymbol{\Sigma} = \mathrm{var}(\mathbf{y}^*) = \mathbf{R}^{-1} + \sigma_\delta^2\boldsymbol{\Phi}$. The estimating equations for the fixed and random effects can be obtained via Fisher scoring. After some algebra, $\widehat{\boldsymbol{\beta}} = \left(\mathbf{X}'\widehat{\boldsymbol{\Sigma}}^{-1}\mathbf{X}\right)^{-1}\mathbf{X}'\widehat{\boldsymbol{\Sigma}}^{-1}\mathbf{y}^*$ and the estimating equations must be solved iteratively until convergence. The final working trait vector $\mathbf{y}^*$ and the MLE of the covariance matrix $\boldsymbol{\Sigma}$ can be calculated numerically, such as from the function glmmPQL in the R package MASS [39]. Replacing $\boldsymbol{\Sigma}$ with its MLE, we have the test statistic

$$\mathrm{Q} = \left(\mathbf{y}^* - \mathbf{X}\widehat{\boldsymbol{\beta}}\right)'\widehat{\boldsymbol{\Sigma}}^{-1}\mathbf{GWG}'\widehat{\boldsymbol{\Sigma}}^{-1}\left(\mathbf{y}^* - \mathbf{X}\widehat{\boldsymbol{\beta}}\right).$$

Under H_0: $\tau = 0$, the variance of residual is

$$\text{var}\left(\mathbf{y}^* - \mathbf{X}\widehat{\boldsymbol{\beta}}\right) = \text{var}\left(\mathbf{y}^* - \mathbf{X}\left(\mathbf{X}'\widehat{\boldsymbol{\Sigma}}^{-1}\mathbf{X}\right)^{-1}\mathbf{X}'\widehat{\boldsymbol{\Sigma}}^{-1}\mathbf{y}^*\right)$$
$$= \widehat{\boldsymbol{\Sigma}} - \mathbf{X}\left(\mathbf{X}'\widehat{\boldsymbol{\Sigma}}^{-1}\mathbf{X}\right)^{-1}\mathbf{X}' = \mathbf{P}_0.$$

The statistic Q is a quadratic form of $\left(\mathbf{y}^* - \mathbf{X}\widehat{\boldsymbol{\beta}}\right)$ and follows a mixture of chi-square distributions [36] under H_0. Thus,

$$Q \sim \sum_{i=1}^{q} \lambda_i \chi^2_{1,i}.$$

Following the same rationale as described above, λ_i are the eigenvalues of the matrix $\mathbf{W}^{\frac{1}{2}}\mathbf{G}'\widehat{\boldsymbol{\Sigma}}^{-1}\mathbf{P}_0\widehat{\boldsymbol{\Sigma}}^{-1}\mathbf{G}\mathbf{W}^{\frac{1}{2}}$ and $\chi^2_{1,i}$ represents a chi-square distribution with one degree of freedom. The p-values can be calculated by Davies' method [37]. The algorithm has been implemented in R and the software is available in Yan et al. [40].

2.3 SKAT for Multiple Correlated Traits in Family Samples

In genetic studies of complex human diseases, multiple correlated traits are usually collected. Because of this relatedness, jointly testing the association of these correlated traits with genetic markers may increase the power to detect causative genes underlying diseases. The SKAT has been extended to test for the association of multiple correlated traits per subject in the context of family-based samples. The method uses kernel machine regression and is again based on a linear mixed model framework. Here, the null hypothesis being tested is that the group of genetic markers is not associated with any traits, and the alternative hypothesis is that they are associated with at least one of the traits. For the sake of simplicity, we consider a data set containing m individuals and two correlated phenotypes for illustration. The model with correlation among phenotypes and familial correlation is

$$\mathbf{y} = \mathbf{X}\boldsymbol{\beta} + \mathbf{G}\boldsymbol{\gamma} + \mathbf{h} + \boldsymbol{\varepsilon}.$$

Following the same rationale as described for the single continuous trait, the model under null hypothesis is

$$\mathbf{y} = \mathbf{X}\boldsymbol{\beta} + \mathbf{h} + \boldsymbol{\varepsilon},$$

where $\mathbf{y}$ is a vector of continuous trait (i.e., $\mathbf{y} = (y_{11}, y_{12}, y_{21}, y_{22}, \ldots, y_{m1}, y_{m2})$ where m is the number of samples). $\mathbf{X}\boldsymbol{\beta}$ is the fixed effects of covariates, $\mathbf{h}$ is the random effect of correlated phenotypes corresponding to the polygenic contribution, and $\boldsymbol{\varepsilon}$ is the random effect of correlated phenotypes corresponding to the random environmental contribution. Since we consider two correlated phenotypes per sample,

$$\mathbf{h} \sim N\left(0,\ \mathbf{\Phi} \otimes \begin{pmatrix} \sigma_{G1}^2 & \sigma_{G12} \\ \sigma_{G12} & \sigma_{G2}^2 \end{pmatrix}\right)$$

$$\boldsymbol{\varepsilon} \sim N\left(0,\ \mathbf{I} \otimes \begin{pmatrix} \sigma_{E1}^2 & \sigma_{E12} \\ \sigma_{E12} & \sigma_{E2}^2 \end{pmatrix}\right)$$

$$\mathrm{var}(\mathbf{y}) = \mathbf{\Phi} \otimes \begin{pmatrix} \sigma_{G1}^2 & \sigma_{G12} \\ \sigma_{G12} & \sigma_{G2}^2 \end{pmatrix} + \mathbf{I} \otimes \begin{pmatrix} \sigma_{E1}^2 & \sigma_{E12} \\ \sigma_{E12} & \sigma_{E2}^2 \end{pmatrix} = \mathbf{\Sigma}$$

where $\mathbf{\Phi}$ is twice the $m \times m$ kinship matrix obtained either from familial relationship and $\otimes$ is the kronecker product. $\sigma_{G1}^2, \sigma_{G2}^2, \sigma_{G12}, \sigma_{E1}^2, \sigma_{E2}^2$ and σ_{E12} represent the polygenic variances of the first and second traits, the polygenic covariance between the two traits, the environmental variances of the first and second traits, and the environmental covariance between the two traits, which can be estimated from the data, by employing the classic optimization methods such as Nelder-Mead method [41] and quasi-Newton method [42–45], and then the test statistic Q can be constructed,

$$\widehat{\boldsymbol{\beta}} = \left(\mathbf{X}'\widehat{\mathbf{\Sigma}}^{-1}\mathbf{X}\right)^{-1}\mathbf{X}'\widehat{\mathbf{\Sigma}}^{-1}\mathbf{y},$$

$$\widehat{\mathbf{\Sigma}} = \mathbf{\Phi} \otimes \begin{pmatrix} \widehat{\sigma}_{G1}^2 & \widehat{\sigma}_{G12} \\ \widehat{\sigma}_{G12} & \widehat{\sigma}_{G2}^2 \end{pmatrix} + \mathbf{I} \otimes \begin{pmatrix} \widehat{\sigma}_{E1}^2 & \widehat{\sigma}_{E12} \\ \widehat{\sigma}_{E12} & \widehat{\sigma}_{E2}^2 \end{pmatrix}.$$

Replacing $\widehat{\boldsymbol{\beta}}$ and $\widehat{\mathbf{\Sigma}}$ with their MLE, we have test statistics,

$$\mathrm{Q} = \left(\mathbf{y} - \mathbf{X}\widehat{\boldsymbol{\beta}}\right)'\widehat{\mathbf{\Sigma}}^{-1}\mathbf{GWG}'\widehat{\mathbf{\Sigma}}^{-1}\left(\mathbf{y} - \mathbf{X}\widehat{\boldsymbol{\beta}}\right).$$

Under null hypothesis, the variance of residual is

$$\mathrm{var}\left(\mathbf{y} - \mathbf{X}\widehat{\boldsymbol{\beta}}\right) = \widehat{\mathbf{\Sigma}} - \mathbf{X}\left(\mathbf{X}'\widehat{\mathbf{\Sigma}}^{-1}\mathbf{X}\right)^{-1}\mathbf{X}' = \mathbf{P}_0.$$

The statistic Q is a quadratic form of $\left(\mathbf{y} - \mathbf{X}\widehat{\boldsymbol{\beta}}\right)$ and follows a mixture of chi-square distributions [36] under H_0. Thus,

$$\mathrm{Q} \sim \sum_{i=1}^{q} \lambda_i \chi_{1,i}^2,$$

where λ_i is the eigenvalues of the matrix $\mathbf{W}^{\frac{1}{2}}\mathbf{G}'\widehat{\mathbf{\Sigma}}^{-1}\mathbf{P}_0\widehat{\mathbf{\Sigma}}^{-1}\mathbf{G}\mathbf{W}^{\frac{1}{2}}$ [33]. Again, the p-values can be calculated by Davies' method [37] using the function davies from R package CompQuadForm. The algorithm has been implemented in R and the software is available in Yan et al. [46].

3 Conclusive Remarkers

The above methods are based on kernel machine (KM) regression. As set-based methods, KM shares the advantages of other set-based methods, such as improved power by testing a set of genetic variants jointly and by reducing the multiple testing penalty.

Because KM is a score test, the estimates of fixed effect coefficients and the covariance matrix under the null hypothesis are independent of the genetic variants. Therefore, for a genome-wide analysis, the linear mixed model under the null hypothesis only needs to be fitted once and the total computation time is greatly reduced.

The KM framework is general and flexible. For example, non-genetic covariates can be easily incorporated into the model; the kinship matrix applicable to any relationships (such as grandparents-grandchildren and uncles-nephews) can be directly obtained from familial relationships or estimated from genome-wide genotype data.

References

1. Mardis ER (2008) The impact of next-generation sequencing technology on genetics. Trends in Genetics: TIG 24(3):133–141. https://doi.org/10.1016/j.tig.2007.12.007
2. Metzker ML (2010) Sequencing technologies - the next generation. Nat Rev Genet 11 (1):31–46. https://doi.org/10.1038/nrg2626
3. Wellcome Trust Case Control Consortium (2007) Genome-wide association study of 14,000 cases of seven common diseases and 3,000 shared controls. Nature 447 (7145):661–678. https://doi.org/10.1038/nature05911
4. Hunter DJ, Kraft P, Jacobs KB et al (2007) A genome-wide association study identifies alleles in FGFR2 associated with risk of sporadic postmenopausal breast cancer. Nat Genet 39 (7):870–874. https://doi.org/10.1038/ng2075
5. Yeager M, Orr N, Hayes RB et al (2007) Genome-wide association study of prostate cancer identifies a second risk locus at 8q24. Nat Genet 39(5):645–649. https://doi.org/10.1038/ng2022
6. Hindorff LA, Sethupathy P, Junkins HA et al (2009) Potential etiologic and functional implications of genome-wide association loci for human diseases and traits. Proc Natl Acad Sci U S A 106(23):9362–9367. https://doi.org/10.1073/pnas.0903103106
7. Manolio TA, Brooks LD, Collins FS (2008) A HapMap harvest of insights into the genetics of common disease. J Clin Invest 118 (5):1590–1605. https://doi.org/10.1172/JCI34772
8. Schork NJ, Murray SS, Frazer KA et al (2009) Common vs. rare allele hypotheses for complex diseases. Curr Opin Genet Dev 19 (3):212–219. https://doi.org/10.1016/j.gde.2009.04.010
9. Li B, Leal SM (2008) Methods for detecting associations with rare variants for common diseases: application to analysis of sequence data. Am J Hum Genet 83(3):311–321. https://doi.org/10.1016/j.ajhg.2008.06.024
10. Liu JZ, McRae AF, Nyholt DR et al (2010) A versatile gene-based test for genome-wide association studies. Am J Hum Genet 87 (1):139–145. https://doi.org/10.1016/j.ajhg.2010.06.009
11. Wu MC, Kraft P, Epstein MP et al (2010) Powerful SNP-set analysis for case-control genome-wide association studies. Am J Hum Genet 86(6):929–942. https://doi.org/10.1016/j.ajhg.2010.05.002
12. Neale BM, Sham PC (2004) The future of association studies: gene-based analysis and replication. Am J Hum Genet 75 (3):353–362. https://doi.org/10.1086/423901

13. Han F, Pan W (2010) A data-adaptive sum test for disease association with multiple common or rare variants. Hum Hered 70(1):42–54. https://doi.org/10.1159/000288704
14. Hoffmann TJ, Marini NJ, Witte JS (2010) Comprehensive approach to analyzing rare genetic variants. PLoS One 5(11):e13584. https://doi.org/10.1371/journal.pone.0013584
15. Lin WY, Lou XY, Gao G et al (2014) Rare variant association testing by adaptive combination of P-values. PLoS One 9(1):e85728. https://doi.org/10.1371/journal.pone.0085728
16. Lin WY, Yi N, Lou XY et al (2013) Haplotype kernel association test as a powerful method to identify chromosomal regions harboring uncommon causal variants. Genet Epidemiol 37(6):560–570. https://doi.org/10.1002/gepi.21740
17. Lin WY, Yi N, Zhi D et al (2012) Haplotype-based methods for detecting uncommon causal variants with common SNPs. Genet Epidemiol 36(6):572–582. https://doi.org/10.1002/gepi.21650
18. Madsen BE, Browning SR (2009) A groupwise association test for rare mutations using a weighted sum statistic. PLoS Genet 5(2):e1000384. https://doi.org/10.1371/journal.pgen.1000384
19. Morgenthaler S, Thilly WG (2007) A strategy to discover genes that carry multi-allelic or mono-allelic risk for common diseases: a cohort allelic sums test (CAST). Mutat Res 615(1–2):28–56. https://doi.org/10.1016/j.mrfmmm.2006.09.003
20. Zawistowski M, Gopalakrishnan S, Ding J et al (2010) Extending rare-variant testing strategies: analysis of noncoding sequence and imputed genotypes. Am J Hum Genet 87(5):604–617. https://doi.org/10.1016/j.ajhg.2010.10.012
21. Yi N, Liu N, Zhi D et al (2011) Hierarchical generalized linear models for multiple groups of rare and common variants: jointly estimating group and individual-variant effects. PLoS Genet 7(12):e1002382. https://doi.org/10.1371/journal.pgen.1002382
22. Wu MC, Lee S, Cai T et al (2011) Rare-variant association testing for sequencing data with the sequence kernel association test. Am J Hum Genet 89(1):82–93. https://doi.org/10.1016/j.ajhg.2011.05.029
23. Yan Q, Tiwari HK, Yi N et al (2014) Kernel-machine testing coupled with a rank-truncation method for genetic pathway analysis. Genet Epidemiol 38(5):447–456. https://doi.org/10.1002/gepi.21813
24. Falk CT, Rubinstein P (1987) Haplotype relative risks: an easy reliable way to construct a proper control sample for risk calculations. Ann Hum Genet 51(Pt 3):227–233
25. Ott J (1989) Statistical properties of the haplotype relative risk. Genet Epidemiol 6(1):127–130. https://doi.org/10.1002/gepi.1370060124
26. Spielman RS, McGinnis RE, Ewens WJ (1993) Transmission test for linkage disequilibrium: the insulin gene region and insulin-dependent diabetes mellitus (IDDM). Am J Hum Genet 52(3):506–516
27. Terwilliger JD, Ott J (1992) A haplotype-based 'haplotype relative risk' approach to detecting allelic associations. Hum Hered 42(6):337–346
28. Almasy L, Blangero J (1998) Multipoint quantitative-trait linkage analysis in general pedigrees. Am J Hum Genet 62(5):1198–1211. https://doi.org/10.1086/301844
29. Rabinowitz D, Laird N (2000) A unified approach to adjusting association tests for population admixture with arbitrary pedigree structure and arbitrary missing marker information. Human heredity 50(4):211–223. doi:22918
30. Yu J, Pressoir G, Briggs WH et al (2006) A unified mixed-model method for association mapping that accounts for multiple levels of relatedness. Nat Genet 38(2):203–208. https://doi.org/10.1038/ng1702
31. Kang HM, Sul JH, Service SK et al (2010) Variance component model to account for sample structure in genome-wide association studies. Nat Genet 42(4):348–354. https://doi.org/10.1038/ng.548
32. Zhang Z, Ersoz E, Lai CQ et al (2010) Mixed linear model approach adapted for genome-wide association studies. Nat Genet 42(4):355–360. https://doi.org/10.1038/ng.546
33. Chen H, Meigs JB, Dupuis J (2013) Sequence kernel association test for quantitative traits in family samples. Genet Epidemiol 37(2):196–204. https://doi.org/10.1002/gepi.21703
34. Schifano ED, Epstein MP, Bielak LF et al (2012) SNP set association analysis for familial data. Genet Epidemiol 36:797–810. https://doi.org/10.1002/gepi.21676
35. Oualkacha K, Dastani Z, Li R et al (2013) Adjusted sequence kernel association test for rare variants controlling for cryptic and family relatedness. Genet Epidemiol 37(4):366–376. https://doi.org/10.1002/gepi.21725

36. Yuan KH, Bentler PM (2010) Two simple approximations to the distributions of quadratic forms. Br J Math Stat Psychol 63 (Pt 2):273–291. https://doi.org/10.1348/000711009X449771
37. Davies R (1980) The distribution of a linear combination of chi-square random variables. J R Stat Soc Ser C Appl Stat 29:323–333
38. Breslow NE, Clayton DG (1993) Approximate inference in generalized linear mixed models. J Amer Statist Assoc 88:9–25
39. Venables WN, Ripley BD, Venables WN (2002) Modern applied statistics with S. Statistics and computing, 4th edn. Springer, New York
40. Yan Q, Tiwari HK, Yi N et al (2015) A sequence kernel association test for dichotomous traits in family samples under a generalized linear mixed model. Hum Hered 79(2):60–68. https://doi.org/10.1159/000375409
41. Nelder JA, Mead R (1965) A simplex-method for function minimization. Comput J 7 (4):308–313
42. Broyden CG (1969) A new double-rank minimisation algorithm. Preliminary report. Not Am Math Soc 16(4):670
43. Fletcher R (1970) A new approach to variable metric algorithms. Comput J 13(3):317. https://doi.org/10.1093/comjnl/13.3.317
44. Goldfarb D (1970) A family of variable-metric methods derived by variational means. Math Comput 24(109):23. https://doi.org/10.2307/2004873
45. Shanno DF (1970) Conditioning of quasi-newton methods for function minimization. Math Comput 24(111):647. https://doi.org/10.2307/2004840
46. Yan Q, Weeks DE, Celedon JC et al (2015) Associating multivariate quantitative phenotypes with genetic variants in family samples with a novel kernel machine regression method. Genetics 201(4):1329–1339. https://doi.org/10.1534/genetics.115.178590

Chapter 10

Methods for Polygenic Traits

Raha Pazoki

Abstract

An important aspect of public health is disease prediction and health promotion through better targeting of preventive strategies. Well-targeted preventive strategies will eventually decrease burden of diseases and thus precise prediction plays a crucial role in public health. Many investigators put efforts into finding models that improve prediction using known risk factors of diseases. Recently with the overwhelming load of genetic loci discovered for complex diseases through genome-wide association studies (GWAS), much of attention has been focused on the role of these genetic loci to improve prediction models. Genetic loci in solo explain little variance of diseases. It is thus necessary to create new genetic parameters that combine the effect of as many genetic loci as possible. Such new parameters aim to better distinguish individuals who will develop a disease from those who will not. In this chapter, various polygenic methods that use multiple genetic loci to directly or indirectly improve precision of genetic prediction are discussed.

Key words Genetic prediction, Genetic risk score, Genome-wide polygenic score, GWAS, SNP

1 Introduction

Human diseases can be caused by defects in both genetic and environmental factors [1]. For many years, genetic diseases were thought to be monogenic (monolocus/Mendelian disorders) caused by defects in single genes. Monogenic diseases can clearly be traced in families while demonstrating distinct autosomal recessive, autosomal dominant, or X-linked inheritance [2]. In contrast, the concept of polygenic susceptibility implies that many different genes with small effects impact heritability of a trait [3–5].

Human genome consists of more than 25,000 protein-coding genes [6]. According to Online Mendelian Inheritance in Man (OMIM), by November 10th 2016, disorders in 3266 genes have been linked to monogenic diseases. In contrast to monogenic diseases, disorders in a considerably lower number of genes ($n = 500$) have been linked to complex (polygenic) diseases [7–10]. Despite remarkable advancement in gene discovery for monogenic and complex diseases, biologic function of most of these genes is not yet well understood [6]. Further work has to be done to illuminate

Evangelos Evangelou (ed.), *Genetic Epidemiology: Methods and Protocols*, Methods in Molecular Biology, vol. 1793, https://doi.org/10.1007/978-1-4939-7868-7_10, © Springer Science+Business Media, LLC, part of Springer Nature 2018

clinical utility of the knowledge produced by recent gene discoveries achieved through genome-wide association studies (GWAS) for complex diseases. Various clinical dimensions of genetic studies including disease prevention, pharmacogenomics, and gene therapy can particularly have significant impact on patient care and disease burden. An essential element in disease prevention is predicting risk of diseases in order to be able to launch preventive strategies for high risk groups [11]. Preventive strategies for complex diseases can be as simple as lifestyle modification or as invasive as surgical interventions. For many complex diseases, such as cancers or cardiovascular diseases, prior prediction is crucial to increase survival. A prediction model with higher precision can better classify population into high risk and low risk groups and help make more accurate clinical decisions that are beneficial for patients and society.

2 Genetic Prediction of Diseases

Genetic factors are considered to have added value in prediction of complex diseases. Family history is an easily recognizable genetic factor [1]. Many complex diseases aggregate in families and family history is considered one of the most important predictors of complex diseases [1, 12–16]. Although family history is an important factor in disease prediction, it is often neglected in patient's records and is very much affected by recall bias or lack of detailed information regarding clinical aspects of family history such as exact clinical type of the event that is occurred in families years ago [1]. Recent GWAS have revealed numerous genetic variants/loci in the form of single nucleotide polymorphism (SNP) associated with various complex diseases. These loci can putatively increase precision of prediction models [11]. By definition, genetic information obtained from human samples are not expected to be vulnerable to recall bias and to missing information that accompanies family history. Addition of SNP-based information to family history has improved prediction of complex diseases such as coronary heart disease and prostate cancer [17–19]. Very recent models have demonstrated that prediction models that are based on SNP associations are powerful in predicting less common complex diseases [20, 21]. Results provided by including robust (i.e., genome-wide significant) SNP-associations in prediction models show significant added value in several cases [18, 22].

3 Genetic Risk Scores (GRS)

Despite recognized possibility for genetic information to improve disease prediction, most current prediction models omit genetic information [18]. One of the limitations is that genetic susceptibility identified so far through GWAS explains little variance of complex diseases and traits [23, 24]. Nevertheless, GWAS provide a very large and growing number of SNPs through international collaborations which aim to continually increase sample sizes for GWAS. To benefit from such a large number of SNPs provided by GWAS, various methods have been developed to better capture genetic basis of complex diseases [25]. These methods also aim to introduce new genetic determinants that explain greater variance of diseases compared to single-SNP methods. An example is to create a combined effect of multiple SNPs for which several statistical methods have been proposed. One naive but popular method is the so-called genetic risk score (GRS) analysis which combines the effect of a panel of selected SNPs [17, 25–34] that are associated with a given trait. The calculation is performed by summing up the effect of SNPs defined as weighted sum of risk alleles ($GRS = \sum_{i=1}^{k} wiXi$) where k is the number of bi-allelic SNPs, w_i is GWAS effect estimate from regression coefficients for ith SNP, and X_i is the number of risk alleles each individual carries for ith SNP.

Historically, the most initial equation to calculate GRS did not include the weighting part of the model and was simply a sum of total risk alleles an individual carried for a set of SNPs (un-weighted GRS). The main assumption of such an approach is that all selected SNPs have equal effects on the trait. This is an incorrect assumption since results from well-performed GWAS demonstrate that the effect estimates of various SNPs are not equal and therefore this method has lost popularity over time.

The first step in the construction of GRS is to select a suitable panel of SNPs. Construction of GRS is based on a conservative approach to select a robust set of SNPs showing strong evidence of association with the trait of interest. These are usually genome-wide significant SNPs, i.e., SNPs with association P-value less than 5×10^{-8}. This approach includes a relatively small subset of SNPs that are highly associated with the trait and may not capture much of the genetic variance in the trait (resembling the tip of the iceberg). Increasing sample sizes of GWAS will result in identification of more robust SNP-disease associations and consequently in long-term a greater number of SNPs will be available to construct GRS.

When constructing GRS, several important quality steps need to be considered. In most of the current large-scale GWAS, the most significant SNP associations are independent of each other. Nonetheless, when selecting SNPs to construct GRS, it is often the case that investigators create their set of SNPs from multiple sources. In such instances, a final set of SNPs may include highly correlated or even similar SNPs. It is therefore important to refine the subset of SNPs to obtain a selection of independent SNPs.

The main source of correlation between SNPs is linkage disequilibrium (LD) that is non-random association between alleles at two or more loci along a chromosomal segment. Studies take various LD thresholds represented by correlation coefficient (*R*-squared value; r^2) as low as 0.1 below which two SNPs can be called independent of each other. All SNPs with *R*-squared values below this pre-determined threshold are considered independent and are allowed to be included in the construction of GRS.

Advent of imputation methods allowed predicting alleles at non-genotyped loci. Since this process is accompanied with uncertainties, at any genetic locus the imputed genotypes are not exactly equal to the true genotypes. The greater the uncertainty in imputation, the lower the correlation between the imputed genotypes and the true genotypes. The uncertainty under the imputation process necessitates an additional level of quality control at the SNP selection process to construct GRS. Most imputation platforms provide a correlation coefficient (*R*-squared value; r^2) index to quantify imputation quality. This index represents the correlation between the predicted genotype and the true genotype reflecting how reliable the genotype prediction is. This *R*-squared value is used to filter and focus on SNPs with best imputation quality.

Some investigators take more conservative approach and refine their subset of SNPs even further by adding a plausibility index to quality control steps (for example, by selecting SNPs showing evidence of involvement in biological pathways) [35]. The advantage is to increase the true positivity value of the set of selected SNPs and to increase the likelihoods of finding a predictive genetic risk score. The limitation of plausibility filtering is the fact that important genetic information may be lost by removing novel SNPs for which scientists do not have any previously described biological knowledge.

The second step in the construction of GRS is allocation of weights to each SNP. These weights should represent the strength of the SNP-trait association (the effect estimates per copy of risk allele) provided by a previously published GWAS (from which the subset of SNP is selected; this is often called the *training sample*). GRS is usually constructed in a secondary study (i.e., the *target sample*). The target sample needs to be independent of the original GWAS from which the weights are obtained. Due to differences in genotyping such as different genotyping platforms as well as strand differences across studies, the allele coding in the target sample may not necessarily be the same as the training sample. Thus at this stage, it is essential to properly allocate the weights to the correct allele. For instance, if each copy of the C allele of a given SNP in the training sample increases height of an individual by 0.5 cm, effort needs to be taken to reassure that a weight of 0.5 is assigned to the C allele of that SNP in the target sample. Assigning this weight to the other allele will cause error in the construction of GRS.

After a proper SNP selection and weight assignment, GRS can be calculated for each individual in the study using the equation mentioned in the beginning of this section ($GRS = \sum_{i=1}^{k} wiXi$). A properly calculated GRS provides an index for each individual in the study representing their combined genetic risk for developing a certain disease. Many studies have constructed their GRS of interest and have investigated their effect on various traits. A good example is GRS calculated for cardiovascular traits (Table 1). Several cardiovascular GRS demonstrate increased risk of cardiovascular events. Their prediction value beyond traditional risk factors is however not significant in most cases and few studies demonstrated an improved predictive value by GRS beyond traditional risk factors of cardiovascular disease. Table 1 provides an overview of studies investigating cardiovascular GRS.

4 Genome-Wide Polygenic Score

A recently developed entity as a continuation of GRS is polygenic score [39] also called genome-wide polygenic score (GPS) [24] or polygenic risk score. The idea of GPS is based on the fact that current hypotheses suggest the heritability of complex traits may be captured by thousands of SNPs with small effects [24] including variants that are not genome wide significant rather than using merely robust SNPs with a genome-wide significant effect [40]. GPS that is developed by Purcell et al. [39] aggregates the effect of a much larger number of SNPs (compared with GRS) across the genome. Purcell et al. applied this method for the first time in 2009 to give insight into polygenic variation contributing to the risk of schizophrenia and bipolar disorder [39]. The basic calculation model of GPS is comparable to GRS where an in-aggregate effect of SNPs is being calculated:

$$\mathrm{GPS} = \left(\sum_{i=1}^{k} wiXi\right)/k$$

where k is the number of bi-allelic SNPs across the whole genome, w_i is the estimate of the regression coefficients for ith SNP (provided by previously published GWAS), and X_i is the number of risk alleles individuals carry for ith SNP.

GPS aims to summarize the collective effect of thousands of associated SNPs regardless of robustness [39]. The difference between the two methods is that GRS is a weighted *sum* of risk alleles for a *limited* number of *robust* SNPs, whereas GPS calculates a weighted *average* of SNP effects across the *whole genome* for each individual. Regardless of the method used, GRS and GPS are based on a common foundation to create a score that represents the effect of a collection of SNPs.

Table 1
Overview of the studies investigating combined SNP effects to predict cardiovascular events

Author	Selected SNPs	N SNPs	Predicted outcome	Genetic risk score prediction value
Morrison et al. [27]	SNPs of coronary heart disease	116	Coronary heart disease	Little improvement of prediction among black ethnicity
Kathiresan et al. [28]	SNPs of HDL & LDL	9	A first cardiovascular event	No significant improvement in clinical risk prediction; Significant improvement in risk reclassification
Ripatti et al. [29]	Cardiovascular SNPs	13	A first cardiovascular event	Identification of 20% of individuals who were at 70% risk of a first coronary event
Andreassi et al. [33]	Coronary artery/myocardial infarction SNPs	48	Major adverse cardiac events	Genetic risk score increases major adverse cardiac events
Lluis-Ganella et al. [32]	Coronary artery disease but not cardiovascular risk factors	8	Coronary heart disease	Genetic risk score improved re-classification among individuals with intermediate coronary risk
Patel et al. [34]	Coronary artery/myocardial infarction SNPs	11	Prevalent/incident myocardial infarction and death	Genetic risk score was associated with prevalent but not incident myocardial infarction
Vaarhorst et al. [31]	Coronary heart disease	29		
Ganna et al. [36]	Coronary heart disease and intermediate cardiovascular traits	395	Coronary artery disease	Genetic risk score was association with coronary heart disease and improved net reclassification index Up to 5% beyond traditional risk factors

Krarup et al. [30]	Coronary artery disease	45	Myocardial infarction	Genetic risk score increased risk of myocardial infarction; no improvement in net reclassification index (NRI) Or integrated discrimination improvement (IDI)
de Vries et al. [37]	Coronary heart disease	152	Incident coronary heart disease	Genetic risk score did not improve risk prediction
Tada et al. [17]	Coronary heart disease	27 vs. 50	A first coronary artery event	Genetic risk score improved risk prediction of coronary heart disease
Hindieh et al. [38]	Coronary artery/myocardial infarction SNPs	30	Severity of coronary heart disease in acute coronary syndrome	Genetic risk score was associated with the severity of coronary heart disease

As for GRS, the first step in GPS is to allocate a selection of SNPs. This step is quite straightforward and usually uses a set of SNPs and their effects from summary statistics of a previously published GWAS. This set should consist of SNP names, coded allele, effect estimates, and *P*-values for association tests per SNP.

The second step is to apply necessary quality control and filtering in the target sample (the sample in which GPS is being calculated). Purcell et al. [39] applied several layers of genome-wide filtering such as minor allele frequency of greater than 2%, genotyping rate threshold greater than 99%, pair-wise LD threshold of 0.25 within a sliding window of 200 SNPs. Filtering based on LD is considered essential since linked genotypes may negatively impact accuracy of prediction [41]. GPS have been used for multiple studies such as schizophrenia [39], body mass index [42], and cardiovascular diseases [43] demonstrating that inclusion of weekly associated markers can improve prediction of diseases. Purcell et al.'s method is implemented in plink genomic tool [44, 45].

5 Mendelian Randomization Studies

An important aspect in disease prediction and prevention is developing strategies that help decrease burden of diseases. If a risk factor is in causal relationship with a disease, reducing or eradicating such factor will decrease risk of disease. Causal inference is thus important and insightful to pinpoint the key causal factors in disease occurance. It is at the same time a complex process in biology given that investigators deal with many known and unknown factors confounding and interacting with each other in occurrence of a trait/disease [46]. Animal/plant studies are widely used for biologic causal inference where a certain intervention/treatment is imposed to their biologic environment and any impact of such intervention is observed and followed. Similarly in human randomized controlled trials (RCTs), participants are randomized into two or more groups of intervention (treatment) and control. In RCTs the beneficial effect of a certain intervention or treatment or procedure is examined on human subjects. RCTs are substantially limited to be used in disease aetiology [47] as it is unethical to expose humans to potentially harmful exposures. A solution to this limitation has been provided by the so-called Mendelian randomization studies that investigate causality using genetic data. Development of GWAS in recent years has led to the identification of genetic loci for numerous traits and diseases providing an optimal environment for Mendelian randomization studies to grow, develop, and to be used as a causal inference tool similar to RCTs. Mendelian randomization is grounded on the basis of Mendel's second law (genotypes are randomly assigned at gamete formation). Mendelian randomization studies use SNPs identified

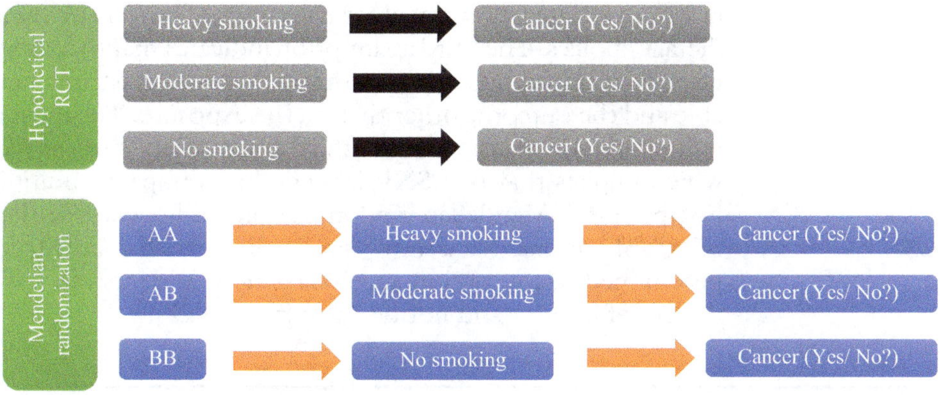

Fig. 1 Comparison of RCT and Mendelian randomization

by GWAS [48] as an *instrumental variable* to resemble randomization in RCTs in order to reduce confounding and draw causal inference [47].

Figure 1 illustrates a schematic diagram of a hypothetical RCT in which subjects are randomized into three groups and are exposed to various levels of smoking. Risk of developing cancer is then compared in each group. This RCT is not suitable to be performed on human subjects due to ethical reasons. Instead of performing an RCT as illustrated in Fig.1 a hypothetical SNP (genotypes are specifiedd as AA, AB, and BB) can be used to randomize human participants into three different genotype groups. The SNP must be robustly associated with levels of smoking in human subjects according to previous well-performed GWAS. In a scenario where association between the SNP and smoking status is additive and robust (i.e., identified in GWAS with large sample size, providing narrow confidence interval and genome-wide significance), carriers of the AA genotype, consisting of two smoking risk alleles, represent the "*heavy smoking*" group, carriers of the AB genotype represent the "*moderate smoking*" group, and carriers of the BB genotype, consisting of no smoking risk alleles, represent the "*no smoking*" group. Based on Mendel's second law, these genotype groups are randomly assigned at conception and therefore this model resembles randomization in an actual RCT. In this scenario, if the A allele increases risk of cancer, it implies that smoking is causal to cancer as if it would be resulted from an RCT. For a Mendelian randomization study to validly draw causal inference, several assumptions regarding the *instrumental variable* (SNP/genetic variant) must hold [47, 48]. The first assumption necessitates a robust association between the instrumental variable and exposure (SNP and smoking in the above example). The second assumption indicates that instrumental variable should not by any means be associated with a potentially confounding variable (e.g., alcohol consumption). In the example above, the SNP should not be associated with any other risk factor of cancer such as specific dietary choices. The third assumption indicates that there should be no evidence of biological pathway between instrumental variable and the outcome other that via the exposure. The most important source of violation of the third assumption is called *pleiotropy* which implies that one SNP/genetic locus impacts multiple phenotypes [49]. Mendelian randomization studies exclude the possibility of reverse causation since the genetic architecture is determined at conception and thus genetic variants can only cause disease of interest and not be a result of it [47].

6 Conclusion

Research into genetic prediction models is increasingly moving toward exploitation of polygenic variation to investigate their prediction value for complex diseases. Polygenic methods are also used to draw causal inference. It is important to investigate the clinical utility of polygenic prediction models. Cost-effectiveness studies are required to estimate the benefits of using such tools in patient care and treatment as well as in primary and secondary prevention. Focus on translation of these information into public health policy and clinical practice is an essential next step.

References

1. Guttmacher AE, Collins FS, Carmona RH (2004) The family history--more important than ever. N Engl J Med 351:2333–2336
2. Reyna BA, Pickler RH (1999) Patterns of genetic inheritance. Neonatal Netw 18:7–10
3. Maher BS (2015) Polygenic scores in epidemiology: risk prediction, etiology, and clinical utility. Curr Epidemiol Rep 2:239–244
4. Cotsapas C, Hafler DA (2013) Immune-mediated disease genetics: the shared basis of pathogenesis. Trends Immunol 34:22–26
5. Dudbridge F (2016) Polygenic epidemiology. Genet Epidemiol 40:268–272
6. Antonarakis SE, Beckmann JS (2006) Mendelian disorders deserve more attention. Nat Rev Genet 7:277–282
7. Amberger J, Bocchini CA, Scott AF, Hamosh A (2009) McKusick's online Mendelian inheritance in man (OMIM). Nucleic Acids Res 37: D793–D796
8. Amberger JS, Bocchini CA, Schiettecatte F, Scott AF, Hamosh A (2015) OMIM.org: online Mendelian inheritance in man (OMIM (R)), an online catalog of human genes and genetic disorders. Nucleic Acids Res 43: D789–D798
9. Hamosh A et al (2002) Online Mendelian inheritance in man (OMIM), a knowledgebase of human genes and genetic disorders. Nucleic Acids Res 30:52–55
10. Hamosh A, Scott AF, Amberger JS, Bocchini CA, McKusick VA (2005) Online Mendelian inheritance in man (OMIM), a knowledgebase of human genes and genetic disorders. Nucleic Acids Res 33:D514–D517
11. Jostins L, Barrett JC (2011) Genetic risk prediction in complex disease. Hum Mol Genet 20:R182–R188
12. Yang Q et al (1998) Family history score as a predictor of breast cancer mortality: prospective data from the cancer prevention study II, United States, 1982-1991. Am J Epidemiol 147:652–659
13. Li R et al (2000) Family risk score of coronary heart disease (CHD) as a predictor of CHD: the atherosclerosis risk in communities (ARIC) study and the NHLBI family heart study. Genet Epidemiol 18:236–250
14. Leander K, Hallqvist J, Reuterwall C, Ahlbom A, de Faire U (2001) Family history of coronary heart disease, a strong risk factor for myocardial infarction interacting with other cardiovascular risk factors: results from the

Stockholm Heart Epidemiology Program (SHEEP). Epidemiology 12:215–221

15. Graffagnino C, Gasecki AP, Doig GS, Hachinski VC (1994) The importance of family history in cerebrovascular disease. Stroke 25:1599–1604
16. Friedlander Y et al (2001) Family history as a risk factor for early onset myocardial infarction in young women. Atherosclerosis 156:201–207
17. Tada H et al (2016) Risk prediction by genetic risk scores for coronary heart disease is independent of self-reported family history. Eur Heart J 37:561–567
18. Muller B et al (2016) Improved prediction of complex diseases by common genetic markers: state of the art and further perspectives. Hum Genet 135:259–272
19. Chen H et al (2016) Adding genetic risk score to family history identifies twice as many high-risk men for prostate cancer: results from the prostate cancer prevention trial. Prostate 76:1120–1129
20. Stower H (2012) Complex disease: Family history versus SNPs for disease predictions. Nat Rev Genet 13:827–827
21. Do CB, Hinds DA, Francke U, Eriksson N (2012) Comparison of family history and SNPs for predicting risk of complex disease. PLoS Genet 8:e1002973
22. Manson JE, Bassuk SS (2015) Biomarkers of cardiovascular disease risk in women. Metabolism 64:S33–S39
23. Maher B (2008) Personal genomes: the case of the missing heritability. Nature 456:18–21
24. Selzam S et al (2016) Predicting educational achievement from DNA. Mol Psychiatry 22:267–272
25. Sebastiani P, Solovieff N, Sun J (2012) Naïve Bayesian classifier and genetic risk score for genetic risk prediction of a categorical trait: not so different after all! Front Genet 3:26
26. Drenos F, Whittaker JC, Humphries SE (2007) The use of meta-analysis risk estimates for candidate genes in combination to predict coronary heart disease risk. Ann Hum Genet 71:611–619
27. Morrison AC et al (2007) Prediction of coronary heart disease risk using a genetic risk score: the atherosclerosis risk in communities study. Am J Epidemiol 166:28–35
28. Kathiresan S et al (2008) Polymorphisms associated with cholesterol and risk of cardiovascular events. N Engl J Med 358:1240–1249
29. Ripatti S et al (2010) A multilocus genetic risk score for coronary heart disease: case-control and prospective cohort analyses. Lancet 376:1393–1400
30. Krarup NT et al (2015) A genetic risk score of 45 coronary artery disease risk variants associates with increased risk of myocardial infarction in 6041 Danish individuals. Atherosclerosis 240:305–310
31. Vaarhorst AAM et al (2012) Literature-based genetic risk scores for coronary heart disease; the CAREMA prospective-cohort study. Circulation: Cardiovascular Genetics 5(2):202–209
32. Lluis-Ganella C et al (2012) Assessment of the value of a genetic risk score in improving the estimation of coronary risk. Atherosclerosis 222:456–463
33. Andreassi MG et al (2012) Individual and summed effects of high-risk genetic polymorphisms on recurrent cardiovascular events following ischemic heart disease. Atherosclerosis 223:409–415
34. Patel RS et al (2012) Association of a Genetic Risk Score with Prevalent and Incident Myocardial Infarction in subjects undergoing coronary angiography. Circ Cardiovasc Genet 5:441–449
35. Li X et al (2013) Genome-wide association study identifies TH1 pathway genes associated with lung function in asthmatic patients. *J Allergy Clin Immunol* 132:313–20.e15
36. Ganna A et al (2013) Multilocus genetic risk scores for coronary heart disease prediction. Arterioscler Thromb Vasc Biol 33:2267–2272
37. de Vries PS et al (2015) Incremental predictive value of 152 single nucleotide polymorphisms in the 10-year risk prediction of incident coronary heart disease: the Rotterdam study. Int J Epidemiol 44:682–688
38. Hindieh W et al (2016) Association between family history, a genetic risk score, and severity of coronary artery disease in patients with premature acute coronary syndromes. Arterioscler Thromb Vasc Biol 36:1286–1292
39. Purcell SM et al (2009) Common polygenic variation contributes to risk of schizophrenia and bipolar disorder. Nature 460:748–752
40. Chatterjee N, Shi J, Garcia-Closas M (2016) Developing and evaluating polygenic risk prediction models for stratified disease prevention. Nat Rev Genet 17:392–406
41. Vilhjalmsson BJ et al (2015) Modeling linkage disequilibrium increases accuracy of polygenic risk scores. Am J Hum Genet 97:576–592
42. Speliotes EK et al (2010) Association analyses of 249,796 individuals reveal 18 new loci associated with body mass index. Nat Genet 42:937–948
43. Simonson MA, Wills AG, Keller MC, McQueen MB (2011) Recent methods for polygenic analysis of genome-wide data implicate an important effect of common variants on

cardiovascular disease risk. BMC Med Genet 12:146

44. Purcell S et al (2007) PLINK: a tool set for whole-genome association and population-based linkage analyses. Am J Hum Genet 81:559–575
45. Chang CC et al (2015) Second-generation PLINK: rising to the challenge of larger and richer datasets. Gigascience 4:7
46. Rothman KJ, Greenland S (2005) Causation and causal inference in epidemiology. Am J Public Health 95:S144–S150
47. Verduijn M, Siegerink B, Jager KJ, Zoccali C, Dekker FW (2010) Mendelian randomization: use of genetics to enable causal inference in observational studies. Nephrol Dial Transplant 25:1394–1398
48. Burgess S, Thompson SG (2013) Use of allele scores as instrumental variables for Mendelian randomization. Int J Epidemiol 42:1134–1144
49. Solovieff N, Cotsapas C, Lee PH, Purcell SM, Smoller JW (2013) Pleiotropy in complex traits: challenges and strategies. Nat Rev Genet 14:483–495

Chapter 11

Multivariate Methods for Meta-Analysis of Genetic Association Studies

Niki L. Dimou, Katerina G. Pantavou, Georgia G. Braliou, and Pantelis G. Bagos

Abstract

Multivariate meta-analysis of genetic association studies and genome-wide association studies has received a remarkable attention as it improves the precision of the analysis. Here, we review, summarize and present in a unified framework methods for multivariate meta-analysis of genetic association studies and genome-wide association studies. Starting with the statistical methods used for robust analysis and genetic model selection, we present in brief univariate methods for meta-analysis and we then scrutinize multivariate methodologies. Multivariate models of meta-analysis for a single gene-disease association studies, including models for haplotype association studies, multiple linked polymorphisms and multiple outcomes are discussed. The popular Mendelian randomization approach and special cases of meta-analysis addressing issues such as the assumption of the mode of inheritance, deviation from Hardy–Weinberg Equilibrium and gene-environment interactions are also presented. All available methods are enriched with practical applications and methodologies that could be developed in the future are discussed. Links for all available software implementing multivariate meta-analysis methods are also provided.

Key words Meta-analysis, Multivariate methodology, Genetic association studies

1 Introduction

Genetic epidemiology, being the fusion of mainstream epidemiology and statistical genetics, studies the inherited causes of disease by detecting genetic markers of disease susceptibility and identifying gene–gene or gene–environment interactions [1]. Classical epidemiological designs, such as population based case–control or cohort designs, are adopted in genetic association studies (GASs) in order to reduce the amount of genotyping whereas research in families (e.g., segregation and linkage studies) can be used complementary to account for population stratification [2]. However, GASs test one or a few genetic markers. Thus, in complex diseases, which are determined by multiple genetic and environmental determinants, the single variant examined in a genetic association study

Evangelos Evangelou (ed.), *Genetic Epidemiology: Methods and Protocols*, Methods in Molecular Biology, vol. 1793, https://doi.org/10.1007/978-1-4939-7868-7_11, © Springer Science+Business Media, LLC, part of Springer Nature 2018

usually accounts for little hereditability and its small to moderate effect may not be detectable even when large sample sizes are assessed [3]. From 2005, genome-wide association studies (GWASs) appeared, which examine the entire genome at acceptable cost [4]. In GWASs, millions of Single Nucleotide Polymorphisms (SNP) are read in a single scan of the study participants' genome [5]. Nowadays, the number of GWASs increases nearly exponentially ushering into a new era of high-throughput sequencing and discoveries of rare variants underlying susceptibility to polygenic disorders [6] even though the single studies are underpowered to detect small to moderate genetic effects [7]. The statistical issues encountered in analysis of GWAS have been extensively discussed elsewhere [8, 9].

The continuously growing number of published GASs and GWASs [10, 11] necessitate the collection and combination of the available information in a statistical procedure known as meta-analysis [12–14]. In the meta-analytic context, the eligible primary research is synthesized and the potential between studies diversity is investigated using formal statistical methods [12, 13, 15, 16]. Although meta-analysis was initially employed in the field of randomized clinical trials [17, 18], it is nowadays widely used in the synthesis of observational studies [19, 20], as well as in GASs and GWASs [14, 21–26].

Currently, the statistical methodologies for performing meta-analysis of GASs or GWASs are oriented towards the "one gene, one disease" approach. Multivariate approaches for meta-analysis of single gene-disease associations are oriented towards modelling separately the Odds Ratios (ORs) derived from the multiple genotypes in order to infer the genetic model of inheritance [22, 27] which are presented in a unified framework [23, 26]. Additionally, some GASs may report on more than one outcome that are potentially correlated (i.e., diabetes–hypertension). Other studies may report results on haplotypes [28] or on more than one polymorphism, of the same or nearby genes, that are in linkage disequilibrium (LD) [29]. In addition, there has been a dramatic increase in GASs reporting simultaneously on genotype-disease and genotype–phenotype associations (Mendelian Randomization) [30, 31]. In principle, under such circumstances, a multivariate random effects meta-analysis approach taking into account the correlations between the outcomes is necessary [32]. Formal overall tests can be constructed and the pooled estimates have better statistical properties under a missing at random assumption of the reported outcomes [33, 34].

In this chapter, we begin with presenting statistical methods used for robust analysis and genetic model selection in GASs and GWASs. We then discuss briefly the univariate approach for meta-analysis that is widely used in practice in GASs and proceed with illustrating the multivariate methodology. We describe the multivariate meta-analytic methods of haplotype association studies, studies reporting on a gene associated with correlated diseases or phenotypes and studies involving LD associated genes with a single disease or trait. We close with the presentation of the Mendelian Randomization approach and some special models developed to address issues such as the assumption of the mode of inheritance (dominant, recessive, additive and so on), the deviation from Hardy–Weinberg Equilibrium (HWE) and gene–environment interactions. Available software implementations of the described methods are also presented. We need to emphasize that this is a narrative and not a systematic review, but nevertheless, due to the extensive search in the literature we believe that no important publication in the field was neglected.

2 Analysis and Univariate Meta-Analysis of Genetic Association Studies

2.1 Analysis of Genetic Association Studies

The simplest class of association analysis in population based case–control studies involves a binary disease trait and a functional gene with two alleles (A, B) where the second (B) is assumed to be the risk factor for a particular disease. The possible genotypes of a person could be AA, AB and BB. Another situation is when the outcome of interest is continuous, such as Systolic Blood Pressure (SBP), cholesterol levels and so on. In this case, the studies are usually classified as having a cross-sectional design, where a representative sample from the general (or from a high-risk) population is collected, the individuals are genotyped and the mean values of the continuous measure that is under investigation are compared across genotypes. A graphical representation of the most commonly encountered types of associations in genetic epidemiology is presented in Fig. 1.

In GASs or GWASs, there is a variety of methods for analyzing data [35, 36]. Some methods are usually called genetic model-free (GMF), in the sense that they do not rely on pre-specifying the genetic model of inheritance, while others make such assumptions beforehand. For instance, if we compare BB+AB vs. AA genotypes we assume a dominant model of inheritance, the comparison of BB vs. AB+AA corresponds to a recessive model and B vs. A allele implies a co-dominant model. Under a GMF framework, one could calculate the traditional Pearson's chi-square statistic [35, 36] or an exact test, which is, however, computationally intensive. Another option would be to perform a logistic regression using the case/control status as the dependent and the genotype as the independent variable [35]. On the other hand, there are methods that are based on assuming a genetic model beforehand with the Cochran–Armitage trend test (CATT) being the most popular [37, 38]. These methods are powerful under the correct model

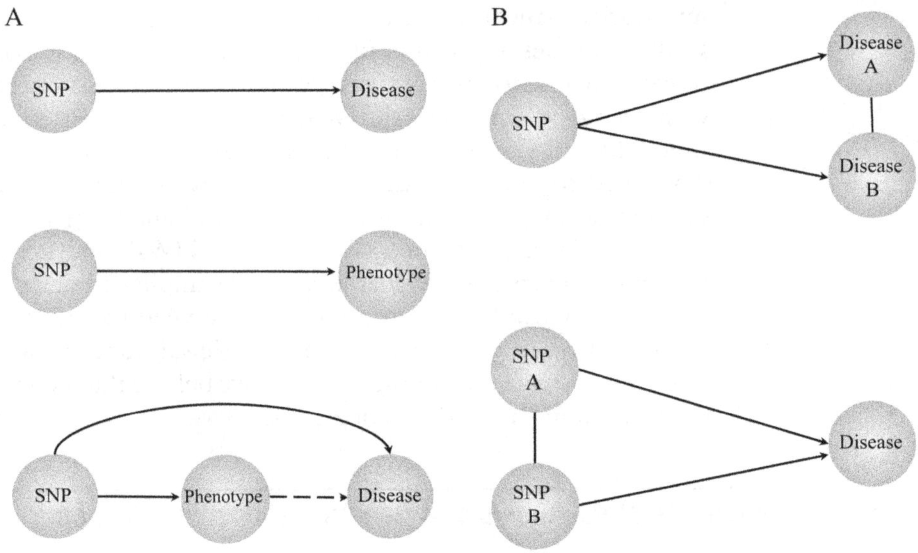

Fig. 1 Types of associations commonly met in genetic epidemiology studies. (**a**) Gene-disease association (upper), gene-phenotype association (middle) and Mendelian randomization (bottom) with the dotted arrow representing the indirectly inferred association of the phenotype with the disease. (**b**) A gene associated with two diseases (upper) and two genes in linkage disequilibrium associated with a single disease

specification but suffer from a decrease in power when the assumption does not hold.

Several robust approaches that detect the true underlying model of inheritance and, at the same time perform the analysis maximizing the power and preserving the nominal type I error rate have been proposed. Some of these robust methods are based on the theory of efficiency robust procedures [39, 40], namely the Maximum Efficiency Robust Test (MERT) and the maximum (MAX) test [41]. MERT is a linear combination of the optimal CATT for the recessive and dominant models whereas MAX tests all three possible models and chooses the one with the largest score. Another category of robust methods exploits the departures from HWE for the selection of the underlying genetic model [42]. In the Genetic Model Selection (GMS) method [43], it was shown that the Transmission Disequilibrium Trend Test (Z_{HWDTT}) [44] is positive under the recessive and negative under the dominant genetic model. On the other hand, Joo and coworkers [45] noted that the probability of correctly excluding the most unlikely genetic model remains high even in the case that the genotype relative risks are small. Thus, they proposed the Genetic Model Exclusion (GME) procedure, in which the dominant or recessive model of inheritance is excluded if $Z_{HWDTT} > 0$ or $Z_{HWDTT} < 0$ respectively, while, when $Z_{HWDTT} = 0$, the additive model is selected. Both GMS and GME have been shown to be robust with power comparable to the MAX test. Finally, a robust approach (MIN2) was suggested by applying the χ^2 test along with the CATT of the additive model of inheritance and subsequently choosing the minimum of the P-values [46]. Two years later, Joo and coworkers [47] derived the joint distribution needed in order to calculate a proper P-value. MIN2 was slightly less powerful than MAX for the recessive model, it outperformed MAX under the additive, whereas for the dominant model both tests performed similarly. Robust methods based on the MERT statistic, the MAX statistic and the MIN2 were recently implemented in Stata [48].

When continuous outcomes are assessed in GASs or GWASs, a linear regression with the value of the trait as the dependent variable and the genotypes as covariates could be performed [35]. Similar considerations concerning model selection can also be applied to quantitative traits under the linear regression formulation [49]. Therefore, some of the robust procedures discussed above such as MAX have been presented in such framework [50]. Moreover, it can easily be shown that MERT can also be used for continuous outcomes. However, this is not the case for the other methods such as the GMS, GME and MIN2, which use explicitly the case–control design and therefore cannot be applied for quantitative traits. Implementation of MAX, MERT, MIN2 and GMS approaches are available in R, SAS and Stata (Table 1).

Table 1
The available software for performing robust analysis of GAS or GWAS

Software	URL	Method	Environment
Coin [51]	http://cran.r-project.org/web/packages/coin/index.html	MAX	R
SNPassoc [52]	http://cran.r-project.org/web/packages/SNPassoc/index.html	MAX	R
RobustSNP [50]	https://sites.google.com/site/honcheongso/software/robustsnp	MAX	R
Rassoc [53]	https://cran.r-project.org/src/contrib/Archive/Rassoc/	MAX/MERT/GMS	R
R macro [45]	http://www.biometrics.tibs.org/datasets/080703P_Rcode.txt	GMS/GME	R
SAS macro [43]	http://biostatistics.oxfordjournals.org/content/9/3/391/suppl/DC1	GMS	SAS
GWAR [48]	http://www.compgen.org/tools/GWAR	MERT/MAX/MIN2	STATA

2.2 Univariate Meta-Analysis of Genetic Association Studies

Usually, the data from a meta-analysis of retrospective case–control studies are depicted in the form of Tables 2 or 3 in the case of continuous outcomes. The majority of meta-analyses of GASs involving one locus with two variants (A vs. B), are conducted by collapsing the genotypes in two categories assuming a particular genetic model and then by performing comparisons either by means of the Odds Ratio (OR, for dichotomous outcomes) or by using the average difference (also known as weighted mean difference-WMD, for continuous outcomes).

After the appropriate effect size y_i for each study ($i = 1, 2 \ldots k$) is calculated, a univariate fixed-effects or random-effects meta-analysis is conducted [12, 13]. In a traditional fixed-effects meta-analysis using summary measures, the assumption usually made is that the individual estimates y_i of the logOR (or the mean difference) of

Table 2
A typical layout of the data used in a meta-analysis of case–control genetic association studies involving a single bi-allelic locus with a dichotomous outcome. The distribution of the various genotypes (AA, AB and BB) is listed for cases and controls, whereas the different studies ($i = 1, 2, \ldots k$) included in the meta-analysis are listed in different rows

Study	Cases			Controls		
1	AA_{11}	AB_{11}	BB_{11}	AA_{01}	AB_{01}	BB_{01}
2	AA_{12}	AB_{12}	BB_{12}	AA_{02}	AB_{02}	BB_{02}
...	...	...	...	...	...	...
k	AA_{1k}	AB_{1k}	BB_{1k}	AA_{0k}	AB_{0k}	BB_{0k}

Table 3
A typical layout of the data used in a meta-analysis of genetic association studies involving a single bi-allelic locus with a continuous outcome. The distribution of the various genotypes (AA, AB and BB) is listed for all participants (N), accompanied by the mean and the standard deviation of the measured continuous outcome in each group. The different studies ($i = 1, 2 \ldots k$) included in the meta-analysis are listed in different rows

	Genotypes					
	AA		AB		BB	
Study	Mean (sd)	*N*	Mean (sd)	*N*	Mean (sd)	*N*
1	y_{AA1} (s_{AA1})	AA_1	y_{AB1} (s_{AB1})	AB_1	y_{BBA1} (s_{BB1})	BB_1
2	y_{AA2} (s_{AA2})	AA_2	y_{AB2} (s_{AB2})	AB_2	y_{BBA2} (s_{BB2})	BB_2
...	...	...	...	...	...	...
k	y_{AAk} (s_{AAk})	AA_k	y_{ABk} (s_{ABk})	AB_k	y_{BBAk} (s_{BBk})	BB_k

each study, are distributed normally with mean equal to the true effect θ and variance σ^2, which is the estimated variance of the logOR (or the mean difference) of the particular contrast of each study [12, 13]. In the presence of heterogeneity, an alternative and perhaps preferable method, is the random-effects method, which assumes that the true effects vary randomly between studies and a random component of the between studies variance (τ^2) is introduced. The most common approach for estimation of τ^2 is the non-iterative method of moments (MM) proposed by [54]. Other methods summarized by [55], include iterative techniques, such as maximum likelihood (ML), restricted maximum likelihood (REML) and empirical Bayes estimation (EB). When heterogeneity is absent, τ^2 is essentially equal to zero and the fixed and random-effects methods coincide. Similar models have also been described in a Bayesian framework [56–58]. Meta-analysis of GASs or GWASs can be implemented by various statistical packages such as STATA, R, METAL, GWAMA, MetABEL and PLINK (Table 4).

3 Multivariate Meta-Analysis of Genetic Association Studies

Univariate meta-analysis presented in the previous section is suitable for one-dimensional parameters. On the other hand, multivariate meta-analysis jointly synthesizes the estimates arising from each study [32, 70, 71]. This modeling framework provides estimates for all the effect sizes, and makes easier the comparison of the results, avoiding multiple comparisons and consequently, the inflation of type I error rate. Moreover, the potential correlation between the estimates is taken into account yielding more robust and precise estimates while the univariate approach ignores such correlation structure [70]. Kirkham and co-workers have demonstrated a notable advantage of a multivariate approach when there is selective non reporting of outcomes reducing bias of the parameter estimates [72]. Overall, multivariate meta-analysis can accommodate, under the missing-at-random assumption, studies reporting only one of the parameters of interest, resulting in borrowing strength from external studies [73].

3.1 The General Multivariate Model

To perform a joint analysis, following the general framework for multivariate meta-analysis [32, 74], we denote by $\mathbf{y}_i$ the vector containing the p different estimates and by $\boldsymbol{\beta}$, the vector of the overall means, given by:

$$\mathrm{y}_i = \begin{pmatrix} \widehat{y}_{1i} \\ \widehat{y}_{2i} \\ \cdots \\ \widehat{y}_{pi} \end{pmatrix}, \upbeta = \begin{pmatrix} \beta_1 \\ \beta_2 \\ \cdots \\ \beta_p \end{pmatrix} \tag{1}$$

Table 4
The available software for performing meta-analysis of GAS or GWAS

Software	URL
Univariate meta-analysis	
METAL [59]	http://csg.sph.umich.edu/abecasis/metal/index.html
GWAMA [60]	http://www.geenivaramu.ee/en/tools/gwama
MetABEL [61]	www.genabel.org/packages/MetABEL
PLINK [62]	https://www.cog-genomics.org/plink2
Multivariate meta-analysis of single gene-disease	
Stata do-file [26]	http://www.compgen.org/tools/multivariate-genetic/
Multivariate meta-analysis of haplotypes/multiple alleles	
Stata do-file [28]	http://www.compgen.org/tools/haplotype
Multivariate meta-analysis of multiple outcomes	
Cpma [63]	https://cran.r-project.org/web/packages/omics/index.html
ASSET [64]	https://dceg.cancer.gov/tools/analysis/asset
CPASSOC [65]	http://hal.case.edu/zhu-web/
PRIMe [66]	https://www.framinghamheartstudy.org/researchers/gwas-pleiotropic-tool.php
TATES [67]	http://ctg.cncr.nl/software/tates
p_ACT_meta [68]	http://csg.sph.umich.edu/boehnke/p_act.php
Stata do-file [69]	http://www.compgen.org/tools/multiple-outcomes
Multivariate meta-analysis of Mendelian randomization	
Stata do-file [30, 31]	http://www2.le.ac.uk/departments/health-sciences/research/gen-epi/reports

In the multivariate random-effects meta-analysis, we assume that $\mathbf{y}_i$ is distributed following a multivariate normal distribution around the true means $\boldsymbol{\beta}$ according to the marginal model:

$$\mathrm{y}_i \sim \mathrm{MVN}(\beta, \Sigma + \mathrm{C}_i) \tag{2}$$

with a within-studies covariance matrix $\mathbf{C}_i$ given by:

$$\mathrm{C}_i = \begin{pmatrix} {s_{1i}}^2 & \rho_{w12i}s_{1i}s_{2i} & \cdots & \rho_{w1pi}s_{1i}s_{pi} \\ \rho_{w12i}s_{1i}s_{2i} & {s_{2i}}^2 & \cdots & \rho_{w2pi}s_{2i}s_{pi} \\ \cdots & \cdots & \cdots & \cdots \\ \rho_{w1pi}s_{1i}s_{pi} & \rho_{w2pi}s_{2i}s_{pi} & \cdots & {s_{pi}}^2 \end{pmatrix} \tag{3}$$

and a between-studies covariance matrix $\boldsymbol{\Sigma}$ given by the following:

$$\boldsymbol{\Sigma} = \begin{pmatrix} {\tau_1}^2 & \rho_{B12}\tau_1\tau_2 & \cdots & \rho_{B1p}\tau_1\tau_p \\ \rho_{B12}\tau_1\tau_2 & {\tau_2}^2 & \cdots & \rho_{B2p}\tau_2\tau_p \\ \cdots & \cdots & \cdots & \cdots \\ \rho_{B1p}\tau_1\tau_p & \rho_{B2p}\tau_2\tau_p & \cdots & {\tau_p}^2 \end{pmatrix} \quad (4)$$

The diagonal elements of $\mathbf{C}_i$ are the study-specific estimates of the variance and are assumed known [32]. The off-diagonal elements of $\mathbf{C}_i$ correspond to the pairwise within-studies covariances (for instance $\rho_{w12i}s_{1i}s_{2i} = \text{cov}(\hat{y}_{1i}, \hat{y}_{2i})$) (see next session). The diagonal elements of $\boldsymbol{\Sigma}$ are the between studies variances, whereas the off-diagonal elements correspond to the between studies covariances that are estimated during the fitting procedure. When the number of the freely estimated parameters increases, a structured specification for $\boldsymbol{\Sigma}$ can be imposed.

The general multivariate method of Eq. (2) can be fitted in any statistical package capable of fitting random-effects weighted regression models with an arbitrary covariance matrix. The Stata command `mvmeta` performs inferences based on either Maximum Likelihood (ML) or Restricted Maximum Likelihood (REML) by direct maximization of the approximate likelihood using a Newton–Raphson algorithm [75]. Alternatively, `mvmeta` can also implement the multivariate version of the DerSimonian and Laird's method of moments [70, 76]. The last option, being non-iterative, is very attractive, particularly in applications in GWAS. A command with the same name (`mvmeta`) and functionality is also available in R. The particular model, being general can also be fitted using software for generalized mixed models. Van Houwelingen and coworkers used such a formulation for multivariate meta-analysis and meta-regression and provided illustrative code in `SAS PROC MIXED` [32], Bagos has shown the same for `gllamm` in STATA [77], whereas R users can use the `metafor` package [78].

3.2 Estimating the Within-Studies Covariances

Several approaches have been proposed in order to deal with the problem of correlated estimates [79]. However, the general case includes a within-study correlation that needs to be computed using individual data [32, 74]. Special cases in which the correlation can be computed analytically using solely the observed summary counts, include studies with multiple treatment arms [73] or multiple outcomes [79], clinical trials with mutually exclusive outcomes [80], dose–response models [81–83] and multivariate modeling of log-odds ratios in genetic association studies [26]. Recently, the problem has also attracted increased interest in GWAS that share overlapping sets of subjects [84, 85], in matched and unmatched case–control studies that use the same group of cases [86, 87] and in multipoint meta-analysis of genetic association studies (*see* Sect. 3.3.2 for details) [29]. In other more general cases however, the correlation cannot be calculated and simulation techniques have been proposed [31, 88].

Table 5
The full table describing the association of binary variables Y_i, X_{1i} and X_{2i} for study i ($i = 1,2, \ldots, k$). We denote the counts as n_{clmi}, with c being the indicator for Y_i, l the indicator for X_{1i} and m the indicator for X_{2i}

		X_{1i}			
		$X_{1i} = 1$		$X_{1i} = 0$	
		X_{2i}			
		$X_{2i} = 1$	$X_{2i} = 0$	$X_{2i} = 1$	$X_{2i} = 0$
Y_i	$Y_i = 1$	n_{111i}	n_{110i}	n_{101i}	n_{100i}
	$Y_i = 0$	n_{011i}	n_{010i}	n_{001i}	n_{000i}

By encompassing all the previous approaches in a unifying framework, a general method for computing the covariance of two correlated log-odds ratios (for instance $\widehat{y}_{1i}$ and $\widehat{y}_{2i}$) was proposed using solely the observed counts of the contingency tables (Table 5) [89]. Briefly, let Y_i, X_{1i} and X_{2i} denote three categorical random variables with two levels (i.e., 0, 1) that are used to classify n_i individuals for study i ($i = 1,2, \ldots, k$). In the general case, the data would be presented in the form of a three-dimensional ($2 \times 2 \times 2$) contingency table (Table 5) where we denote the counts as n_{clmi} with c, l, $m \in \{0, 1\}$ and this table is referred to as partial contingency table. It has been shown that an estimate of the covariance is given by:

$$\widehat{\text{cov}}\left(\widehat{y}_{1i}, \widehat{y}_{2i}\right) = \sum_{c}\sum_{l}\sum_{m}(-1)^{l-m}\left(\frac{n_{clmi}}{n_{cl+i}n_{c+mi}}\right) \quad (5)$$

This method is very simple and straightforward and is based on standard large sample approximations [90, 91].

3.3 Models of Meta-Analysis for a Single Gene-Disease Association

In the majority of the published meta-analyses of GASs [92–94], the data are routinely analyzed in a univariate fashion (Fig. 1a) ignoring the within-studies pairwise correlation of genotype contrasts and a genetic model of inheritance is assumed beforehand. However, a GMF multivariate approach was proposed by Minelli and coworkers [22], according to which the genetic model is inferred from the data. In particular, they introduced the joint (bivariate) modelling of the logarithm of OR_{BB}, which is the OR of BB genotype vs. AA, and λ which is the ratio of $\log OR_{AB}$ (i.e., the OR of AB genotype vs. AA) and the $\log OR_{BB}$, an approach that recognizes the fact that the two ORs are correlated. The value of λ is not restricted, but values equal to 0, 0.5 and 1 correspond to the recessive, co-dominant and dominant genetic model, respectively.

This model imposes a single between studies variance τ^2 and treats λ as fixed-effects parameter [22, 26, 70, 71].

A less parsimonious but more general model was described by Bagos [26], who proposed modelling directly the two logORs ($logOR_{AB}$ and $logOR_{BB}$) as a bivariate response in order to account for the correlation of those estimates [74, 95]. Thus, the vector $\mathbf{y}_i$ described in Eq. (1) contains two different estimates. The estimation of the parameters of the multivariate model depicted in Eq. (2) requires the calculation of the off-diagonal elements of the within-studies covariance matrix (Eq. 3). Since the logORs derived from each genotype (AB and BB) are compared against the same reference AA genotype, their pairwise covariance is calculated as the sum of the inverse quantity of cases and controls carrying AA genotype [26, 89].

A major advantage of the aforementioned approach [26] is that it can be easily fitted using standard software for multivariate meta-analysis [70, 71] (Table 4). The model of Minelli and coworkers [22], on the other hand, although being similar, requires specialised code to be written. Nevertheless, in many practical applications, the parameter estimates of the two models are equivalent. Minelli and coworkers also presented a Bayesian version of their model that uses the prospective likelihood [27]. Finally, Salanti and coworkers [96] extended the method and presented a model that can be used in situations in which some studies assumed a genetic model and presented their results in the form of collapsed genotypes.

The methods presented so far use summary data and a normal approximation. However, we could exploit directly the binary nature of the data and perform the analysis using an ordinary logistic regression. Then, we have two alternatives for modelling, either using the prospective or the retrospective likelihood. In the former case, we treat the case/control status as the dependent variable and the genotypes as covariates in a logistic regression and both fixed and random effects models for such a meta-analysis have been presented [23]. Alternatively, the model may be parameterized assuming a multinomial sampling scheme utilizing the retrospective likelihood. In this case, the genotypes are treated as dependent variables and the case/control status as the predictor in a multinomial (polytomous) logistic regression [97] which can also be employed in a meta-analysis framework [98]. These models are extensions of the general method of multivariate meta-analysis proposed by van Houwelingen and coworkers [95]. Similarly, the methods could be viewed as extensions of the univariate multilevel methods for random effects meta-analysis [55, 99, 100]. These models are expected to perform better compared to the models based on summary data when the normality assumption for logORs is invalid.

Multivariate methods for meta-analysis can be also applied in continuous outcomes as shown in [26]. In such a case, from the three genotypes (AA, AB and BB) we will have the mean value of the trait (y_{AA}, y_{AB} and y_{BB}) and the standard deviation (sd_{AA}, sd_{AB} and sd_{BB}) (Table 3). The bivariate method, can be easily applied if we denote the pairwise differences of the outcomes arising from individuals carrying the two risk genotypes (AB, BB) from the reference genotype AA. It is straightforward to show that the two differences are distributed normally with mean equal to the difference of the means and variance equal to the sum of the variances, whereas the covariance can also be easily derived [26]. Therefore, the bivariate GMF methods can easily be used without any further change. Stata programs for fitting the meta-analysis models described in this section are available at http://www.compgen.org/tools/multivariate-genetic (Table 4).

3.3.1 Models of Meta-Analysis of Haplotype Association Studies

The analysis of haplotypes allows the simultaneous evaluation of multiple potentially causal variants or they may be a proxy for untyped causal markers. Haplotypes are the combination of closely linked alleles on a chromosome and are important in the investigation of the genetic basis of a disease since the SNP under study may not always be the true susceptibility allele. Instead, it may be a SNP which is in LD with the unknown disease [101]. A major problem in haplotype analyses (and hence the meta-analyses derived from them) is that in order for the analysis to be performed we need to reconstruct or infer the haplotypes, usually with an approach based on missing data imputation [102–104].

A commonly used approach that is based on traditional univariate methods for meta-analysis of aggregated data for binary traits is to consider separately the effect of the jth haplotype against the $j - 1$ remaining ones. However, this method is prone to an increased type I error rate due to multiple comparisons, especially as the number of haplotypes increases [105, 106]. In order to overcome this drawback, we can perform a multivariate meta-analysis modelling simultaneously the logORs derived from comparing haplotypes $j = 2,3, \ldots, r$ against a reference haplotype ($j = 1$). Thus, the vector $\mathbf{y}_i$ described in Eq. (1) contains now $r - 1$ different estimates. Again here, the elements of the within-studies covariance matrix are calculated as the sum of the inverse quantity of cases and controls carrying the reference haplotype. This method allows an overall test for the haplotype disease association with increased precision as the single marker tests may be underpowered, depending on the degree of LD and the allele frequencies [107]. Other methods that exploit directly the binary nature of the data (logistic, multinomial logistic and poisson regression) or methods for assessing continuous traits have been previously described in detail [28]. These methods assume that the haplotypes are directly observed. However, they can be easily extended to deal with such an uncertainty by weighting the inferred haplotypes by their probability [108, 109]. Although we eliminated our scheme for the analysis of haplotype-association studies, this approach can be also used to account for genes with multiple alleles. Implementing meta-analysis of haplotypes using Stata is straightforward (Table 4).

3.3.2 Models of Meta-Analysis for Multiple Linked Polymorphisms

A closely related situation to the meta-analysis of haplotypes is encountered when multiple linked loci (polymorphisms of the same gene or from different ones) are considered (Fig. 1b). This scenario approximates the concept of network meta-analysis [110] (Fig. 2). Several methods for multilocus association have been proposed [111–113]. A major shortcoming of such methods is that we need to have access to individual patients' data (IPD) in order to specify the joint distribution of the genotypes from several linked polymorphisms. Bayesian methods have also been proposed for meta-analysis of published studies reporting various correlated markers, either involving a continuous trait [114], or a

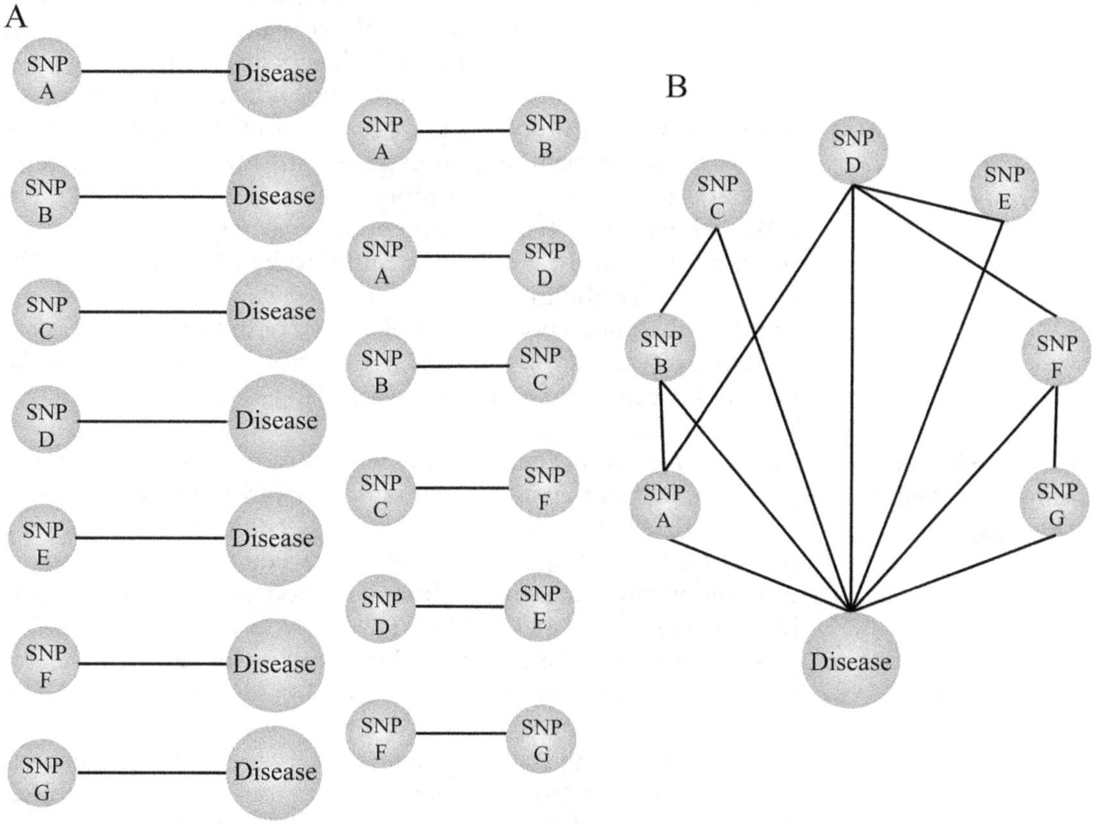

Fig. 2 (**a**) Reviews on the role of multiple polymorphisms in a disease (**b**) A network with the same data. SNPs in linkage disequilibrium are shown with links between the nodes. Each association may have data from several studies that may be combined in a meta-analysis

dichotomous outcome (case–control studies) [115]. However, these approaches assume a genetic model in advance and induce an extra complexity in the analysis using a complicated parameterization and MCMC algorithms. Recently, a Bayesian semiparametric approach which models the observed genotype group frequencies conditional to the case/control status and uses pairwise LD measurements between markers as prior information to make posterior inference on adjusted effects was introduced [116]. The model allows to make inference on the genetic model of inheritance while overlapping sets of SNPs between studies are handled by incorporating prior information on LD between markers obtained by HapMap [117] or other public databases. The main drawback of this model is the assumption of a common LD structure that restricts the combination of ethnically different populations.

A more general and easily applicable method for multivariate meta-analysis of multiple polymorphisms that are in LD has been proposed in a frequentist framework [29]. This model is a direct extension of the bivariate meta-analysis of GAS [26] where the logORs (discrete outcomes) or mean differences (continuous outcomes) derived from candidate polymorphisms are modelled simultaneously as a multivariate response. Exact analytical formulas for the calculation of the within-studies covariances involve the knowledge of the combined genotypes for each study which is rarely the case. Thus, the authors proposed the calculation of probabilities of the combined genotypes using an external estimate for the degree of pairwise LD between the polymorphisms under the assumption of HWE. However, even if this assumption is violated it is used only for the calculation of the covariances, and thus its effect is limited. The assumption that the LD patterns in the populations under study are similar to the ones reported in the literature or in HapMap [117] can be tested by comparing the allele frequencies in the studied populations against the ones reported in HapMap [114, 115].

3.4 Models of Meta-Analysis for Multiple Outcomes

Another frequently encountered scenario is the reporting of multiple correlated outcomes for the same or overlapping sets of participants that are expected to reflect common physiological processes. For example, a hypertension study often measures systolic blood pressure (SBP), diastolic blood pressure (DBP), and hypertension status [118, 119]. Of course, a negative correlation exists in the case of mutually exclusive outcomes [80]. Correlated results also arise from GWASs that reuse the same control samples [85].

Currently, univariate meta-analytical approaches aggregate summary statistics from individual studies into one statistic to test for associations of genetic loci with multiple traits, also termed cross-phenotype (CP) associations. The statistic for Cross Phenotype Meta-Analysis (CPMA) which detects association of a SNP to multiple phenotypes [63] does not reveal which phenotypes the marker is associated with and thus a clustering analysis is necessary. CPMA assumes that the *P*-values for the individual traits come from different non-overarlapping cohorts. An R function 'cpma' is included in the package 'omics' (Table 4) for conducting the analysis. The subset-based approach is the only available method that identifies a subset of traits influenced by selected variants through a selection procedure but this advantage comes with a steep multiple testing price [64]. This method has been implemented in R statistical package called ASSET. Several variations of the O'Brien's linear combination test [120] have been proposed accounting for heterogeneity and correlated outcomes measured in the same individuals [121, 122]. A closely related framework allowing for sample sizes as weights and heterogeneity using solely summary statistics for the estimation of the correlation matrix among test statistics has recently been presented [65]. The software CPASSOC (Cross Phenotype Association) for conducting the analysis can be freely downloaded (Table 4). This approach could be further enriched for testing multiple variants by adopting an interesting method presented by Huang and coworkers [66]. They developed the PRIMe software tool (Table 4) to calculate the Pleiotropy Index (PI) over a region of SNPs where PI indicates the number of traits that have low *P*-values from the individual association test with each trait. However, this method generally finds SNPs that are consistently significantly associated among multiple independent tests for each trait on the same dataset, or via meta-analyses on different datasets. The TATES (Trait-based Association Test that uses Extended Simes procedure) requires only *P*-values obtained in standard univariate GWAS to acquire one trait-based *P*-value while correcting for correlations between components. However, it has not yet been utilized for meta-analysis of GWASs [67]. TATES is available as an open source program (Table 4). Finally, an alternative method was introduced which was based on a multiple-testing adjustment that accounts for the correlation between traits [68], implemented in R (Table 4).

It is well documented, that separate univariate analyses ignore the dependencies between multiple outcomes resulting in low power to detect genetic linkage and association and thus multivariate methods have been proposed [123–125]. An intuitive multivariate method for meta-analysis, for both discrete and continuous multiple outcomes (using log odds-ratios or mean differences), could be formulated extending the general approach for bivariate meta-analysis for two outcomes [26]. Thus, we will have two logORs or mean differences (AB vs. AA and BB vs. AA) for each outcome under a GMF approach that could be modelled simultaneously as a multivariate response. Of course, we could assume the genetic model beforehand and result in a bivariate meta-analysis. The within-studies covariances for discrete outcomes could be calculated using the cross-classification of the genotypes in both outcomes, which are retrieved using a log-linear model with the iterative proportional fitting algorithm under the assumption of no three-way interaction [69]. Because the model is based on the general model for multivariate meta-analysis [32, 71], it could easily be extended to more than two outcomes, it could be fitted using standard software for multivariate meta-analysis [70, 71] and finally, it allows the direct comparison of the parameters estimates using formal techniques. Stata programs are available for the meta-analysis of both discrete and continuous multiple outcomes (Table 4).

3.5 Models of Meta-Analysis Using Mendelian Randomization

In the so-called "Mendelian Randomization" approach, the goal is to model simultaneously the genotype–phenotype and genotype-disease estimates for association (Fig. 1a), deriving thus an indirect estimate of the relationship between phenotype and disease [30, 31]. This approach uses the intermediate metabolites (i.e., a gene product) on the pathway leading from a gene to a disease, and under several assumptions can lead to causal inferences. The methodology is based on the natural randomization process that occurs at conception to determine a person's genotype before birth. Because of the nature of genetic inheritance, by combining the information from genotype-disease and genotype–phenotype studies, it is possible to derive an estimate of the phenotype-disease association that is free of confounding and reverse causation. Plotting the logOR of genotype-disease against the mean genotype–-phenotype difference may help investigators detect departures from the assumptions underlying Mendelian randomization. This graph would be expected to show a monotonic trend if the phenotype is intermediate on the etiologic pathway to disease, and the line should pass through the origin.

A bivariate meta-analysis can be performed in order to capture the correlation structure of genotype-disease and genotype–phenotype associations when some studies provide information on both associations (Fig. 3). Thus, for each study we could calculate the logOR of disease given genotype and the mean difference in phenotype. The within-studies correlation is considered negligible in most studies used in Mendelian randomization as phenotype levels are measured usually in a subsample of the subjects. The between-studies covariance can be estimated using the standard approach described in Sect. 3.1, or by an alternative model that assumes that the heterogeneities on genotype–phenotype and phenotype-disease are independent [30, 31]. Implementation is feasible using source code available in http://www2.le.ac.uk/departments/health-sciences/research/gen-epi/reports or employing a bivariate meta-analysis using the `mvmeta` command in Stata. Later, another extension of this method was presented, which combined the Mendelian randomization with the genetic model-free approach, incorporating all genotype contrasts in a tetravariate

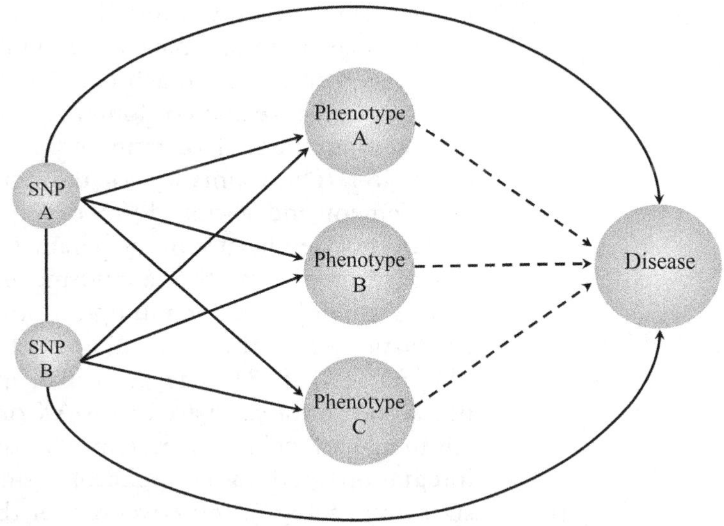

Fig. 3 Graphical representation of a proposed extension of the Mendelian randomization methodology (*see* Fig. 1). This approach incorporates measures of association of the genotype with more than one phenotype as well as with the disease. The dotted lines represent the indirectly inferred associations of the intermediate phenotypes with the disease

model, assuming a common mode of inheritance for both pairs of logORs (that describe the genotype-disease association) and the mean differences (which describe the genotype–phenotype association) [126].

3.6 Special Cases of Meta-Analysis

Apart from the general categories that we described in the previous sections, there are several other special cases where a multivariate meta-analysis procedure can be performed. We will begin with a general procedure for performing efficient meta-analyses when the genetic mode of inheritance is a priori unknown and proceed with adjustments allowing for deviations from HWE under a multivariate framework. We close with presenting multivariate methods for investigating gene-environment interactions.

An important field where a multivariate perspective could be adopted is the meta-analysis of GAS estimating at the same time the most plausible model of inheritance (the robust methods mentioned earlier). Simulation studies have demonstrated that when a test is performed assuming an incorrect model of inheritance, it cannot maintain the nominal type I error rate and in some situations, this procedure results also in a decrease of the power [127–129]. Although most robust methods described in Sect. 2.1 (such as MAX, MERT and MIN2) can be extended to meta-analysis in a univariate fashion [48], a special case can be easily formulated in a multivariate meta-analysis setting very easily. Pereira and coworkers [130], found that by fitting both co-dominant and recessive models and then adjusting the significance by the Bonferroni method may be an optimal approach in most scenarios. A multivariate version of this approach could be to model jointly the odds-ratios for recessive and co-dominant models taking the correlation into account instead of employing the conservative Bonferroni correction. The estimation of the within-studies covariance is a key element and a close-form expression can be easily derived. The overall significance of the parameter estimates can be obtained directly from the multivariate normal distribution. Thus, the parameters are adjusted for multiple testing taking into account the correlation, and thus no adjustment of the P-value is needed [41, 51, 131–133]. The particular approach, even though it is not so powerful compared to MAX or MIN2, has the important advantage of being faster (since it does not require numerical integration) and easily applicable (since it can be fitted in any statistical package). Moreover, under this model, studies reporting data for calculating only one of the estimates can be incorporated in the analysis under a missing at random assumption, allowing borrowing strength.

Another special case can be found in the meta-analysis of GAS taking into account the deviations from Hardy–Weinberg Equilibrium (HWE). Assessing HWE and adjusting the effect sizes are of particular concern in GAS. The control group, which is considered a representative of the general population, is expected to be in HWE and investigators are advised to check the studied sample in order to detect any deviations. However, evaluation studies have shown that most genetic-association studies do not appropriately report deviations from HWE [134–136]. Several approaches have been proposed for dealing with deviations from HWE. The most common approach is to adjust the estimates of the measures of association (logORs) along with their variance, for the degree of deviation from HWE and perform the analysis using the adjusted estimates. Several methods for such adjustments have been proposed during the last years concerning genotype and allele-based contrasts [137–141]. Salanti and coworkers formulated a bayesian methodology that incorporates deviations from HWE using the fixation coefficient in a meta-regression framework [142]. A more general frequentist method could involve the extension of the bivariate genetic model-free approach [26] to model simultaneously the α coefficient instead of the fixation index as a measure for quantifying the departures from HWE [143–145]. The measures for departures from HWE use genotype counts and thus we expect them to be correlated with the logORs; thus, analytical expressions for the calculations of the within-studies covariances can be derived. The particular model can be used to draw simultaneously inferences for both the genetic model of inheritance and the deviations from HWE, whereas adjusts the estimates of genetic association for such deviations. Thompson and coworkers proposed a very similar model in a Bayesian framework incorporating variations in genetic effect size, genetic model, allele frequency in controls and deviations from Hardy–Weinberg equilibrium to improve the estimates [146].

The last issue which we will cover is the meta-analysis of gene–environment interactions. Such studies are particularly appropriate to elucidate the genetic architecture of a trait, explain the remaining heritability and identify genetic contributors with weak effects. A growing interest is observed in the context of GWASs for assessing simultaneously genetic main effect plus gene–environment interaction parameters maximizing the power compared with standard univariate meta-analyses [147]. However, because this particular procedure requires analyses to be conducted within strata of a categorical exposure, in some situations it may result in decreased power compared to analyses that assume a particular form for the interaction term. This drawback is overcome by conducting a joint meta-analysis strategy of the beta coefficients for a SNP's main effect and its interaction with an environmental factor accounting for the covariance between the parameter estimates [148]. The joint meta-analysis method has been implemented in METAL [59]. Individual studies can obtain the required beta and covariance estimates for interaction regression models using QUICKTEST version 0.95 (http://toby.freeshell.org/software/quicktest/) and ProbABEL version 0.1–3 (http://www.genabel.org/packages/ProbABEL). This method performs better when both main and interaction effects are present. Gene–environment interactions were also studied under a Bayesian framework [149] acquiring information from a subset studies that report on these interaction terms.

4 Conclusions

Multivariate meta-analysis takes into account the potential correlation between the effect sizes of different studies and the within and the between-study correlations deriving further robust and precise estimates. It allows the study of the effect of more than one factor on a disease as well as the confounding effect of factors that may be interrelated or associated with the disease. The bias is potentially reduced due to partial reporting. It also provides estimates for all effects within a single modelling framework making easier the comparison of the results. Multivariate approach can be performed even for investigating the association of a single gene with a disease, since the ORs derived from genotype contrasts in genetic association studies are inherently correlated.

This chapter summarized the main methods for multivariate meta-analysis of genetic association studies presented in the literature. We presented and discussed models of meta-analysis for gene-disease association using single nucleotide polymorphisms, multiple alleles, haplotypes, multiple linked polymorphisms, as well as models for multiple outcomes. Furthermore, we discussed methods that seek to maximizing the power by not being restricted to a single genetic mode of inheritance, models dealing with deviations from HWE, and models for meta-analysis of gene–environment interactions. In all cases, we presented the main assumptions underlying these models and discussed their applicability in real-life situations, as well as the available software that is capable of fitting them. Although most methods presented in this review focused on GASs, we should mention that multivariate methods can also be employed for GWASs, particularly since fast and accurate routines of multivariate versions of the non-iterative method of moments (MM) are being available [70, 76], and thus we expect such methods to be widely used in the near future.

Acknowledgments

Niki Dimou and Katerina Pantavou were supported by a scholarship from the IKY Scholarship Programs in the context of the action "Strengthening Post-Doctoral Research" of the Human Resources Development Program, Education and Lifelong Learning, co-financed by the European Social Fund – ESF and the Greek government.

References

1. Burton PR, Tobin MD, Hopper JL (2005) Key concepts in genetic epidemiology. Lancet 366(9489):941–951. https://doi.org/10.1016/S0140-6736(05)67322-9
2. Cordell HJ, Clayton DG (2005) Genetic association studies. Lancet 366 (9491):1121–1131. https://doi.org/10.1016/S0140-6736(05)67424-7
3. Rao DC (2008) An overview of the genetic dissection of complex traits. Adv Genet 60:3–34. https://doi.org/10.1016/S0065-2660(07)00401-4
4. Klein RJ, Zeiss C, Chew EY et al (2005) Complement factor H polymorphism in age-related macular degeneration. Science 308(5720):385–389. https://doi.org/10.1126/science.1109557
5. Manolio TA (2010) Genomewide association studies and assessment of the risk of disease. N Engl J Med 363(2):166–176. https://doi.org/10.1056/NEJMra0905980
6. MacArthrur J, Bowler E, Cerezo M et al (2017) The new NHGRI-EBI catalog of published genome-wide association studies. Nucleic Acids Res 45(D1):D896–D901. https://doi.org/10.1093/nar/gkw1133
7. Mendel S, McCarthy A, Barnett JP et al (2008) The Escherichia coli TatABC system and a Bacillus subtilis TatAC-type system recognise three distinct targeting determinants in twin-arginine signal peptides. J Mol Biol 375(3):661–672. https://doi.org/10.1016/j.jmb.2007.09.087
8. Teo YY (2008) Common statistical issues in genome-wide association studies: a review on power, data quality control, genotype calling and population structure. Curr Opin Lipidol 19(2):133–143. https://doi.org/10.1097/MOL.0b013e3282f5dd77
9. Ziegler A, Konig IR, Thompson JR (2008) Biostatistical aspects of genome-wide association studies. Biom J 50(1):8–28. https://doi.org/10.1002/bimj.200710398
10. Hirschhorn JN, Lohmueller K, Byrne E et al (2002) A comprehensive review of genetic association studies. Genet Med 4(2):45–61.

https://doi.org/10.1097/00125817-200203000-00002
11. Becker KG, Barnes KC, Bright TJ et al (2004) The genetic association database. Nat Genet 36(5):431–432. https://doi.org/10.1038/ng0504-431
12. Normand SL (1999) Meta-analysis: formulating, evaluating, combining, and reporting. Stat Med 18(3):321–359
13. Petiti DB (1994) Meta-analysis decision analysis and cost-effectiveness analysis. In: Monographs in epidemiology and biostatistics, vol 24. Oxford University Press, Oxford
14. Trikalinos TA, Salanti G, Zintzaras E et al (2008) Meta-analysis methods. Adv Genet 60:311–334. https://doi.org/10.1016/S0065-2660(07)00413-0
15. Glass G (1976) Primary, secondary and meta-analysis of research. Educ Res 5:3–8
16. Greenland S (1998) Meta-analysis. In: Rothman KJ, Greenland S (eds) Modern epidemiology. Lippincott Williams & Wilkins, Philadelphia, pp 643–673
17. Chalmers TC, Berrier J, Sacks HS et al (1987) Meta-analysis of clinical trials as a scientific discipline. II: replicate variability and comparison of studies that agree and disagree. Stat Med 6(7):733–744
18. Sacks HS, Berrier J, Reitman D et al (1987) Meta-analyses of randomized controlled trials. N Engl J Med 316(8):450–455. https://doi.org/10.1056/NEJM198702193160806
19. Stroup DF, Berlin JA, Morton SC et al (2000) Meta-analysis of observational studies in epidemiology: a proposal for reporting. Meta-analysis of observational studies in epidemiology (MOOSE) group. JAMA 283(15):2008–2012
20. Nikolopoulos GK, Bagos PG, Bonovas S (2011) Developing the evidence base for cancer chemoprevention: use of meta-analysis. Curr Drug Targets 12(13):1989–1997. doi: BSP/CDT/E-Pub/00218
21. Thakkinstian A, McElduff P, D'Este C et al (2005) A method for meta-analysis of molecular association studies. Stat Med 24(9):1291–1306. https://doi.org/10.1002/sim.2010
22. Minelli C, Thompson JR, Abrams KR et al (2005) The choice of a genetic model in the meta-analysis of molecular association studies. Int J Epidemiol 34(6):1319–1328. https://doi.org/10.1093/ije/dyi169
23. Bagos PG, Nikolopoulos GK (2007) A method for meta-analysis of case–control genetic association studies using logistic regression. Stat Appl Genet Mol Biol 6: Article17. https://doi.org/10.2202/1544-6115.1281
24. Evangelou E, Ioannidis JP (2013) Meta-analysis methods for genome-wide association studies and beyond. Nat Rev Genet 14(6):379–389. https://doi.org/10.1038/nrg34721
25. Evangelou E, Maraganore DM, Ioannidis JP (2007) Meta-analysis in genome-wide association datasets: strategies and application in Parkinson disease. PLoS One 2(2):e196. https://doi.org/10.1371/journal.pone.0000196
26. Bagos PG (2008) A unification of multivariate methods for meta-analysis of genetic association studies. Stat Appl Genet Mol Biol 7(1): Article31. https://doi.org/10.2202/1544-6115.1408
27. Minelli C, Thompson JR, Abrams KR et al (2005) Bayesian implementation of a genetic model-free approach to the meta-analysis of genetic association studies. Stat Med 24(24):3845–3861. https://doi.org/10.1002/sim.2393
28. Bagos PG (2011) Meta-analysis of haplotype-association studies: comparison of methods and empirical evaluation of the literature. BMC Genet 12:8. https://doi.org/10.1186/1471-2156-12-8
29. Bagos PG, Liakopoulos TD (2010) A multipoint method for meta-analysis of genetic association studies. Genet Epidemiol 34(7):702–715. https://doi.org/10.1002/gepi.20531
30. Minelli C, Thompson JR, Tobin MD et al (2004) An integrated approach to the meta-analysis of genetic association studies using Mendelian randomization. Am J Epidemiol 160(5):445–452. https://doi.org/10.1093/aje/kwh228
31. Thompson JR, Minelli C, Abrams KR et al (2005) Meta-analysis of genetic studies using Mendelian randomization—a multivariate approach. Stat Med 24(14):2241–2254. https://doi.org/10.1002/sim.2100
32. van Houwelingen HC, Arends LR, Stijnen T (2002) Advanced methods in meta-analysis: multivariate approach and meta-regression. Stat Med 21(4):589–624. https://doi.org/10.1002/sim.1040
33. Riley RD, Abrams KR, Lambert PC et al (2007) An evaluation of bivariate random-effects meta-analysis for the joint synthesis of two correlated outcomes. Stat Med 26(1):78–97. https://doi.org/10.1002/sim.2524
34. Riley RD, Abrams KR, Sutton AJ et al (2007) Bivariate random-effects meta-analysis and

the estimation of between-study correlation. BMC Med Res Methodol 7:3. https://doi.org/10.1186/1471-2288-7-3

35. Balding DJ (2006) A tutorial on statistical methods for population association studies. Nat Rev Genet 7(10):781–791. https://doi.org/10.1038/nrg1916
36. Langefeld CD, Fingerlin TE (2007) Association methods in human genetics. Methods Mol Biol 404:431–460. https://doi.org/10.1007/978-1-59745-530-5_21
37. Armitage P (1955) Tests for linear trends in proportions and frequencies. Biometrics 11 (3):375–386
38. Cochran WG (1954) Some methods for strengthening the common chi-squared tests. Biometrics 10(4):417–451
39. Gastwirth JL (1985) The use of maximin efficiency robust tests in combining contingency tables and survival analysis. J Am Stat Assoc 80(390):380–384
40. Freidlin B, Podgor MJ, Gastwirth JL (1999) Efficiency robust tests for survival or ordered categorical data. Biometrics 55(3):883–886
41. Freidlin B, Zheng G, Li Z et al (2002) Trend tests for case–control studies of genetic markers: power, sample size and robustness. Hum Hered 53(3):146–152. doi:64976
42. Wittke-Thompson JK, Pluzhnikov A, Cox NJ (2005) Rational inferences about departures from Hardy–Weinberg equilibrium. Am J Hum Genet 76(6):967–986. https://doi.org/10.1086/430507
43. Zheng G, Ng HK (2008) Genetic model selection in two-phase analysis for case–control association studies. Biostatistics 9 (3):391–399. https://doi.org/10.1093/biostatistics/kxm039
44. Song K, Elston RC (2006) A powerful method of combining measures of association and Hardy–Weinberg disequilibrium for fine-mapping in case–control studies. Stat Med 25 (1):105–126. https://doi.org/10.1002/sim.2350
45. Joo J, Kwak M, Zheng G (2010) Improving power for testing genetic association in case--control studies by reducing the alternative space. Biometrics 66(1):266–276. https://doi.org/10.1111/j.1541-0420.2009.01241.x
46. Burton PR, Clayton DG, Cardon LR et al (2007) Genome-wide association study of 14,000 cases of seven common diseases and 3,000 shared controls. Nature 447 (7145):661–678
47. Joo J, Kwak M, Ahn K et al (2009) A robust genome-wide scan statistic of the Wellcome trust case–control consortium. Biometrics 65 (4):1115–1122. https://doi.org/10.1111/j.1541-0420.2009.01185.x
48. Dimou NL, Tsirigos KD, Elofsson A et al (2017) GWAR: robust analysis and meta-analysis of genome-wide association studies. Bioinformatics 33(10):1521–1527. https://doi.org/10.1093/bioinformatics/btx008
49. Lettre G, Lange C, Hirschhorn JN (2007) Genetic model testing and statistical power in population-based association studies of quantitative traits. Genet Epidemiol 31 (4):358–362. https://doi.org/10.1002/gepi.20217
50. So HC, Sham PC (2011) Robust association tests under different genetic models, allowing for binary or quantitative traits and covariates. Behav Genet 41(5):768–775. https://doi.org/10.1007/s10519-011-9450-9
51. Hothorn LA, Hothorn T (2009) Order-restricted scores test for the evaluation of population-based case–control studies when the genetic model is unknown. Biom J 51 (4):659–669. https://doi.org/10.1002/bimj.200800203
52. Gonzalez JR, Armengol L, Sole X et al (2007) SNPassoc: an R package to perform whole genome association studies. Bioinformatics 23(5):644–645. https://doi.org/10.1093/bioinformatics/btm025
53. Zang Y, Fung WK, Zheng G (2010) Simple algorithms to calculate asymptotic null distribution for robust tests in case–control genetic association studies in R. J Stat Softw 33:1–24
54. DerSimonian R, Laird N (1986) Meta-analysis in clinical trials. Control Clin Trials 7 (3):177–188
55. Thompson SG, Sharp SJ (1999) Explaining heterogeneity in meta-analysis: a comparison of methods. Stat Med 18(20):2693–2708
56. Warn DE, Thompson SG, Spiegelhalter DJ (2002) Bayesian random effects meta-analysis of trials with binary outcomes: methods for the absolute risk difference and relative risk scales. Stat Med 21(11):1601–1623. https://doi.org/10.1002/sim.1189
57. Smith TC, Spiegelhalter DJ, Thomas A (1995) Bayesian approaches to random-effects meta-analysis: a comparative study. Stat Med 14(24):2685–2699
58. Sutton AJ, Abrams KR (2001) Bayesian methods in meta-analysis and evidence synthesis. Stat Methods Med Res 10(4):277–303. https://doi.org/10.1177/096228020101000404
59. Willer CJ, Li Y, Abecasis GR (2010) METAL: fast and efficient meta-analysis of genomewide

association scans. Bioinformatics 26 (17):2190–2191. https://doi.org/10.1093/bioinformatics/btq340

60. Magi R, Morris AP (2010) GWAMA: software for genome-wide association meta-analysis. BMC Bioinformatics 11:288. https://doi.org/10.1186/1471-2105-11-288
61. Aulchenko YS, Ripke S, Isaacs A et al (2007) GenABEL: an R library for genome-wide association analysis. Bioinformatics 23 (10):1294–1296. https://doi.org/10.1093/bioinformatics/btm108
62. Purcell S, Neale B, Todd-Brown K et al (2007) PLINK: a tool set for whole-genome association and population-based linkage analyses. Am J Hum Genet 81(3):559–575. https://doi.org/10.1086/519795
63. Cotsapas C, Voight BF, Rossin E et al (2011) Pervasive sharing of genetic effects in autoimmune disease. PLoS Genet 7(8):e1002254. https://doi.org/10.1371/journal.pgen.1002254
64. Bhattacharjee S, Rajaraman P, Jacobs KB et al (2012) A subset-based approach improves power and interpretation for the combined analysis of genetic association studies of heterogeneous traits. Am J Hum Genet 90 (5):821–835. https://doi.org/10.1016/j.ajhg.2012.03.015
65. Zhu X, Feng T, Tayo BO et al (2015) Meta-analysis of correlated traits via summary statistics from GWASs with an application in hypertension. Am J Hum Genet 96(1):21–36. https://doi.org/10.1016/j.ajhg.2014.11.011
66. Huang J, Johnson AD, O'Donnell CJ (2011) PRIMe: a method for characterization and evaluation of pleiotropic regions from multiple genome-wide association studies. Bioinformatics 27(9):1201–1206. https://doi.org/10.1093/bioinformatics/btr116
67. van der Sluis S, Posthuma D, Dolan CV (2013) TATES: efficient multivariate genotype–phenotype analysis for genome-wide association studies. PLoS Genet 9(1):e1003235. https://doi.org/10.1371/journal.pgen.1003235
68. Conneely KN, Boehnke M (2010) Meta-analysis of genetic association studies and adjustment for multiple testing of correlated SNPs and traits. Genet Epidemiol 34 (7):739–746. https://doi.org/10.1002/gepi.20538
69. Dimou NL, Bagos PG (2014) A multivariate method for meta-analysis of multiple outcomes in genetic association studies. Paper presented at the 35th Annual Conference of the International Society for Clinical Biostatistics, Vienna, Austria
70. Jackson D, Riley R, White IR (2011) Multivariate meta-analysis: potential and promise. Stat Med 30(20):2481–2498. https://doi.org/10.1002/sim.4172
71. Mavridis D, Salanti G (2013) A practical introduction to multivariate meta-analysis. Stat Methods Med Res 22(2):133–158. https://doi.org/10.1177/0962280211432219
72. Kirkham JJ, Riley RD, Williamson PR (2012) A multivariate meta-analysis approach for reducing the impact of outcome reporting bias in systematic reviews. Stat Med 31 (20):2179–2195. https://doi.org/10.1002/sim.5356
73. Higgins JP, Whitehead A (1996) Borrowing strength from external trials in a meta-analysis. Stat Med 15(24):2733–2749. https://doi.org/10.1002/(SICI)1097-0258(19961230)15:24<2733::AID-SIM562>3.0.CO;2-0
74. Berkey CS, Hoaglin DC, Antczak-Bouckoms A et al (1998) Meta-analysis of multiple outcomes by regression with random effects. Stat Med 17(22):2537–2550
75. White IR (2009) Multivariate random-effects meta-analysis. Stata J 9:40–56
76. Jackson D, White IR, Thompson SG (2010) Extending DerSimonian and Laird's methodology to perform multivariate random effects meta-analyses. Stat Med 29(12):1282–1297. https://doi.org/10.1002/sim.3602
77. Bagos PG (2015) Meta-analysis in Stata using gllamm. Res Synth Methods 6(4):310–332. https://doi.org/10.1002/jrsm.1157
78. Viechtbauer W (2010) Conducting meta-analyses in R with the metafor package. J Stat Softw 36(3):1–48
79. Gleser LJ, Olkin I (1994) Stochastically dependent effect sizes. In: Cooper HM, Hedges LV (eds) The handbook of research synthesis. Russell Sage Foundation, New York, pp 339–355
80. Trikalinos TA, Olkin I (2008) A method for the meta-analysis of mutually exclusive binary outcomes. Stat Med 27(21):4279–4300. https://doi.org/10.1002/sim.3299
81. Berrington A, Cox DR (2003) Generalized least squares for the synthesis of correlated information. Biostatistics 4(3):423–431. https://doi.org/10.1093/biostatistics/4.3.423
82. Greenland S, Longnecker MP (1992) Methods for trend estimation from summarized dose–response data, with applications to

meta-analysis. Am J Epidemiol 135 (11):1301–1309

83. Berlin JA, Longnecker MP, Greenland S (1993) Meta-analysis of epidemiologic dose-response data. Epidemiology 4(3):218–228

84. Lin DY, Sullivan PF (2009) Meta-analysis of genome-wide association studies with overlapping subjects. Am J Hum Genet 85 (6):862–872. https://doi.org/10.1016/j.ajhg.2009.11.001

85. Zaykin DV, Kozbur DO (2010) *P*-Value based analysis for shared controls design in genome-wide association studies. Genet Epidemiol 34(7):725–738. https://doi.org/10.1002/gepi.20536

86. le Cessie S, Nagelkerke N, Rosendaal FR et al (2008) Combining matched and unmatched control groups in case–control studies. Am J Epidemiol 168(10):1204–1210. https://doi.org/10.1093/aje/kwn236

87. Bagos PG, Dimou NL, Liakopoulos TD et al (2011) Meta-analysis of family-based and case–control genetic association studies that use the same cases. Stat Appl Genet Mol Biol 10(1):Article19

88. Daniels MJ, Hughes MD (1997) Meta-analysis for the evaluation of potential surrogate markers. Stat Med 16(17):1965–1982. https://doi.org/10.1002/(SICI)1097-0258(19970915)16:17<1965::AID-SIM630>3.0.CO;2-M

89. Bagos PG (2012) On the covariance of two correlated log-odds ratios. Stat Med 31 (14):1418–1431. https://doi.org/10.1002/sim.4474

90. Clayton D, Hills M (1993) Statistical models in epidemiology. Oxford University Press, Oxford

91. Agresti A (2002) Categorical data analysis. Wiley series in probability and mathematical statistics. In: Applied probability and statistics, 2nd edn. John Wiley & Sons, New York

92. Attia J, Thakkinstian A, D'Este C (2003) Meta-analyses of molecular association studies: methodologic lessons for genetic epidemiology. J Clin Epidemiol 56(4):297–303

93. Ioannidis JP, Trikalinos TA, Ntzani EE et al (2003) Genetic associations in large versus small studies: an empirical assessment. Lancet 361(9357):567–571. https://doi.org/10.1016/S0140-6736(03)12516-0

94. Ioannidis JP, Trikalinos TA (2005) Early extreme contradictory estimates may appear in published research: the Proteus phenomenon in molecular genetics research and randomized trials. J Clin Epidemiol 58 (6):543–549. https://doi.org/10.1016/j.jclinepi.2004.10.019

95. Van Houwelingen HC, Zwinderman KH, Stijnen T (1993) A bivariate approach to meta-analysis. Stat Med 12(24):2273–2284

96. Salanti G, Higgins JP (2008) Meta-analysis of genetic association studies under different inheritance models using data reported as merged genotypes. Stat Med 27 (5):764–777. https://doi.org/10.1002/sim.2919

97. McCullagh P, Nelder JA (1989) Generalized linear models. Chapman & Hall, London

98. Skrondal A, Rabe-Hesketh S (2003) Multilevel logistic regression for polytomous data and rankings. Psychometrika 68(2):267–287

99. Higgins JP, Whitehead A, Turner RM et al (2001) Meta-analysis of continuous outcome data from individual patients. Stat Med 20 (15):2219–2241. https://doi.org/10.1002/sim.918

100. Turner RM, Omar RZ, Yang M et al (2000) A multilevel model framework for meta-analysis of clinical trials with binary outcomes. Stat Med 19(24):3417–3432

101. Zondervan KT, Cardon LR (2004) The complex interplay among factors that influence allelic association. Nat Rev Genet 5 (2):89–100

102. Marchini J, Cutler D, Patterson N et al (2006) A comparison of phasing algorithms for trios and unrelated individuals. Am J Hum Genet 78(3):437–450. https://doi.org/10.1086/500808

103. Xu H, Wu X, Spitz MR et al (2004) Comparison of haplotype inference methods using genotypic data from unrelated individuals. Hum Hered 58(2):63–68

104. Niu T (2004) Algorithms for inferring haplotypes. Genet Epidemiol 27(4):334–347. https://doi.org/10.1002/gepi.20024

105. Becker T, Cichon S, Jonson E et al (2005) Multiple testing in the context of haplotype analysis revisited: application to case–control data. Ann Hum Genet 69(Pt 6):747–756. https://doi.org/10.1111/j.1529-8817.2005.00198.x

106. Becker T, Knapp M (2004) A powerful strategy to account for multiple testing in the context of haplotype analysis. Am J Hum Genet 75(4):561–570. https://doi.org/10.1086/424390

107. Kaplan N, Morris R (2001) Issues concerning association studies for fine mapping a susceptibility gene for a complex disease. Genet Epidemiol 20(4):432–457. https://doi.org/10.1002/gepi.1012

108. French B, Lumley T, Monks SA et al (2006) Simple estimates of haplotype relative risks in case–control data. Genet Epidemiol 30

(6):485–494. https://doi.org/10.1002/gepi.20161

109. Zaykin DV, Westfall PH, Young SS et al (2002) Testing association of statistically inferred haplotypes with discrete and continuous traits in samples of unrelated individuals. Hum Hered 53(2):79–91. doi:57986
110. Lumley T (2002) Network meta-analysis for indirect treatment comparisons. Stat Med 21 (16):2313–2324. https://doi.org/10.1002/sim.1201
111. Marchini J, Donnelly P, Cardon LR (2005) Genome-wide strategies for detecting multiple loci that influence complex diseases. Nat Genet 37(4):413–417. https://doi.org/10.1038/ng1537
112. Devlin B, Roeder K, Wasserman L (2003) Analysis of multilocus models of association. Genet Epidemiol 25(1):36–47. https://doi.org/10.1002/gepi.10237
113. Shoemaker CA, Pungliya M, Sao Pedro MA et al (2001) Computational methods for single-point and multipoint analysis of genetic variants associated with a simulated complex disorder in a general population. Genet Epidemiol 21(Suppl 1):S738–S745
114. Verzilli C, Shah T, Casas JP et al (2008) Bayesian meta-analysis of genetic association studies with different sets of markers. Am J Hum Genet 82(4):859–872. https://doi.org/10.1016/j.ajhg.2008.01.016
115. Newcombe PJ, Verzilli C, Casas JP et al (2009) Multilocus Bayesian meta-analysis of gene-disease associations. Am J Hum Genet 84(5):567–580. https://doi.org/10.1016/j.ajhg.2009.04.001
116. De Iorio M, Newcombe PJ, Tachmazidou I et al (2011) Bayesian semiparametric meta-analysis for genetic association studies. Genet Epidemiol 35(5):333–340. https://doi.org/10.1002/gepi.20581
117. HapMap http://hapmap.ncbi.nlm.nih.gov/
118. Franceschini N, Fox E, Zhang Z et al (2013) Genome-wide association analysis of blood-pressure traits in African-ancestry individuals reveals common associated genes in African and non-African populations. Am J Hum Genet 93(3):545–554. https://doi.org/10.1016/j.ajhg.2013.07.010
119. Ehret GB, Munroe PB, International Consortium for Blood Pressure Genome-Wide Association Studies et al (2011) Genetic variants in novel pathways influence blood pressure and cardiovascular disease risk. Nature 478 (7367):103–109. https://doi.org/10.1038/nature10405
120. O'Brien PC (1984) Procedures for comparing samples with multiple endpoints. Biometrics 40(4):1079–1087
121. Xu X, Tian L, Wei LJ (2003) Combining dependent tests for linkage or association across multiple phenotypic traits. Biostatistics 4(2):223–229. https://doi.org/10.1093/biostatistics/4.2.223
122. Yang Q, Wu H, Guo CY et al (2010) Analyze multivariate phenotypes in genetic association studies by combining univariate association tests. Genet Epidemiol 34(5):444–454. https://doi.org/10.1002/gepi.20497
123. Yang Q, Wang Y (2012) Methods for analyzing multivariate phenotypes in genetic association studies. J Probab Stat 2012:652569. https://doi.org/10.1155/2012/652569
124. Solovieff N, Cotsapas C, Lee PH et al (2013) Pleiotropy in complex traits: challenges and strategies. Nat Rev Genet 14(7):483–495. https://doi.org/10.1038/nrg3461
125. Shriner D (2012) Moving toward system genetics through multiple trait analysis in genome-wide association studies. Front Genet 3(1). https://doi.org/10.3389/fgene.2012.00001
126. Palmer TM, Thompson JR, Tobin MD (2008) Meta-analysis of Mendelian randomization studies incorporating all three genotypes. Stat Med 27(30):6570–6582. https://doi.org/10.1002/sim.3423
127. Ohashi J, Yamamoto S, Tsuchiya N et al (2001) Comparison of statistical power between 2 * 2 allele frequency and allele positivity tables in case–control studies of complex disease genes. Ann Hum Genet 65 (Pt 2):197–206
128. Ohashi J, Tokunaga K (1999) Selecting a contingency table in a population-based association study: allele frequency or positivity? J Hum Genet 44(4):246–248. https://doi.org/10.1007/s100380050152
129. Matthews AG, Haynes C, Liu C et al (2008) Collapsing SNP genotypes in case–control genome-wide association studies increases the type I error rate and power. Stat Appl Genet Mol Biol 7(1):Article23. https://doi.org/10.2202/1544-6115.1325
130. Pereira TV, Patsopoulos NA, Pereira AC et al (2011) Strategies for genetic model specification in the screening of genome-wide meta-analysis signals for further replication. Int J Epidemiol 40(2):457–469. https://doi.org/10.1093/ije/dyq203
131. Li Q, Yu K, Li Z et al (2008) MAX-rank: a simple and robust genome-wide scan for case-control association studies. Hum Genet 123

(6):617–623. https://doi.org/10.1007/s00439-008-0514-8

132. Gonzalez JR, Carrasco JL, Dudbridge F, Armengol L, Estivill X, Moreno V (2008) Maximizing association statistics over genetic models. Genet Epidemiol 32(3):246–254. https://doi.org/10.1002/gepi.20299
133. Li Q, Zheng G, Li Z et al (2008) Efficient approximation of *P*-value of the maximum of correlated tests, with applications to genome-wide association studies. Ann Hum Genet 72 (Pt 3):397–406. https://doi.org/10.1111/j.1469-1809.2008.00437.x
134. Trikalinos TA, Salanti G, Khoury MJ et al (2006) Impact of violations and deviations in Hardy–Weinberg equilibrium on postulated gene-disease associations. Am J Epidemiol 163(4):300–309. https://doi.org/10.1093/aje/kwj046
135. Salanti G, Amountza G, Ntzani EE et al (2005) Hardy–Weinberg equilibrium in genetic association studies: an empirical evaluation of reporting, deviations, and power. Eur J Hum Genet 13(7):840–848. https://doi.org/10.1038/sj.ejhg.5201410
136. Minelli C, Thompson JR, Abrams KR et al (2008) How should we use information about HWE in the meta-analyses of genetic association studies? Int J Epidemiol 37 (1):136–146. https://doi.org/10.1093/ije/dym234
137. Zaykin DV, Meng Z, Ghosh SK (2004) Interval estimation of genetic susceptibility for retrospective case–control studies. BMC Genet 5:9. https://doi.org/10.1186/1471-2156-5-9
138. Schaid DJ, Jacobsen SJ (1999) Biased tests of association: comparisons of allele frequencies when departing from Hardy–Weinberg proportions. Am J Epidemiol 149(8):706–711
139. Lathrop GM (1983) Estimating genotype relative risks. Tissue Antigens 22(2):160–166
140. Sato Y, Suganami H, Hamada C et al (2006) The confidence interval of allelic odds ratios under the Hardy–Weinberg disequilibrium. J Hum Genet 51(9):772–780. https://doi.org/10.1007/s10038-006-0020-6
141. Zintzaras E (2008) Variance estimation of allele-based odds ratio in the absence of Hardy–Weinberg equilibrium. Eur J Epidemiol 23 (5):323–326. https://doi.org/10.1007/s10654-008-9242-6
142. Salanti G, Higgins JP, Trikalinos TA et al (2007) Bayesian meta-analysis and meta-regression for gene-disease associations and deviations from Hardy–Weinberg equilibrium. Stat Med 26(3):553–567. https://doi.org/10.1002/sim.2575
143. Lindley D (1988) Statistical inference concerning Hardy–Weinberg equilibrium. Bayesian Stat 3:307–326
144. Pereira C, Rogatko A (1984) The Hardy--Weinberg equilibrium under a Bayesian perspective. Revista Brasileira de Genética 7 (4):689–707
145. Weir BS (1970) Equilibria under inbreeding and selection. Genetics 65(2):371–378
146. Thompson J, Minelli C, Abrams K et al (2008) Combining information from related meta-analyses of genetic association studies. J R Stat Soc Ser C Appl Stat 57(1):103–115
147. Aschard H, Hancock DB, London SJ et al (2011) Genome-wide meta-analysis of joint tests for genetic and gene–environment interaction effects. Hum Hered 70(4):292–300
148. Manning AK, LaValley M, Liu CT et al (2011) Meta-analysis of gene–environment interaction: joint estimation of SNP and SNP× environment regression coefficients. Genet Epidemiol 35(1):11–18
149. Salanti G, Higgins JP, White IR (2006) Bayesian synthesis of epidemiological evidence with different combinations of exposure groups: application to a gene–gene–environment interaction. Stat Med 25(24):4147–4163. https://doi.org/10.1002/sim.2689

Chapter 12

Methods of Analysis and Meta-Analysis for Identifying Differentially Expressed Genes

Panagiota I Kontou, Athanasia Pavlopoulou, and Pantelis G. Bagos

Abstract

Microarray approaches are widely used high-throughput techniques to assess simultaneously the expression of thousands of genes under certain conditions and study the effects of certain treatments, diseases, and developmental stages. The traditional way to perform such experiments is to design oligonucleotide hybridization probes that correspond to specific genes and then measure the expression of the genes in order to determine which of them are up- or down-regulated compared to a condition that is used as a control. Hitherto, individual experiments cannot capture the bigger picture of how a biological system works and, therefore, data integration from multiple experimental studies and external data repositories is necessary to understand the function of genes and their expression patterns under certain conditions. Therefore, the development of methods for handling, integrating, comparing, interpreting and visualizing microarray data is necessary. The selection of an appropriate method for analysing microarray datasets is not an easy task. In this chapter, we provide an overview of the various methods developed for microarray data analysis, as well as suggestions for choosing the appropriate method for microarray meta-analysis.

Key words Gene expression, Microarrays, Differentially expressed genes, Meta-analysis, Statistical tests, Multiple comparisons

1 Introduction

Gene expression microarrays have been used in various applications, including the identification of novel genes associated with certain diseases (most notably cancers), tumor classification, and prediction of patient outcome.

In a microarray experiment, the mRNA levels of thousands of genes are measured simultaneously in tissue samples. One basic method for preparing microarrays is spotting arrays on plates. Each spot on a microarray plate is designed to contain multiple identical copies of single DNA strands, fragments or oligonucleotides that represent specific gene coding regions, and are referred to as "probes." Each spot or a set of spots corresponds to one gene. The order of the probes on the chip is stored in a computer

Evangelos Evangelou (ed.), *Genetic Epidemiology: Methods and Protocols*, Methods in Molecular Biology, vol. 1793,
https://doi.org/10.1007/978-1-4939-7868-7_12,

database so that results can be obtained easily. Probes are designed in such a way that they are uniquely complementary to purified RNA or DNA fragments which are fluorescently or radioactively prelabeled. The probes are then hybridized to their corresponding target sequences. The more RNA or DNA fragments get attached to a spot, the higher the radioactive signal; thus, the intensity of a set of spots represents the expression of a gene. After thorough washing to remove non-specific binding sequences, the raw microarray data are obtained by laser scanning or autoradiographic imaging. Microarrays can be fabricated using various technologies.

In **spotted microarrays**, the probes, which are oligonucleotides, cDNA or small fragments of PCR products that correspond to mRNAs, are "spotted" onto the surface. Spotted microarrays are "customizable", since the researcher can choose the probes for each experimental study [1]. In **oligonucleotide microarrays**, with Agilent and Affymetrix being the most popular platforms, the probes are short sequences designed to be complementary to parts of the target sequence so that a gene is represented by a set of probes (probe-set) instead of a single probe. Contrary to spotted microarrays, the probes are synthesized directly onto the surface. The length of the oligo sequences depends on the specific experimental needs [2].

Dual channel (or two-color) microarrays are typically hybridized with cDNA prepared from two samples to be compared (e.g., diseased tissue versus healthy tissue). These samples are labeled with two different fluorophores (e.g., Cy3 and Cy5) with different emission intensity. Relative signal intensities of each fluorophore are used to measure differential gene expression [3]. In **single-channel (or one-color) microarrays**, contrary to dual-channel microarrays, the samples to be compared are labeled with a single fluorophore. Relative signal intensities for each probe or probe-set reflect the expression level of the labeled target sequence. The main representatives of single-channel microarray platforms are Affymetrix, Illumina and Agilent [4].

The selection of a microarray platform is done on the basis of cost, chip availability for the species under analysis, genome coverage, the starting amount of RNA quality array manufacturing, the validity and availability of software tools for image analysis and intra platform variability [5, 6].

After hybridization, **image analysis** is performed [7], followed by pre-filtering/masking for microarray signal correction. Background signal adjustment is also recommended before scaling. **Normalization** is performed to adjust microarray data for effects that are attributed to technology variations [8]. Typical normalization methods include the rank invariant normalization [9], quantile [10] and LOWESS/LOESS methods [9]. For many types of commercial arrays, suites of R-BioConductor-based packages [11], such as RMA (Robust Multi-array Average expression measure) [12] and MAS 5.0 Algorithm [13], are used to perform consecutive background adjustments and data normalization.

After pre-processing and normalization (and potentially some other steps, such as filtering, imputation of missing values and standardization), we usually end up with an expression matrix that contains the expression values for each probe. The objectives of an analysis may be classified into three broad classes: identification of differentially expressed genes (DEGs), classification /class prediction and clustering.

Clustering of microarray data seeks to group genes based on specific features in a biologically meaningful manner. Clustering operates in an unsupervised manner. There are clustering methods that require the number of clusters to be defined beforehand and methods where the number of clusters is automatically defined. There are several clustering methods available, the most popular being the Unweighted Pair Group Method with Arithmetic Mean (UPGMA), as well as other hierarchical clustering methods for tree-based representations. Evolutionary tree-based algorithms such as Neighbor Joining could be also applied in clustering. In the widely used *k*-means algorithm, the number of clusters is pre-defined. Another popular clustering algorithm, the Self-Organizing Map (SOM) [14], produces ordered low-dimensional representations of an input data space, and is particularly well suited for exploratory data analysis. Most of the aforementioned methods are implemented in BioConductor [11], Expander [15] and Hierarchical Clustering Explorer (HCE) [16].

Classification of microarray data refers to class prediction from gene expression patterns. In classification, the classes, two or more, (e.g., healthy individuals vs. diseased), are predefined and a classifier is built to discriminate between the classes in future applications [17, 18], most notably screening and diagnosis [19]. A wide variety of supervised methods have been designed for classification, including Neural Networks [20], Support Vector Machines [21], Graphical Models [22], genetic algorithms [23], nearest neighbour classifiers and many other statistical methods such as shrunken centroids [24] and Partial Least Squares and Discriminant analysis [25]. Due to the large number of features given as input to the various classifiers, a subsequent problem is to select the subset of features that can be used efficiently by the classifier. This problem is known as **feature selection** in machine learning and statistics [26]. A great number of feature selection methods tailored for microarray studies have been developed. Comparison of such methods in gene expression classification can be found in several excellent reviews and evaluation studies [27–29].

The topic of this review is the description of methodologies for the **identification of DEGs.** The main objective is to identify which genes are differentially expressed, that is, up- or down-regulated, under different conditions. Ideally, the identification of

DEGs is a simple procedure reduced to a statistical test for the equality of means (e.g., *t*-test, see below). Microarray datasets, however, are characterised by several key distinctive features such as small number of samples, large number of variables and excessive amount of noise; therefore, several advanced statistical methods have been proposed to handle these issues efficiently. Moreover, the generation of similar datasets from various laboratories highlight the need for combining these datasets in order to increase the sample size. This approach, which is termed "meta-analysis" in the medical literature, has been increasingly popular during the last years, and a variety of meta-analysis methods have been developed. In this review, we explore the statistical methods for analysis and meta-analysis of DEGs arising from microarray experiments by focusing on the simple case of comparing only two classes (disease-healthy, treated-non treated etc.). First, the analysis methods for detecting DEGs, starting with the well-known *t*-test, as well as the various modifications of these methods proposed for different microarray datasets, are described. Afterwards, the methods for meta-analysis of microarray datasets are presented. Moreover, the related software implementation methods are listed, as well as the novel variants of these methods. Examples of microarray data analysis and meta-analysis are also presented.

2 Methods

2.1 Methods of Analysis of Differentially Expressed Genes

Earlier microarray publications assessed differential expression merely in terms of fold-change (FC), with a FC $\pm$ 2 being considered as a reliable cut-off value. However, FC cut-off values do not take intra-dataset variability into account or ensure reproducibility. Moreover, the FC-based ranking is not adequate, since a gene with larger variance in expression values has a higher probability of having a larger statistic value. It is also suggested that FC-based methods result in lists of DEGs that are more reproducible. However, reproducibility does not signify accuracy, and the question of whether to use FC to identify DEGs is essentially biological, rather than statistical [30].

2.1.1 t-Test

The *t*-test assesses whether the means of two groups have statistically significant differences. The **one sample *t*-test** is a statistical method used to determine the mean difference between the sample and the known or hypothesized value of the population mean. The null hypothesis assumes that there are no significant differences between the sample and the population mean. In real life applications, however, the one sample *t*-test is used for testing statistical differences in paired observations, either measuring the same sample (for instance, an individual before and after treatment) or, more generally, samples that are somehow grouped (matched observations):

$$\bar{X}_1 - \bar{X}_2 = \bar{X}_D \tag{1}$$

To calculate the value of the one sample *t*-test, we use the formula:

$$t = \frac{\bar{X}_D}{S_D/\sqrt{n}} \tag{2}$$

In this analysis, subscripts 1 and 2 denote the two conditions, the mean difference of which is assumed to be zero according to the null hypothesis. The *t*-statistic is compared against a *t*-distribution with $n - 1$ degrees of freedom.

The **two sample *t*-test** is used to compare two independent population means. The null hypothesis here assumes that the means of two populations are equal. The *t*-statistic assuming equal variances can be calculated as follows:

$$t = \frac{\bar{X}_1 - \bar{X}_2}{S_p\sqrt{\frac{1}{n_1} + \frac{1}{n_2}}} \tag{3}$$

where the pooled variance S_p is given by the formula:

$$S_p = \sqrt{\frac{(n_1 - 1)S_1{}^2 + (n_2 - 1)S_2{}^2}{n_1 + n_2 - 2}} \tag{4}$$

The *t*-statistic is compared against a *t*-distribution with $n_1 + n_2 - 2$ degrees of freedom.

In the case of unequal variances, the appropriate *t*-statistic to test the equality of population means is calculated as:

$$t = \frac{\bar{X}_1 - \bar{X}_2}{S_{\bar{X}_1 - \bar{X}_2}} \tag{5}$$

where

$$S_{\bar{X}_1 - \bar{X}_2} = \sqrt{\frac{S_1{}^2}{n_1} + \frac{S_2{}^2}{n_2}} \tag{6}$$

However, in this case the asymptotic distribution is difficult to obtain, and a reasonable approximation is to use a *t*-distribution with degrees of freedom (d.f.) given by the formula:

$$\text{d.f.} = \frac{\left(S_1{}^2/n_1 + S_2{}^2/n_2\right)^2}{\left(S_1{}^2/n_1\right)^2/(n_1-1) + \left(S_2{}^2/n_2\right)^2/(n_2-1)} \tag{7}$$

A drawback of the *t*-test in microarray data analysis is that most microarray experiments contain only a few samples in each group (n_1 and n_2) the assumption of normality does not hold. Thus, several alternatives to the *t*-test have been proposed in the literature.

2.1.2 Resampling Methods

Bootstrap [31, 32] is a statistical method for estimating the sampling distribution of an estimator by sampling with replacement from the original sample. Bootstrap provides an ideal alternative method when no formula for the sampling distribution is available or when available formulas make inappropriate assumptions (e.g., small sample size, non-normal distribution). The accuracy of bootstrapping depends on the number of observations in the original sample and the number of replications. A crudely estimated sampling distribution is adequate to calculate, for instance, a standard error; a better estimate is needed for constructing a 95% confidence interval. There are various methods for constructing a Bootstrap confidence interval from the resampled statistics, such as the normal approximation method, the bias corrected method, the percentile method and the t-percentile method [33]. Generally, replications of the order of 1000 produce very accurate estimates, although more may be needed for the accurate estimation of *p*-values. Only 50–200 replications are needed for estimating standard errors, though this may have implications in meta-analysis (see below). Various methods have been proposed for estimating the adequate number of replications [34, 35]. The Bootstrap has been applied in microarray experiments and empirical evidence suggests that it produces accurate estimates, at least for moderate sample sizes [36]. For really small sample sizes (i.e., <10), various modifications to the standard bootstrap method have been proposed [37, 38].

A conceptually different resampling method is the **permutation** test. This is a type of statistical significance test where the distribution of the test statistic under the null hypothesis is obtained by calculating all possible values of the test statistic following rearrangements of the labels on the observations. If under the null hypothesis the labels are exchangeable, then the resulting tests generate exact significance levels. Confidence intervals can then be derived from the tests. The theory has evolved from the works of Fisher and Pitman in the 1930s (reviewed in Kaiser [39]). For small samples, all possible permutations can be evaluated; however, for sample sizes >15, a random sample of the permutation is used instead, hence the name Monte Carlo permutation. An important assumption underlying a permutation test is that under the null hypothesis the observations are exchangeable. Thus, a consequence of this is that tests of difference in location (e.g., *t*-test) require equal variance. In this respect, the permutation *t*-test has the same weakness as the classical Student's *t*-test (i.e., the Behrens–Fisher problem). In general, since the permutation computes a *p*-value by counting the times the test statistic is larger than the observed one, a large number of replications are required (typically of the order of 1000 or more). Permutation tests have been used for the analysis of microarray data [40]. In the case sample sizes are very small, the number of distinct permutations can be severely restricted, and combining the permutation-derived test statistics for each gene has been proposed. However, since the null distribution of the test statistics under permutation is not the same for all genes, this can have a negative impact on *p*-value estimation [41].

Bootstrap and permutation methods are readily available in major statistical packages like Stata [42] and R [43]. There are various implementations of the Bootstrap available in Stata (*bootstrap* command) and in R (*boot* command). Permutation can be also performed using the *permute* and *permtest* (for paired observations) commands in Stata, as well as the *perm* command in R. In the Supplement at http://www.compgen.org/tools/microarrays we give examples of performing bootstrapping and permutation *t*-test is Stata.

2.1.3 Bayesian Methods

The **Bayesian** methods provide an intuitively appealing framework for handling most of the problems encountered in the analysis of microarray data. Several Bayesian methods have been developed that replace *t*-test, which is one of the simplest and widely used statistical methods in microarray expression data analysis. These Bayesian methods share some common features but have also marked differences according to various criteria, especially in the prior distribution for the hyperparameters. Moreover, some of these methods are oriented towards hypothesis testing by relying on the Bayes Factor to compare the null against the alternative hypothesis [44–47]; other methods are oriented towards parameter estimation and compute credible intervals for the parameters of interest, for example the difference of the means [48, 49]. One of the advantages of the *t*-test is that its simplicity allows in many cases a closed-form expression to be derived, especially for the Bayes Factor [44–47], whereas other methods rely on Markov Chain Monte Carlo (MCMC) to sample from the posterior distribution [48, 49]. Another major advantage of the Bayesian methods is that within the Bayesian framework, one cannot only incorporate the uncertainty regarding the parameters and the small sample size, but also multiple testing, which is very important in microarray analysis [44, 50, 51].

There are several software implementations available of the aforementioned Bayesian methods. For instance, the Bayes Factor method of Rouder and coworkers [45], which is known as the Jeffreys–Zellner–Siow (JZS) *t*-test, is available as a web-calculator (http://pcl.missouri.edu/bayesfactor), as well as an R package (https://cran.r-project.org/web/packages/BayesFactor/index.html). The Savage–Dickey (SD) *t*-test, proposed by Wetzels and coworkers [48], is inspired by the JZS *t*-test and retains its key concepts. It is, however, applicable to a wider range of statistical problems, since it allows researchers to test order restrictions and applies to two-sample situations with unequal variance. The SD *t*-test is also implemented into an R package that uses WinBUGS (http://www.ruudwetzels.com/sdtest). Finally, the BEST (Bayesian Estimation Supersedes the *t*-test) software package, which provides a Bayesian alternative to *t*-test, providing much richer information than a simple *p*-value, such as complete distributions of credible values for the effect size, difference of mean between groups, difference of standard deviations, and the normality of the data within the groups [49]. The BEST package is implemented in R (http://www.indiana.edu/~kruschke/BEST/) and is also available as an online calculator (http://sumsar.net/best_online/). Moreover, the BEST method is implemented in the Bayesian First Aid package (https://github.com/rasmusab/bayesian_first_aid) that aims to provide user friendly Bayesian alternatives to the most widely used estimation commands.

2.1.4 Penalized t-Test

As we have already mentioned, the ordinary *t*-test is not recommended for microarray experiments because a large *t*-statistic can be driven by an unrealistically small value for S^2. Genes with small sample variances, possibly due to a very small sample size, have a good chance of giving a large *t*-statistic even if they are not expressed differentially. Alternative methods have been proposed in order to alleviate such problems, namely, **penalized**, **moderated** or **regularized *t*-tests**. Most of these methods are characterized by an empirical Bayesian justification, and hence share a lot of common features with the Bayesian methods; other methods mainly consist of ad-hoc rules. In any case, all of these methods apply certain types of modification to the denominator in the *t*-test formula by increasing the variance [52]. Thus, they all have the same interpretation as an ordinary *t*-statistic, except that the standard errors have been moderated across genes. Baldi and Long were among the first to discuss Bayesian methods for the *t*-test in the context of microarray experiments [53, 54] and they preferred to develop an empirical Bayesian regularized *t*-test method with variance equal to:

$$S^2_{\text{Cyber-T}} = \frac{\nu_0 {\sigma_0}^2 + (n-1)S^2}{\nu_0 + n - 2} \tag{8}$$

This method is implemented in the web-server Cyber-T (http://cybert.ics.uci.edu/) and in R (http://cybert.ics.uci.edu/). The parameter ν_0 represents the degree of confidence in the background variance ${\sigma_0}^2$ versus the empirical variance. In Cyber-T, the value of ν_0 is user defined; the smaller the n value, the larger the ν_0 value. A simple rule of thumb is to assume that $K > 2$ is needed to properly estimate the standard deviation and keep $n + \nu_0 = K$. This allows a more flexible treatment of situations in which the number n of available data points varies from gene to gene. The default value of K is 10. In particular, by using this approach, the empirical variance depends on ν_0 "pseudo-observations" with a background variance ${\sigma_0}^2$. For σ_0, one could use the standard deviation of the entire dataset or of particular categories of genes. Cyber-T uses a flexible approach under which the background standard deviation is estimated by pooling together all the neighbouring genes contained in a window of size w (the default value of w is 101, corresponding to 50 genes in the immediate neighbourhood of the gene under consideration).

Another empirical Bayesian method is the method of Lönnstedt and Speed [55] which uses the moderated variance:

$$S^2_{\text{LS}} = a + S^2 \tag{9}$$

where the penalty a is estimated from the mean and standard deviation of the sample variances S. Later, Smyth [56] provided a variant of this formula, which is implemented in the well-known *limma* (linear models for microarray data) package:

$$S^2_{limma} = \frac{\nu_0 {\sigma_0}^2 + nS^2}{\nu_0 + n} \tag{10}$$

Here, d_0 and s_0 are estimated from the data with the method of moments using an empirical Bayesian approach. The *limma* method is one of the most widely used methods for analysing DEGs, and it is available as a Bioconductor package in R (http://bioinf.wehi.edu.au/limma). Tusher et al. [57] and Efron et al. [58] also used a penalized t-statistics:

$$S_{\text{SAM}} = a + S \tag{11}$$

This differs slightly from the previous statistics in that the penalty a is applied to the sample standard deviation S rather than to the sample variance S^2. Tusher et al. [57] in the so-called "Significance Analysis of Microarrays (SAM)" method, chose a to minimize the coefficient of variation of the absolute t-values while Efron et al. [58], used a as the 90th percentile of the S values.

These choices are based on empirical rather than theoretical considerations. SAM is one of the oldest and most widely-used methods and it is available as an Excel plugin at http://statweb.stanford.edu/~tibs/SAM/, as well as implemented in several R packages (*samr*, *ema*).

Ranking Analysis of Microarray data (RAM) uses another type of regularization, which is based on the observation that even when the sample size is small, the fudging effect using the modified *t*-statistic is still quite strong [59]. In particular, small sample size often leads to an unreasonably large value of a that dominates the test statistic and consequently reduces the power of the analysis. Thus, the authors proposed the following:

$$S_{\mathrm{RAM}} = \begin{cases} 1 + S \text{ if } \bar{X}_D > S < 1 \\ S \text{ otherwise} \end{cases} \tag{12}$$

RAM is based on the comparisons between a set of ranked *t*-statistics and a set of ranked *Z*-values (a set of ranked estimated null scores) yielded by a "randomly splitting" (RS) approach instead of the permutation approach used by SAM. Results obtained from simulated and real microarray data revealed that RAM is more efficient in the identification of DEGs under undesirable conditions such as small sample size, a large fudge factor, or mixture distribution of noises compared to SAM.

The regularised *t*-statistics have many desired properties. In particular, they are easily computed, have a natural interpretation, and are less computationally intensive compared to the full Bayesian methods and the resampling approaches. Moreover, simulation studies [30] have shown that regularised *t*-statistics are superior to the ordinary *t*-statistic for detecting DEGs, even when the sample size is very small ($n < 10$). The penalized *t*-statistics, on the other hand, can also be extended in several ways to apply to more general experimental situations. A disadvantage is that the null distribution of the modified *t*-statistic is not standard. Baldi and Long [53], as well as Smyth [56], rely on a modified *t*-distribution with adjusted degrees of freedom. On the other hand, methods such as SAM use permutations in order to calculate False Discovery Rate (FDR, see below).

2.1.5 Other Methods

As we have already mentioned, earlier microarray publications estimated differential expression of genes based solely on FC The moderated *t*-tests, on the other hand, borrow information across genes; they perform better, providing estimates of statistical significance and results more in line with FC rankings. However, even these contemporary statistical tests permit genes with relatively small FCs to be considered statistically significant probably due to *t*-statistic formula's very small denominator.

Hence, it is becoming increasingly necessary in the literature that DEGs meet both *p*-value and FC criteria. Several authors require that genes satisfy an acceptable level of statistical significance and then rank significant genes by FC with an arbitrarily set cut-off. There are also authors who first apply a FC cut-off and then rank genes according to their *p*-value. Other authors declare genes as differentially expressed on the basis that they simultaneously show a FC larger than a given threshold value and satisfy the criterion for *p*-value. Such combined criteria are suggested to identify more biologically relevant sets of genes and even provide a much better inter-platform agreement compared to FC and *p*-values alone [60].

TREAT (*t*-tests relative to a threshold) is used to introduce statistical formalism to these approaches. This method is an extension of the empirical Bayesian moderated *t*-statistic presented by Smyth (i.e., *limma*), and can be used to test whether the true differential gene expression is greater than a given threshold value. By including the FC threshold value of interest in a formal hypothesis test, the methods achieve reliable *p*-values for identifying genes with differential expression that is biologically relevant [60]. TREAT has been shown to perform well in both real and simulated data.

Similar considerations have led to the development of the weighted average difference (WAD) method for ranking DEGs [61]. The authors observed that some genes which are falsely declared to be highly differentially expressed tend to display lower expression levels. In this way, the "true" DEGs cannot be identified because the relative error is increased at lower signal intensities. WAD uses the average gene expression difference and relative average signal intensity in a way such that highly expressed genes are top ranked on the average for the different conditions:

$$\mathrm{WAD} = (\bar{X}_1 - \bar{X}_2)\frac{\bar{X} - \min_p(\bar{X})}{\max_p(\bar{X}) - \min_p(\bar{X})} \tag{13}$$

where $\bar{X} = (\bar{X}_1 + \bar{X}_2)/2$and the max (or min) indicates the maximum (or minimum) value, respectively, in an average expression vector of $\bar{X}$ among the p genes analysed (on a log scale). WAD was compared to several other methods and the results showed that it outperforms them in terms of both sensitivity and specificity.

Finally, the RankProduct (RP) method is based on calculating rank products from replicate experiments, in a fast and simple way. This method seeks to alleviate the above-mentioned problems by relying on biologically significant FC, providing at the same time an estimate of the statistical significance. The RP method is essentially a non-parametric method for detecting DEGs in microarray experiments [62, 63]. The genes are ranked according to FC and then analysis is performed separately for up-regulated and under-regulated genes. For instance, concerning the up-regulated gene g with $i = 1, 2, \ldots, k$ replicates, the rank product will be given by the geometric mean:

$$\mathrm{RP}_g^{\mathrm{up}} = \left(\Pi_k r_{g,i}^{\mathrm{up}}\right)^{1/k} \tag{14}$$

The RP method is available as an R package (RankProd), and also supported by the webserver RankProdIt (http://strep-microarray.sbs.surrey.ac.uk/RankProducts/).

The use of exact calculation and permutation methods have been proposed to determine the statistical significance. These approaches have serious limitations as they are computationally demanding. Approximation methods have been also proposed but these usually provide inaccurate estimates in the tail of the p-value distribution. Lately, however, a method to determine upper bounds and accurate approximate p-values of the RP statistic has been developed, decreasing the computational time significantly. The R code for this method is available at http://www.ru.nl/publish/pages/726696/rankprodbounds.zip [64].

The RP method has been reported to perform more reliably and consistently compared to SAM, even on highly noisy data. In realistic simulated microarray datasets, RP is more robust and accurate for sorting genes based on differential expression compared to t-statistics, especially for replicate numbers $n < 10$. This method performs particularly well on data contaminated by abnormal random noise and heterogeneous samples. RP, however, assumes equal measurement variance for all genes and tends to give overly optimistic p-values when this assumption does not apply. Therefore, appropriate variance-stabilizing normalization should be performed on the data prior to calculating the RP values. If applicable, another rank-based variant of RP, that is, average ranks, provides a suitable alternative with comparable performance.

2.2 Meta-Analysis of Microarrays

Meta-analysis is the statistical technique for combining data from multiple independent but related studies [65]. In particular, meta-analysis can be used to identify a treatment effect that is consistent among studies. In case the treatment effect varies among studies, meta-analysis may be used to identify the cause for this variation. Hypotheses cannot be inferred and validated based solely on the results of a single study, as the results typically vary between studies; instead, data across studies should be combined [66]. Meta-analysis applies universal formulas to a number of different studies. Nowadays, GEO (http://www.ncbi.nlm.nih.gov/geo/) and ArrayExpress (https://www.ebi.ac.uk/arrayexpress/) databases provide the option to compare the normalized raw data across many experiments and organisms, allowing in this way comparative gene expression profiling.

In this section, we provide a practical guide that could enable the reader to make informed decisions on how to conduct a meta-analysis of microarray data.

Issue 1: Selection of Appropriate Microarray Datasets

The first, and most critical, step in an experimental study is to clearly state objectives. Meta-analysis enables the identification of DEGs among multiple samples in order to improve classification within and across platforms, detect redundancy across diverse datasets, identify differentially co-expressed genes, and infer networks of genetic interactions. The second step of meta-analysis is to set eligibility criteria, either biological (e.g., tissue type, disease) or technical (e.g., one-channel versus two-channel detection, density of microarrays, technological platform). Based on these criteria, literature searches are preformed, using appropriate key terms, to retrieve relevant studies. These studies can be complemented by microarray data available in public databases that conform to the MIAME (Minimum Information About a Microarray Experiment) guidelines.

Issue 2: Data Acquisition from Studies

The genes found to be differentially expressed in a given study constitute the published gene lists (PGLs) which are either included in the main text or provided as supplementary material. The gene expression data matrices (GEDM) contain preprocessed expression values of every probe-set and sample for one gene. The published GEDM cannot be used directly as input for meta-analysis because of the different algorithms used for processing raw data in the original studies, which may generate heterogeneous, non-comparable results.

Issue 3: Preprocessing of Datasets from Diverse Platforms

To enable consistent analysis of all datasets, bias introduced by the preprocessing algorithms should be eliminated. To this end, feature-level extraction output (FLEO) files, such as CEL files, should be obtained and converted to GEDM suitable for meta-analysis. Multiple studies from the same platform should be preprocessed using a single algorithm. In case the studies are conducted on different platforms, it is recommended to be preprocessed with comparable algorithms in order to be combinable.

Issue 4: Promiscuous Hybridization between Probes and Genes

The datasets are annotated using UniGene or RefSeq gene identifiers, collectively referred to as GeneIDs. Multiple probes can hybridize with the same GeneID, as UniGene represents a cluster of sequences that correspond to a unique gene. Conversely, one non-specific probe can cross-hybridize with multiple GeneIDs due to imperfect specificity. There are also probes with inadequate sequence information that cannot hybridize with any GeneID. One approach to resolve the "many-to-many" relationships between probes and genes is to include in the meta-analysis only probes that are associated with a single gene, and exclude the promiscuous probes that are associated with more than one gene; however, important information can be lost. Averaging the expression profiles prior to meta-analysis is not recommended either, given that probe binding affinity differences affect the gene expression measurements. It is therefore recommended to apply descriptive statistics, thereby reducing the "many-to-many" into "one-to-one" relationship between probe and GeneID for each study [66–68].

Issue 5: Choosing a Meta-Analysis Technique

The choice of meta-analysis techniques depends on the type of response (e.g., binary, continuous, survival). In this review, we focus on the two-class comparison of microarrays where the objective is to identify genes expressed differentially between two different conditions. In such cases as this, there are three broad categories of statistical methods for meta-analysis that make use of effect sizes, p-values and ranks.

2.2.1 Effect Size

The first statistical method is a standard approach for meta-analysis using fixed or random effects. In principle, any suitable effect size can be used in meta-analysis; in practice, however, most authors advocate the standardized mean difference:

$$d_i = \frac{X_{1i} - X_{2i}}{S_{pi}} \tag{15}$$

X_{1i} and X_{2i} are the means of the two groups under comparison in the ith study, and S_{pi} is the pooled standard deviation given by:

$$S_{pi} = \sqrt{\frac{(n_{1i} - 1)S_{1i}^2 + (n_{2i} - 1)S_{2i}^2}{n_{1i} + n_{2i} - 2}} \tag{16}$$

In research synthesis, the sample estimate of the standardized mean difference is referred to as Cohen's d [69]. Nevertheless, d has the tendency to overestimate the absolute value in small samples. This bias introduced by d can be corrected using the so-called Hedges' g, which generates an unbiased estimate. A correction factor, called J, is employed to convert from d to Hedges' g. Although there is an exact formula for J, researchers often use an approximation given by $g_i = Jd_i = d_i - 3d_i/(4n_i - 9)$. The estimated variance of d is given by:

$$\text{var}(d_i) = s_i^2 = \left(\frac{1}{n_{1i}} + \frac{1}{n_{2i}}\right) + \frac{d_i^2}{2(n_{1i} + n_{2i})} \tag{17}$$

When g is used, $\text{var}(g) = J^2\text{var}(d)$. In any case, it is straightforward to obtain a pooled estimate of d (or g):

$$\hat{d} = \frac{\sum_{i=1}^{k} w_i d_i}{\sum_{i=1}^{k} w_i} \tag{18}$$

This is the well-known inverse-variance estimate used in meta-analysis with $w_i = 1/s_i^2$ [65, 70]. The above method assumes homogeneity of the effect across studies, which is a rather weak assumption. In the case of between-study heterogeneity, we hypothesize that the true effect varies between studies, $d_i \sim N(d, s_i^2 + \tau^2)$ and, therefore, an additive component of the between studies variance (τ^2) needs to be estimated (random-effects model). The most commonly used method for estimating τ^2 is the non-iterative method of moments proposed by DerSimonian and Laird [71], even though there are several alternative methods including iterative procedures [72]. In case $\tau^2 = 0$, the random-effects and the fixed-effects estimates coincide. In the random-effects case, the weights are calculated by:

$$w_i = \left(\tau^2 + s_i^2\right)^{-1} \tag{19}$$

and subsequently Eq. (18) is applied in order to obtain the overall estimate. In any case, inferences about the overall effect are based on the normal approximation since:

$$\mathrm{var}\left(\hat{d}\right) = \frac{1}{\sum_{i=1}^{k} w_i} \tag{20}$$

In the case of a matched design (e.g., use of same individuals before and after treatment), there is a very similar formula, except that the natural unit of deviation is the standard deviation of the difference scores, and so this is the value that is likely to be reported or calculated from the data.

As we have already noted, this approach is based on common practices in meta-analysis and thus it was advocated early in the literature [73, 74]. However, to handle the problem of small sample size and non-normal data, most authors suggest a type of correction for calculating the statistical significance. Therefore, instead of relying on the normal approximation, they propose the permutation test. Although Choi and coworkers [73] suggest permutations to calculate *p*-values, a faster solution is offered in the Bioconductor package *GeneMeta*, which assumes a normal distribution on the *z*-scores after checking the reliability of this hypothesis by a *Q–Q* plot. In general, all the aforementioned resampling methods can be used, with bootstrapping being, probably, the most advantageous since it requires a smaller number of replications. The bootstrap or the permutation methods can also be used in different settings. One option would be to perform an analysis for each study separately, obtain a corrected estimate of variance and then use this in order to calculate the weights for the meta-analysis. Another option would be to perform the analysis in a single step using the resampling strategy (bootstrap or permutation) in a stratified manner, in which the studies are treated as strata.

Following another approach, inference could be based on the ratio of means instead of the standardized difference [75]. This approach has the distinct advantage that uses a measure related to the well-known FC. Thus, the statistic would be:

$$\gamma_i = \log\left(\frac{X_{1i}}{X_{2i}}\right) \tag{21}$$

with estimated variance equal to:

$$\mathrm{var}(\gamma_i) = s_i^2 = \frac{1}{n_{1i}}\frac{S_{1i}^2}{X_{1i}^2} + \frac{1}{n_{2i}}\frac{S_{2i}^2}{X_{2i}^2} \tag{22}$$

All the standard methods reported above can be easily used with this effect size and its variance. The ratio of means has also been used for data other than gene expression, and, in general, it performs well even in small samples [76]. Lately, the ratio of geometric means has also been proposed, especially for skewed data, and its application in the meta-analysis of gene expression data could be also investigated [77]. The points mentioned above regarding bootstrap and permutation are also applicable to this effect size.

The aforementioned methods, since they are standard methods for meta-analysis, can be easily extended to a Bayesian framework [78]. Several studies have been performed to this end, and source code to fit the model is available [79, 80]. In general, Conlon and coworkers [79, 80] use in their models a structure similar to the one Gotardo and coworkers use in their model for single studies; an additional level is added though to account for multiple studies. The main problem with the Bayesian methods is the increased computational complexity and time needed to perform the analysis, especially when a large number of genes is investigated which perhaps limit their applicability. The WinBUGS code to fit the models of Conlon and coworkers is available at http://people.math.umass.edu/~conlon/research/BayesPoolMicro/.

Finally, another promising approach is to use the moderated effect sizes calculated by methods such as *limma*, instead of the typical effect sizes, in the traditional meta-analysis. This is a two-step method relying in the first step on an advanced method for regularized *t*-test [81]. Then, provided that that $t = d\sqrt{n}$, a traditional random effects meta-analysis is performed. Another modification of this work is that instead of using the approximation for the variance of d, the exact calculation given by Hedges is used. This approach is implemented in the R package *metaMA* (https://cran.r-project.org/web/packages/metaMA/index.html).

Several major meta-analysis methods for DEG analysis, including fixed effects and random effects methods, as well as methods for combining p-values and ranks (see next sections), are implemented in R packages, such as *GeneMeta* and *metaMA*. The most complete package, however, is *MetaDE*, which also offers functionality for preprocessing the data, as well as for displaying the results graphically [82]. Stata lacks a meta-analysis command dedicated to microarrays, but several of the methods mentioned here can be easily implemented. As a proof of concept, we describe in the Appendix several approaches for performing random effects meta-analysis. One approach consists of performing the analysis for each study separately (using bootstrap or permutation) and then combine the results in the usual way. Another approach would be to perform meta-analysis in a single step and run the bootstrap or permutation simulation as a wrapper method; both bootstrap and permutation should be then performed in a stratified manner treating the studies as strata.

2.2.2 Ranks

Another class of methods for meta-analysis consists of methods that combine ranks. There are several different approaches, the common denominator of which is that if the same gene is repeatedly at the top of the list ordered by up- or down-regulated genes in replicate experiments, the gene is more likely to be declared as differentially expressed. The Rank Product method, which we have already described in the context of a single study, uses FC to rank genes and calculates the products of ranks across samples and studies [83]. A similar method, Rank Sum, uses the sum of ranks instead, but all other calculations are identical. The RankProd software is available at: https://www.bioconductor.org/packages/release/bioc/html/RankProd.html.

A related method, termed METRADISC (Meta-analysis of Rank Discovery Dataset), is based on the same principle, but it is more general [84, 85]. The ranking within each study is performed with any available method (FC, t-test, p-value etc.) and then the average rank of a particular gene across studies is calculated. The overall mean can be weighted or unweighted; the weighted overall mean resembles the traditional methods for meta-analysis. The between-study heterogeneity of the study-specific ranks can also be computed. METRADISC is implemented in R (http://www.inside-r.org/node/155959) and it is also available as a stand-alone application (http://biomath.med.uth.gr/). The methods that use ranks are quite robust and can combine studies using different methods. However, the statistical inferences are based on Monte Carlo permutation tests, which may be time-consuming.

The rank-based methods offer several advantages compared to traditional approaches, including the FC criterion, fewer assumptions under the model, and robustness with noisy data and/or low numbers of replicates. These methods overcome heterogeneity across multiple datasets and combine them to achieve increased sensitivity and reliability. Of particular note, these methods do not require the simultaneous normalization of multiple datasets using the same technique, solving in this way a key issue in microarray meta-analysis pre-processing. Moreover, the rank-based methods transform the actual expression values into ranks, and thus they can integrate datasets produced by a wide variety of platforms (Affymetrix oligonucleotide arrays, two-color cDNA arrays etc.). Finally, the rank-based methods are quite general and therefore can be applied to different types of data, such as proteomics or genetic association data.

2.2.3 Combination of p-values

Another class of methods that is popular in meta-analysis of microarray studies [86] involves combination of *p*-values. It is widely accepted that Fisher's seminal work on the combination of *p*-values [87] was the origin of meta-analysis [88]. Fisher noted that since *p*-values from *k* independent samples are uniform random variables, the sum of their logarithm will follow a χ^2 distribution with 2 *k* degrees of freedom:

$$U = -2\sum_{i=1}^{k} \log(p_i) = -2\log\left(\Pi_{i=1}^{k} p_i\right) \quad (23)$$

Bailey and Gribskov, in a different context, showed that the same probability can be calculated easily with their QFAST algorithm without relying on the χ^2 distribution [89]. Edgington suggested to use the sum of the *p*-values in order to obtain a pooled estimate [90].

$$p = \frac{\left(\sum_{i=1}^{k} p_i\right)^k}{k!} \quad (24)$$

Later, the same author suggested the use of a contrast such as [91]

$$\bar{p} = \frac{\sum_{i=1}^{k} p_i}{k} \quad (25)$$

in which case $U = (0.5 - \bar{p})\sqrt{12}$ follows a $N(0,1)$ distribution. A more sophisticated method was presented by Zaykin and coworkers, the so-called truncated product method (TPM). Their procedure was to use the product of only those *p*-values less than a specific cut-off value (τ) to evaluate the probability of such a product, or a smaller value, under the overall hypothesis that all k hypotheses are true [92]. The formula used is:

$$W = \Pi_{i=1}^{k} (p_i)^{I(p_i \leq \tau)} \tag{26}$$

The authors provide an explicit formula for this p-value:

$$P(W \leq w) = \sum_{i=1}^{k} \binom{k}{r} (1-\tau)^{k-r} \left(w \sum_{s=0}^{r-1} \frac{(r\log\tau - \log w)^s}{s!} I(w \leq \tau^r) + \tau^r I(w > \tau^r) \right) \tag{27}$$

where r is the number of p_i's less than τ. Zaykin et al. also showed by simulation that this formula is quite robust for detecting deviations from the overall hypothesis. Of particular note, when $\tau = \min$, p results in the well-known Sidak's correction, and when $\tau = 1$, W becomes $W = \Pi_{i=1}^{k} p_i$. This method provides Fisher's combined p-value without the need of looking up the cumulative probability from the tail of a chi-square distribution:

$$P(W \leq w) = w \sum_{i=0}^{k-1} \frac{(-\log w)^i}{i!} \tag{28}$$

Interestingly, this is the exact formula from the QFAST method of Bailey and Gribskov, presented independently few years earlier. Source code for implementing TPM can be obtained from http://statgen.ncsu.edu/zaykin/tpm/. The different approaches for combining p-values have been compared in several evaluation studies [93, 94]. Most of the methods presented in this section are implemented in the *metap* command available in Stata and R.

Nevertheless, combining p-values presents serious problems relative to combining effect sizes, as in the case of testing different null hypotheses. Moreover, in the combination of p-value, the direction of the association is not taken into consideration and therefore all p-values have to be one-sided, otherwise up- and down-regulated genes have to be combined separately. Finally, these methods cannot quantify the magnitude of the association (the effect size), and, most importantly, do not account for between-studies heterogeneity. A method developed by Stouffer partially overcomes these limitations, by combining the equivalent Z-scores instead of p-values [95]:

$$\bar{Z} = \frac{\sum_{i=1}^{k} Z_i}{\sqrt{k}} \tag{29}$$

This method does not account for the differences in the size of studies. Thus, a weighted variant can be formulated:

$$\bar{Z} = \frac{\sum_{i=1}^{k} \sqrt{w_i} Z_i}{\sqrt{\sum_{i=1}^{k} w_i^2}} \quad (30)$$

with weights being proportional to the square-root of the sample size for each study

$$w_i = \sqrt{n_i} \quad (31)$$

Yet, this method does not account for between-studies variability and, also, recent evidence from genetic association studies [96] suggests that this weighting scheme is suboptimal. Zhou and coworkers [96] demonstrated that the optimal weights are proportional to $(1/n_{1i} + 1/n_{2i})^{-1}$, providing the foundation in this way for a random effects meta-analysis (even without the actual effect sizes). Notably, the peculiarity of microarray experiments allows the (non available) effect sizes to be estimated accurately as follows: from the Z-statistic a hypothetical effect size, d^*, is calculated that would correspond to the same significance level:

$$Z_i = d_i^* / se(d_i^*) \Rightarrow d_i^* = Z_i se(d_i^*) \quad (32)$$

The standard error of this hypothetical effect size is given from Eq. (17). Thus, the formula for d^* is:

$$d_i^* = Z_i \sqrt{\left(\frac{n_{1i} + n_{2i}}{n_{1i} + n_{2i} - Z_i^2/2}\right)\left(\frac{1}{n_{1i}} + \frac{1}{n_{2i}}\right)} \quad (33)$$

Using this (hypothetical) effect size and its variance, standard methods for random effects meta-analysis can be applied easily. This approach requires only the Z-score, which can be either acquired directly or calculated from the p-value, the direction of association, and the number of replicates for each condition. This simple approach, inherits all the desirable properties of the method of Stouffer and, at the same time, performs optimal weighting, quantifies the association and enables random-effects meta-analysis in order to account for between-studies heterogeneity. If the original data are analysed with standard methods, the estimated d's are accurate. If, however, a modified version of the t-test or a resampling method for the statistical significance is used, some discrepancies may be expected; nevertheless, the Z-score and the statistical significance (p-value) of the overall effect are accurate. A Stata program that implements this method and compares it against other methods for combining p-values is given in the Supplement.

2.3 Multiple Comparisons

A typical microarray experiment measures the expression of several thousand genes simultaneously across different conditions. When investigating for potential DEGs between two conditions, each gene is treated independently and a t-test (or any other test described above) usually is performed on each gene separately. The incidence of false positives (i.e., genes falsely declared as DEGs) is proportional to the number of tests performed and the critical significance level (p-value cut-off). When a t-test is performed, the null hypothesis (H_0) is usually the hypothesis of no difference between the gene's expression level, whereas the alternative hypothesis (H_1) is that the expression levels differ. If the p-value is less than the chosen significance level, then the null hypothesis is rejected. Assuming the null hypothesis holds, in case 10,000 genes are tested at a 5% level of significance, 500 genes might be declared as significant, by chance alone. Thus, it is important to correct the p-value when performing a statistical test on a group or genes. This is the case for multiple testing correction methods.

Multiple-comparison correction methods take as input a list of p-values and an uncorrected critical p-value and calculate a corrected overall p-value for rejection of null hypotheses. These methods are clasified into two categories, the ones that control the family-wise error rate (FWER) and the ones that control the False Discovery Rate (FDR). In general, a FWER-controlling method defines a corrected p-value for a set of true null hypotheses. Usually, this level of significance is lower than the uncorrected p-value. The most common procedure to control the FWER is the Bonferroni correction [97], where the critical value (α) for an individual test is calculated by dividing the FWER (usually 0.05) by the number of tests. Thus, for 10,000 genes (i.e., number of tests), the critical value for an individual test would be $\alpha = 0.05/10000 = 5 \times 10^{-6}$; genes with p-value $<5 \times 10^{-6}$ are declared as differentially expressed. Thus, the corrected p-value from Bonferroni correction is given by:

$$p_{\mathrm{cor}(i)} = p_{(i)}/n \tag{34}$$

The Bonferroni correction is easily applied and intuitive, but it is very conservative. Another commonly used method is the method of Sidak [98]:

$$p_{\mathrm{cor}(i)} = 1 - \left(1 - p_{(i)}\right)^{1/n} \tag{35}$$

Other popular methods used for multiple testing correction in microarray analysis and meta-analysis are the methods proposed by Holland et al. [99] and Holm [100].

Benjamini and Hochberg [101] proposed a method which controls the FDR instead of the FWER. FDR-controlling procedures are designed to control the expected proportion of rejected null hypotheses that were incorrect rejections ("false discoveries"). FDR-controlling procedures provide less stringent control of Type I errors compared to FWER-controlling procedures, which control the probability of at least one Type I error. Thus, FDR-controlling procedures have greater power (i.e., they detect more differences as statistically significant), at the cost of increased rates of Type I errors. In this method, the *p*-values of each gene are ranked from the smallest to the largest. In this way, the smallest *p*-value has a rank of $i = 1$, then next smallest has $i = 2$, etc. Then, each individual *p*-value is compared against its Benjamini–Hochberg critical value, $(i/n)Q$, where i is the rank, n is the total number of tests, and Q is the chosen FDR. The largest *p*-value, $p < (i/n)Q$, is significant, Moreover, all of the *p*-values smaller than this are also significant, as well as the ones that aren't less than their Benjamini–Hochberg critical value:

$$p_{\mathrm{cor}(i)} = \frac{i}{n} p_{(i)} \tag{36}$$

Other popular multiple comparison correction methods which control FDR in microarray analysis and meta-analysis are the methods proposed by Benjamini and Yekutieli [102], Benjamini and Liu [103, 104], Benjamini, Krieger and Yekutieli [105]. The methods described above are implemented in the *multproc* command in Stata and in *multcomp* package in R.

3 Closing Remarks

Microarray experiments enable researches to analyze a vast amount of genetic information in a single experimental run. Therefore, the expression of multiple genes can be measured simultaneously under specific conditions. The use of DNA microarrays is very promising towards understanding genes' effect on diseases, drug discovery and development. Microarray experiments combined with bioinformatics analysis can reveal a great deal of information about a biological system and its dynamics. Such approaches though, like any other emerging technologies, come with shortcoming and disadvantages.

One of the main problems concerning microarray experiments is the lack of standardization. As a result, the data collected from different microarray platforms cannot be compared accurately, or even be replicated. In an evaluation study, Ioannidis and coworkers found that a large proportion of published studies could not be reproduced, either partially or completely [106]. This was mainly attributed to data unavailability and incomplete data annotation or specification of data processing and analysis. The authors called for stricter publication rules that will enforce public data availability and explicit description of data processing and analysis. The issue of comparing data generated by different platforms have long been under investigation [107] and filtering of probes has been shown to significantly improve intra-platform data comparability [108].

Methods for combining different datasets in a meta-analysis can help researchers to alleviate some of the problems mentioned above [109]. However, issues mentioned earlier such as the lack of standardization remain important obstacles for the development of such methods. In this chapter, we presented the available methods and provided information about the various available implementations of these statistical methods. In the recent literature, there are various studies that compare the different methods [110–112]. Notably, the lack of standardization is also apparent in the literature pertinent to studies in meta-analysis of microarrays, since different methods and combinations of these methods have been used in the recent literature. We have shown that, especially in the case of meta-analysis of effect sizes, various combinations of methods can be used. The final choice depends on the available software, the number of genes analysed, the number of studies and the different platforms to be combined. We have also shown that a meta-analysis of *p*-values can be performed under a random-effects method. It is also worth mentioning that, apart from the commonly used DerSimonian and Laird estimator, there are many available methods for calculating the between-studies variance in a random-effects meta-analysis; some of these methods are better suited for small and heterogeneous samples [113]. Moreover, there are available approximate Bayesian methods for meta-analysis that do not rely on simulations, and hence faster [114]. Taken together, the points above suggest that there is plenty of room for improvements in microarray meta-analysis methodology and software, both in terms of accuracy and speed. A recent systematic search in PubMed, resulted in the empirical evaluation of 333 articles based on microarray meta-analysis studies [115]. The results of this evaluation were very interesting, since, apart from the three general classes of methods presented earlier (effect size, rank, *p*-values), a large proportion of the published studies was found to be conducted using the "inappropriate" method of pooling datasets. This is a well-known issue in the meta-analysis literature, and this approach of pooling datasets in order to simply create a larger one is not recommended, since it can lead to various types of bias. Vote counting, in which one counts the number of studies in which a gene was declared significant, is another commonly used approach that is not recommended either.

In this chapter, we presented a review on the methodological issues pertaining to microarray data analysis and meta-analysis. The relative microarray databases and available software were also presented. Moreover, statistical methods of microarray data analysis were illustrated by a case study.

References

1. Bammler T, Beyer RP, Bhattacharya S et al (2005) Standardizing global gene expression analysis between laboratories and across platforms. Nat Methods 2(5):351–356. https://doi.org/10.1038/nmeth754
2. Pease AC, Solas D, Sullivan EJ et al (1994) Light-generated oligonucleotide arrays for rapid DNA sequence analysis. Proc Natl Acad Sci U S A 91(11):5022–5026
3. Tang T, Francois N, Glatigny A et al (2007) Expression ratio evaluation in two-colour microarray experiments is significantly improved by correcting image misalignment. Bioinformatics 23(20):2686–2691. https://doi.org/10.1093/bioinformatics/btm399
4. Suarez E, Burguete A, McLachlan GJ (2009) Microarray data analysis for differential expression: a tutorial. P R Health Sci J 28 (2):89–104
5. Bosotti R, Locatelli G, Healy S et al (2007) Cross platform microarray analysis for robust identification of differentially expressed genes. BMC Bioinformatics 8(Suppl 1):S5. https://doi.org/10.1186/1471-2105-8-S1-S5
6. Tan PK, Downey TJ, Spitznagel EL Jr et al (2003) Evaluation of gene expression measurements from commercial microarray platforms. Nucleic Acids Res 31(19):5676–5684
7. Yang YH, Buckley MJ, Speed TP (2001) Analysis of cDNA microarray images. Brief Bioinform 2(4):341–349
8. Quackenbush J (2002) Microarray data normalization and transformation. Nat Genet 32 (Suppl):496–501. https://doi.org/10.1038/ng1032
9. Tseng GC, Oh MK, Rohlin L et al (2001) Issues in cDNA microarray analysis: quality filtering, channel normalization, models of variations and assessment of gene effects. Nucleic Acids Res 29(12):2549–2557
10. Bolstad BM, Irizarry RA, Astrand M et al (2003) A comparison of normalization methods for high density oligonucleotide array data based on variance and bias. Bioinformatics 19(2):185–193
11. Reimers M, Carey VJ (2006) Bioconductor: an open source framework for bioinformatics and computational biology. Methods Enzymol 411:119–134. https://doi.org/10.1016/S0076-6879(06)11008-3
12. Irizarry RA, Hobbs B, Collin F et al (2003) Exploration, normalization, and summaries of high density oligonucleotide array probe level data. Biostatistics 4(2):249–264. https://doi.org/10.1093/biostatistics/4.2.249
13. Pepper SD, Saunders EK, Edwards LE et al (2007) The utility of MAS5 expression summary and detection call algorithms. BMC Bioinformatics 8:273. https://doi.org/10.1186/1471-2105-8-273
14. Tamayo P, Slonim D, Mesirov J et al (1999) Interpreting patterns of gene expression with self-organizing maps: methods and application to hematopoietic differentiation. Proc Natl Acad Sci U S A 96(6):2907–2912
15. Shamir R, Maron-Katz A, Tanay A et al (2005) EXPANDER–an integrative program suite for microarray data analysis. BMC Bioinformatics 6:232. https://doi.org/10.1186/1471-2105-6-232
16. Seo J, Shneiderman B (2002) Interactively exploring hierarchical clustering results. Computer 35(7):80–86. https://doi.org/10.1109/mc.2002.1016905
17. Golub TR, Slonim DK, Tamayo P et al (1999) Molecular classification of cancer: class discovery and class prediction by gene expression monitoring. Science 286(5439):531–537. doi:7911 [pii]
18. Radmacher MD, McShane LM, Simon R (2002) A paradigm for class prediction using gene expression profiles. J Comput Biol 9 (3):505–511
19. Simon R, Radmacher MD, Dobbin K et al (2003) Pitfalls in the use of DNA microarray data for diagnostic and prognostic classification. J Natl Cancer Inst 95(1):14–18
20. Khan J, Wei JS, Ringner M et al (2001) Classification and diagnostic prediction of cancers using gene expression profiling and artificial neural networks. Nat Med 7(6):673–679
21. Furey TS, Cristianini N, Duffy N et al (2000) Support vector machine classification and validation of cancer tissue samples using microarray expression data. Bioinformatics 16 (10):906–914
22. Bura E, Pfeiffer RM (2003) Graphical methods for class prediction using dimension reduction techniques on DNA microarray data. Bioinformatics 19(10):1252–1258
23. Ooi C, Tan P (2003) Genetic algorithms applied to multi-class prediction for the analysis of gene expression data. Bioinformatics 19(1):37–44
24. Tibshirani R, Hastie T, Narasimhan B et al (2002) Diagnosis of multiple cancer types by shrunken centroids of gene expression. Proc Natl Acad Sci U S A 99(10):6567–6572. https://doi.org/10.1073/pnas.082099299

25. Nguyen DV, Rocke DM (2002) Tumor classification by partial least squares using microarray gene expression data. Bioinformatics 18 (1):39–50
26. Guyon I, Elisseeff A (2003) An introduction to variable and feature selection. J Mach Learn Res 3:1157–1182
27. Saeys Y, Inza I, Larrañaga P (2007) A review of feature selection techniques in bioinformatics. Bioinformatics 23(19):2507–2517
28. Li T, Zhang C, Ogihara M (2004) A comparative study of feature selection and multiclass classification methods for tissue classification based on gene expression. Bioinformatics 20 (15):2429–2437
29. Ma S, Huang J (2008) Penalized feature selection and classification in bioinformatics. Brief Bioinform 9(5):392–403
30. Witten D, Tibshirani R (2007) A comparison of fold-change and the t-statistic for microarray data analysis. Analysis 1776:58–85
31. Efron B (1982) The jackknife, the bootstrap and other resampling plans, vol 38. SIAM, Philadelphia
32. Efron B, Tibshirani R (1993) An introduction to the bootstrap. Chapman & Hall/CRC, Boca Raton, FL
33. Efron B (1987) Better bootstrap confidence intervals. J Am Stat Assoc 82(397):171–185
34. Andrews DW, Buchinsky M (2000) A three-step method for choosing the number of bootstrap repetitions. Econometrica 68 (1):23–51
35. Davidson R, MacKinnon JG (2000) Bootstrap tests: how many bootstraps? Econome Rev 19(1):55–68
36. Meuwissen TH, Goddard ME (2004) Bootstrapping of gene-expression data improves and controls the false discovery rate of differentially expressed genes. Genet Sel Evol 36 (2):191–205. https://doi.org/10.1051/gse:2003058
37. Jiang W, Simon R (2007) A comparison of bootstrap methods and an adjusted bootstrap approach for estimating the prediction error in microarray classification. Stat Med 26 (29):5320–5334. https://doi.org/10.1002/sim.2968
38. Neuhauser M, Jockel KH (2006) A bootstrap test for the analysis of microarray experiments with a very small number of replications. Appl Bioinforma 5(3):173–179. doi:535 [pii]
39. Kaiser J (2007) An exact and a Monte Carlo proposal to the fisher–pitman permutation tests for paired replicates and for independent samples. Stata J 7(3):402–412
40. Tsai CA, Chen YJ, Chen JJ (2003) Testing for differentially expressed genes with microarray data. Nucleic Acids Res 31(9):e52
41. Yang H, Churchill G (2007) Estimating p-values in small microarray experiments. Bioinformatics 23(1):38–43. doi:btl548 [pii]
42. StataCorp (2013) Stata statistical software: release. StataCorp LP, College Station, TX, p 13
43. R Core Team (2016) R: a language and environment for statistical computing. R Foundation for Statistical Computing, Vienna, Austria
44. Gottardo R, Pannucci JA, Kuske CR et al (2003) Statistical analysis of microarray data: a Bayesian approach. Biostatistics 4 (4):597–620. https://doi.org/10.1093/biostatistics/4.4.597
45. Rouder JN, Speckman PL, Sun D et al (2009) Bayesian t tests for accepting and rejecting the null hypothesis. Psychon Bull Rev 16 (2):225–237. https://doi.org/10.3758/PBR.16.2.225
46. Gönen M, Johnson WO, Lu Y et al (2005) The Bayesian two-sample t test. Am Stat 59 (3):252–257
47. Wang M, Liu G (2015) A simple two-sample Bayesian t-test for hypothesis testing. Am Stat 70(2):195–201
48. Wetzels R, Raaijmakers JGW, Jakab E et al (2009) How to quantify support for and against the null hypothesis: a flexible WinBUGS implementation of a default Bayesian t test. Psychon Bull Rev 16(4):752–760. https://doi.org/10.3758/PBR.16.4.752
49. Kruschke JK (2013) Bayesian estimation supersedes the t test. J Exp Psychol Gen 142 (2):573–603. https://doi.org/10.1037/a0029146
50. Gonen M (2010) The Bayesian t-test and beyond. Methods Mol Biol 620:179–199. https://doi.org/10.1007/978-1-60761-580-4_4
51. Fox RJ, Dimmic MW (2006) A two-sample Bayesian t-test for microarray data. BMC Bioinformatics 7:126. doi:1471-2105-7-126 [pii]
52. Kooperberg C, Aragaki A, Strand AD et al (2005) Significance testing for small microarray experiments. Stat Med 24 (15):2281–2298
53. Baldi P, Long AD (2001) A Bayesian framework for the analysis of microarray expression data: regularized t -test and statistical inferences of gene changes. Bioinformatics 17 (6):509–519

54. Kayala MA, Baldi P (2012) Cyber-T web server: differential analysis of high-throughput data. Nucleic Acids Res 40(Web Server issue):W553–W559. https://doi.org/10.1093/nar/gks420
55. Lönnstedt I, Speed T (2002) Replicated microarray data. Stat Sin 12:31–46
56. Smyth GK (2005) Limma: linear models for microarray data. In: Bioinformatics and computational biology solutions using R and bioconductor. Springer, New York, pp 397–420
57. Tusher VG, Tibshirani R, Chu G (2001) Significance analysis of microarrays applied to the ionizing radiation response. Proc Natl Acad Sci U S A 98(9):5116–5121. https://doi.org/10.1073/pnas.091062498
58. Efron B, Tibshirani R, Storey JD et al (2001) Empirical Bayes analysis of a microarray experiment. J Am Stat Assoc 96(456):1151–1160
59. Tan YD, Fornage M, Fu YX (2006) Ranking analysis of microarray data: a powerful method for identifying differentially expressed genes. Genomics 88(6):846–854. doi:S0888-7543(06)00237-0 [pii]
60. McCarthy DJ, Smyth GK (2009) Testing significance relative to a fold-change threshold is a TREAT. Bioinformatics 25(6):765–771
61. Kadota K, Nakai Y, Shimizu K (2008) A weighted average difference method for detecting differentially expressed genes from microarray data. Algorithms Mol Biol 3:8. https://doi.org/10.1186/1748-7188-3-8
62. Breitling R, Armengaud P, Amtmann A et al (2004) Rank products: a simple, yet powerful, new method to detect differentially regulated genes in replicated microarray experiments. FEBS Lett 573(1-3):83–92. https://doi.org/10.1016/j.febslet.2004.07.055
63. Breitling R, Herzyk P (2005) Rank-based methods as a non-parametric alternative of the T-statistic for the analysis of biological microarray data. J Bioinforma Comput Biol 3(05):1171–1189
64. Heskes T, Eisinga R, Breitling R (2014) A fast algorithm for determining bounds and accurate approximate p-values of the rank product statistic for replicate experiments. BMC Bioinformatics 15(1):1
65. Normand SL (1999) Meta-analysis: formulating, evaluating, combining, and reporting. Stat Med 18(3):321–359
66. Ramasamy A, Mondry A, Holmes CC et al (2008) Key issues in conducting a meta-analysis of gene expression microarray datasets. PLoS Med 5(9):e184
67. Shi L, Reid LH, MACQ Consortium et al (2006) The microarray quality control (MAQC) project shows inter- and intraplatform reproducibility of gene expression measurements. Nat Biotechnol 24 (9):1151–1161. https://doi.org/10.1038/nbt1239
68. Zeeberg BR, Riss J, Kane DW et al (2004) Mistaken identifiers: gene name errors can be introduced inadvertently when using excel in bioinformatics. BMC bioinformatics 5:80. https://doi.org/10.1186/1471-2105-5-80
69. Cohen J (1988) Statistical power analysis for the behavioral sciences, 2nd edn. L. Erlbaum, Hillsdale, New Jersey
70. Petiti DB (1994) Meta-analysis decision analysis and cost-effectiveness analysis. In: Monographs in epidemiology and biostatistics, vol 24. Oxford University Press, Oxford
71. DerSimonian R, Laird N (1986) Meta-analysis in clinical trials. Control Clin Trials 7:177–188
72. Thompson SG, Sharp SJ (1999) Explaining heterogeneity in meta-analysis: a comparison of methods. Stat Med 18(20):2693–2708
73. Choi JK, Yu U, Kim S et al (2003) Combining multiple microarray studies and modeling interstudy variation. Bioinformatics 19(Suppl 1):i84–i90
74. Stevens JR, Doerge RW (2005) Combining affymetrix microarray results. BMC Bioinformatics 6:57. doi:1471-2105-6-57 [pii]
75. Hu P, Greenwood CM, Beyene J (2009) Using the ratio of means as the effect size measure in combining results of microarray experiments. BMC Syst Biol 3:106. https://doi.org/10.1186/1752-0509-3-106
76. Friedrich JO, Adhikari NK, Beyene J (2008) The ratio of means method as an alternative to mean differences for analyzing continuous outcome variables in meta-analysis: a simulation study. BMC Med Res Methodol 8(1):1
77. Friedrich JO, Adhikari NK, Beyene J (2012) Ratio of geometric means to analyze continuous outcomes in meta-analysis: comparison to mean differences and ratio of arithmetic means using empiric data and simulation. Stat Med 31(17):1857–1886. https://doi.org/10.1002/sim.4501
78. Sutton AJ, Abrams KR (2001) Bayesian methods in meta-analysis and evidence synthesis. Stat Methods Med Res 10(4):277–303
79. Conlon EM, Song JJ, Liu A (2007) Bayesian meta-analysis models for microarray data: a comparative study. BMC Bioinformatics 8:80. doi:1471-2105-8-80 [pii]

80. Conlon EM, Song JJ, Liu JS (2006) Bayesian models for pooling microarray studies with multiple sources of replications. BMC Bioinformatics 7:247. doi:1471-2105-7-247 [pii]
81. Marot G, Foulley JL, Mayer CD et al (2009) Moderated effect size and P-value combinations for microarray meta-analyses. Bioinformatics 25(20):2692–2699. https://doi.org/10.1093/bioinformatics/btp444
82. Wang X, Kang DD, Shen K et al (2012) An R package suite for microarray meta-analysis in quality control, differentially expressed gene analysis and pathway enrichment detection. Bioinformatics 28(19):2534–2536. doi: bts485 [pii]
83. Hong F, Breitling R, McEntee CW et al (2006) RankProd: a bioconductor package for detecting differentially expressed genes in meta-analysis. Bioinformatics 22 (22):2825–2827. doi:btl476 [pii]
84. Zintzaras E, Ioannidis JP (2008) Meta-analysis for ranked discovery datasets: theoretical framework and empirical demonstration for microarrays. Comput Biol Chem 32 (1):38–46. doi:S1476-9271(07)00119-3 [pii]
85. Zintzaras E, Ioannidis JP (2012) METRADISC-XL: a program for meta-analysis of multidimensional ranked discovery oriented datasets including microarrays. Comput Methods Prog Biomed 108 (3):1243–1246. https://doi.org/10.1016/j.cmpb.2012.08.001
86. Hess A, Iyer H (2007) Fisher's combined p-value for detecting differentially expressed genes using Affymetrix expression arrays. BMC Genomics 8:96. doi:1471-2164-8-96 [pii]
87. Fisher RA (1946) Statistical methods for research workers, 10th edn. Oliver and Boyd, Edinburgh
88. Jones DR (1995) Meta-analysis: weighing the evidence. Stat Med 14(2):137–149
89. Bailey TL, Gribskov M (1998) Combining evidence using p-values: application to sequence homology searches. Bioinformatics 14(1):48–54
90. Edgington ES (1972) An additive method for combining probability values from independent experiments. J Psychol 80(2):351–363
91. Edgington ES (1972) A normal curve method for combining probability values from independent experiments. J Psychol 82 (1):85–89
92. Zaykin DV, Zhivotovsky LA, Westfall PH et al (2002) Truncated product method for combining P-values. Genet Epidemiol 22 (2):170–185. https://doi.org/10.1002/gepi.0042
93. Loughin TM (2004) A systematic comparison of methods for combining p-values from independent tests. Comput Stat Data Anal 47 (3):467–485
94. Cousins RD (2007) Annotated bibliography of some papers on combining significances or p-values. arXiv preprint arXiv:07052209
95. Stouffer SA, Suchman EA, De Vinney L et al (1951) Studies in social psychology in world war II. In: The American soldier: adjustment during army life, vol Vol. 1. Princeton University Press, Princeton
96. Zhou B, Shi J, Whittemore AS (2011) Optimal methods for meta-analysis of genome-wide association studies. Genet Epidemiol 35(7):581–591. https://doi.org/10.1002/gepi.20603
97. Dudoit S, Yang YH, Callow MJ, et al (2000) Statistical methods for identifying differentially expressed genes in replicated cDNA microarray experiments. Technical report # 578
98. Sidak Z (1967) Rectangular confidence regions for the means of multivariate normal distributions. J Am Stat Assoc 62:626–633
99. Holland BS, Copenhaver MD (1987) An improved sequentially rejective bonferroni test procedure. Biometrics 43(2):417–423
100. Holm S (1979) A simple sequentially rejective multiple test procedure. Scand J Stat 6:65–70
101. Benjamini Y, Hochberg Y (1995) Controlling the false discovery rate: a practical and powerful approach to multiple testing. J R Stat Soc B Methodol 57(1):289–300
102. Benjamini Y, Yekutieli D (2001) The control of the false discovery rate in multiple testing under dependency. Ann Stat 29:1165–1188
103. Benjamini Y, Liu W (1999) A distribution-free multiple test procedure that controls the false discovery rate. Tel Aviv University, Tel Aviv
104. Benjamini Y, Liu W (1999) A step-down multiple hypotheses testing procedure that controls the false discovery rate under independence. J Stat Plan Inference 82 (1):163–170
105. Benjamini Y, Krieger AM, Yekutieli D (2006) Adaptive linear step-up procedures that control the false discovery rate. Biometrika 93 (3):491–507. https://doi.org/10.1093/biomet/93.3.491
106. Ioannidis JP, Allison DB, Ball CA et al (2009) Repeatability of published microarray gene expression analyses. Nat Genet 41 (2):149–155

107. Jarvinen AK, Hautaniemi S, Edgren H et al (2004) Are data from different gene expression microarray platforms comparable? Genomics 83(6):1164–1168. https://doi.org/10.1016/j.ygeno.2004.01.004

108. Hwang KB, Kong SW, Greenberg SA et al (2004) Combining gene expression data from different generations of oligonucleotide arrays. BMC Bioinformatics 5:159. doi:1471-2105-5-159 [pii]

109. Moreau Y, Aerts S, De Moor B et al (2003) Comparison and meta-analysis of microarray data: from the bench to the computer desk. Trends Genet 19(10):570–577. doi: S0168952503002336 [pii]

110. Chang LC, Lin HM, Sibille E et al (2013) Meta-analysis methods for combining multiple expression profiles: comparisons, statistical characterization and an application guideline. BMC Bioinformatics 14:368. https://doi.org/10.1186/1471-2105-14-368

111. Hong F, Breitling R (2008) A comparison of meta-analysis methods for detecting differentially expressed genes in microarray experiments. Bioinformatics 24(3):374–382

112. Campain A, Yang YH (2010) Comparison study of microarray meta-analysis methods. BMC Bioinformatics 11:408. https://doi.org/10.1186/1471-2105-11-408

113. Thorlund K, Wetterslev J, Awad T et al (2011) Comparison of statistical inferences from the DerSimonian–Laird and alternative random-effects model meta-analyses–an empirical assessment of 920 Cochrane primary outcome meta-analyses. Res Synth Methods 2(4):238–253

114. Abrams K, Sanso B (1998) Approximate Bayesian inference for random effects meta-analysis. Stat Med 17(2):201–218

115. Tseng GC, Ghosh D, Feingold E (2012) Comprehensive literature review and statistical considerations for microarray meta-analysis. Nucleic Acids Res 40 (9):3785–3799. https://doi.org/10.1093/nar/gkr1265

Chapter 13

A Primer in Mendelian Randomization Methodology with a Focus on Utilizing Published Summary Association Data

Niki L. Dimou and Konstantinos K. Tsilidis

Abstract

Mendelian randomization (MR) is becoming a popular approach to estimate the causal effect of an exposure on an outcome overcoming limitations of observational epidemiology. The advent of genome-wide association studies and the increasing accumulation of summarized data from large genetic consortia make MR a powerful technique. In this review, we give a primer in MR methodology, describe efficient MR designs and analytical strategies, and focus on methods and practical guidance for conducting an MR study using summary association data. We show that the analysis is straightforward utilizing either the MR-base platform or available packages in R. However, further research is required for the development of specialized methodology to assess MR assumptions.

Key words Mendelian randomization, Summarized data, Instrumental variable, Causal inference

1 Introduction

Mendelian randomization (MR) is a technique that uses genetic variants to make causal inferences about the effect of an exposure on an outcome. MR is a special case of the instrumental variable (IV) methodology, initially introduced in econometrics, where genetic variants are used as IVs [1]. This approach is based on the principle of the random assignment of an individual's genotype from his or her parental genotypes that occurs at conception, and is analogous to the random allocation of a treatment in randomized controlled trials. The reason for utilising the MR approach is to overcome residual confounding, reverse causation or exposure measurement error, which occur frequently in observational studies and may bias their results [2]. Genetic variants are, in general, not associated with environmental confounders. Reverse causality is not an issue in genetic epidemiology, as the genotype does not usually change through life. Finally, genotypes may index the tendency for

Evangelos Evangelou (ed.), *Genetic Epidemiology: Methods and Protocols*, Methods in Molecular Biology, vol. 1793, https://doi.org/10.1007/978-1-4939-7868-7_13,

lifetime concentrations of an environmental exposure and may thus circumvent exposure measurement error that is frequent when exposures are evaluated at one point in time in observational studies [3].

The use of MR is growing rapidly in popularity during the last 5 years [4]. MR studies have demonstrated causal effects of obesity and low-density lipoprotein cholesterol with cardiovascular disease, but lack of causal effects for high-density lipoprotein cholesterol and C-reactive protein [5–7]. Recent studies have also identified a number of potential causal associations between obesity and related metabolic traits with several cancers [8–11].

Many review articles on MR exist, which include descriptions of MR assumptions and evaluation methods [12–14], commentaries on available study designs [15], statistical models for deriving a causal effect [16, 17], and guidance for the reporting of the MR findings [18, 19]. Many of the aforementioned issues have been recently presented in a unified framework [20]. We seek to complement existing literature by contributing a review article to guide an interested reader to conduct an MR study with publicly available data. We begin with a general description of IV assumptions, MR statistical estimators and study designs when individual level data are available. We then switch to specific MR approaches used when summarized data are available. In particular, we describe general guidelines on the selection of IVs, statistical approaches for the estimation of causal effects and the assessment of IV assumptions. We proceed with demonstration of the MR-base platform [21], an online database of summary genetic association data and a tool to perform MR analyses, as well as popular R packages. We close with a discussion of the advantages and limitations of the MR approach.

2 IV Assumptions in MR

MR studies must fulfil IV assumptions. These assumptions are that (1) the genetic variant (G) is associated with the exposure (X); (2) the genetic variant is not associated with any confounder (U) of the exposure-outcome association; and (3) the genetic variant is conditionally independent of the outcome (Y) given the exposure and confounders (Fig. 1) [22, 23].

For the first assumption to hold, it necessitates the use of genetic variants as IVs that are strongly associated with the exposure. This is the only assumption that can be formally tested and could be satisfied if genome-wide statistically significant variants are selected as candidate IVs. The second assumption is violated if the IVs are associated with confounders, although genes are not in general correlated with environmental confounders. The third assumption implies that all causal pathways from the genetic variants to the outcome pass through the exposure, and that there are

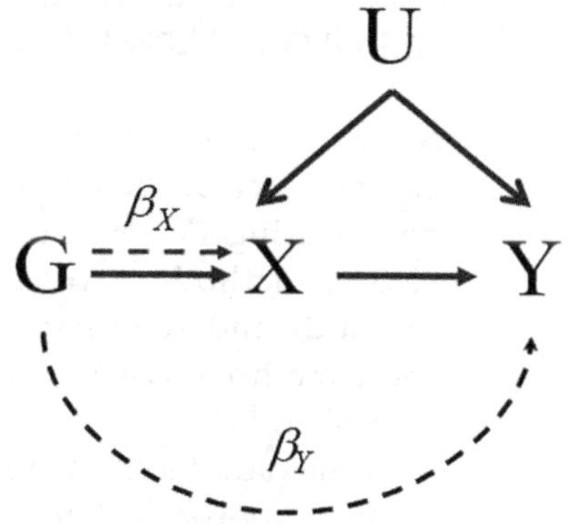

Fig. 1 Directed acyclic graph (DAG) for the instrumental variable assumptions in Mendelian randomization. The exposure (X) is causally associated with the outcome (Y) if: (1) the genetic variant (G) is associated with X; (2) G is independent of any confounding factors (U), and (3) there is no association between G and Y, except through X. The dashed lines represent the coefficient from the regression of the outcome on G (β_Y) and the coefficient from the regression of the exposure on G (β_X)

no alternative pathways [23]. The second and third assumptions are not testable, but we could get some intuition of their validity based on existing biological knowledge. The second assumption is violated when population stratification exists, which is a type of confounding due to different ancestry. It often occurs in genetic epidemiology, when the population under analysis can be decomposed into different ancestries that have different allele frequencies for the genetic variant under study and different risks for the outcome under study. The third assumption can be violated by numerous phenomena including pleiotropy, linkage disequilibrium (LD), population stratification, and gene-environment or gene-gene interactions. There is evidence in the literature that several genetic variants have pleiotropic effects, which means that they are associated with several different phenotypes. Pleiotropy is often categorized as "balanced" if the average pleiotropic effects of the IVs that contribute in an MR analysis are zero or "directional" eitherwise. LD refers to the phenomenon that some genetic variants are jointly inherited due to their physical proximity on a chromosome. Overall, there is no way to prove that the second and third MR assumptions definitively hold. However, it is often possible to find empirical evidence suggesting that the putative IVs are invalid. One of the best ways to indirectly evaluate MR assumptions is if there is high reproducibility of the MR causal estimates in different studies.

3 MR Estimators Using Individual Level Data

Several methods have been proposed for the estimation of the causal effect of the exposure on both continuous and binary outcomes using IVs, which include the ratio of the regression coefficients method, several two-stage methods, likelihood-based methods and semi-parametric models. A thorough overview of these methods as well as guidelines for their use have been recently published [17].

The ratio method, also known as the Wald method [24], is the simplest approach. The causal effect can be expressed as a ratio with nominator the coefficient from the regression of the outcome on the IV (β_Y) and denominator the coefficient from the regression of the exposure on the IV (β_X) (Fig. 1). Confidence intervals for the ratio estimator can be calculated using a normal approximation, which however may be suboptimal when normality assumptions are violated particularly when small sample sizes are available. Alternatively, one could use the Fieller's theorem (https://sb452.shinyapps.io/fieller/) [3, 25], bootstrapping [26], Anderson-Rubin test statistic [27] or the conditional likelihood ratio test statistic [28]. This approach can be extended to account for binary outcomes by simply employing log-linear or logistic regression models. The ratio method for calculating the MR estimator can be performed for single IVs. The sample size required under the ratio method for making causal inferences can be very large [29], and methods that can incorporate multiple IVs are preferable.

Two-stage methods are widely used in MR and are formulated in two separate regression stages: the first-stage involves a regression of the exposure on the IVs, and the second-stage a regression of the outcome on the predicted values of the exposure from the first stage. The first-stage regression model can incorporate multiple IVs. The causal estimate is the second-stage regression coefficient. However, although this estimate is valid, the standard error is estimated imprecisely as the variability of the first-stage regression is not accounted for. Thus, an alternative formula for the calculation of the variance of the two-stage estimator has been presented when the size of the error terms do not differ across values of the independent variables (homoscedasticity assumption) [30], or alternatively robust standard errors can be reported. Binary outcomes can also be accounted for by using log-linear or logistic regression models in the second-stage regression, although these methods have been criticized as the residuals from the second-stage regression may be correlated with the IVs [30]. Under a similar perspective, the "control function" estimator [31] follows the same principle as the two-stage estimator but also includes the estimated residuals from the first-stage regression in the second-stage.

As already pointed out, two-stage methods do not account for the variance of the first-stage regression, and likelihood-based methods are preferable since the two stages are performed simultaneously. These involve full information maximum likelihood (FIML) or limited information maximum likelihood (LIML) models [32] and Bayesian methods [33]. Finally, there are also semi-parametric methods, which make a parametric assumption for the model relating the exposure to the outcome, but make no assumption on the distribution of the errors. These methods include the generalized method of moments (GMM) [34, 35], continuous updating estimator (CUE) [36] and structural mean models (SMM) [37–39]. However, a drawback with all these semi-parametric models is that a unique causal estimate may not be estimated when binary outcomes are assessed. It should also be noted that with a single IV, causal estimates obtained via the ratio, two-stage methods, LIML, GMM and SMM coincide [17].

4 MR Study Designs Using Individual Level Data

When data on the IV(s), exposure, and outcome are available for all participants in a single sample, estimation of the causal effect is straightforward using the appropriate method(s) described in the previous sections. However, in practice, in the era of large scale genome-wide association studies (GWAS), exposure data may not always be available. This may be the case, when the exposure is a biomarker difficult or prohibitively expensive to measure in tens of thousands of disease cases and controls. Therefore, efficient designs of MR studies were recently proposed [40]. A "subsample" IV estimation design can be used, when data on the IV-exposure association are available for a subset of participants but data on the IV-outcome association are available for all participants in the same dataset. A "two-sample" IV estimation design can also be used, when data for the association between the IV and exposure and the IV and outcome are available from different independent datasets. Simulation studies suggest that subsample IV designs obtain statistical power estimates comparable with studies with complete exposure data [40]. In particular, it was shown that power exceeds 90% even when exposure data was available for 20% of the total sample size. Overall, power for MR studies is most efficiently increased by increasing the sample size of the gene-outcome association. Employing two-sample designs does not result in efficiency loss under the assumption that the two samples are selected randomly from the same underlying population.

5 MR Estimators Using Summary Association Data

In the previous sections, we discussed MR study designs and estimation methods of the causal effect when individual level data on the genetic variant(s), exposure and outcome are available. If individual-level data are not available, then valid statistical inference can still be obtained from summarized data on the associations between the genetic variants with the exposure and the outcome. The increasing number of publicly available summary data from GWAS is a valuable source for estimating the causal effect of the exposure on an outcome with greater precision. By using summarized data, one can avoid additional complications arising from confidentiality agreements, especially when it comes to large consortia. Moreover, accumulating evidence from GWAS involving multiple genetic variants can be used to derive an overall causal effect more efficiently [41]. Efficient designs described in Sect. 4 could be adopted. The subsequent sections will focus on details for designing and conducting summary data MR studies.

5.1 Selection of the IVs

Genetic variants used as IVs are selected on the basis of a strong association with the exposure of interest. Robustly and highly statistically significant variants can be selected if individual level data are available from GWAS. Alternatively, the GWAS Catalog, which is a curated repository of accumulating evidence from publicly available GWAS, is a valuable source for identifying summary gene-exposure associations [42]. There is a trade-off in including only genetic variants as IVs with a genome-wide significant association with the exposure, risking an underpowered estimate, or including all available variants with any association with the exposure, risking a biased estimate due to potential violation of the third MR assumption. The current safest recommendation is to select instruments that are genome-wide significantly associated with the exposure.

5.2 Estimation Methods

Two main statistical methods have been proposed for the estimation of causal effects when summarized data are available: the likelihood-based method and the inverse-variance weighted (IVW) method [43].

Let us denote the estimate of association for the genetic variant $k = 1,\ldots,K$ with the exposure by $\widehat{\beta}_{Xk}$ with standard error σ_{Xk}, and the estimate of association with the outcome by $\widehat{\beta}_{Yk}$ with standard error σ_{Yk}. Under the likelihood-based method assuming linearity of the exposure-outcome association, the causal effect $\left(\widehat{\beta}_L\right)$ is estimated by the following model:

$$\begin{aligned} \widehat{\beta}_{Xk} &\sim N(\xi_k, \sigma^2_{Xk}) \\ \widehat{\beta}_{Yk} &\sim N(\beta_L \xi_k, \sigma^2_{Yk}) \end{aligned} \tag{1}$$

The parameters of the model in Eq. (1) can be estimated under standard likelihood or Bayesian approaches. This basic model is valid for two-sample designs. Modification is required to account for the correlation structure of gene-exposure and gene-outcome associations if they are estimated in the same or overlapping participants [43].

Another approach is based on the idea to combine the ratio estimates of the causal effects $\frac{\widehat{\beta_{Yk}}}{\beta_{Xk}}$ from each genetic variant by employing an IVW meta-analysis [44]. The variance of the ratio estimate can be approximately estimated using the Delta method, as $\frac{\sigma^2_{Yk}}{\widehat{\beta^2_{Xk}}}$ [45]. Further terms could be also incorporated to account for the uncertainty in the gene-exposure association. Thus, the IVW estimate can be expressed as:

$$\widehat{\beta}_{\mathrm{IVW}} = \frac{\sum_k \widehat{\beta}_{Xk} \widehat{\beta}_{Yk} \sigma^{-2}_{Yk}}{\sum_k \widehat{\beta}^2_{Xk} \sigma^{-2}_{Yk}} \tag{2}$$

with an approximated standard error given by:

$$\mathrm{se}(\widehat{\beta}_{\mathrm{IVW}}) = \sqrt{\frac{1}{\sum_k \widehat{\beta}^2_{Xk} \sigma^{-2}_{Yk}}} \tag{3}$$

Thus, the IVW method is a weighted average of the causal effects derived from the genetic variants k. Of course, if only one IV is available Eq. (2) is simplified to the classical ratio estimator. If the IVs are not in LD (uncorrelated IVs), the causal estimate obtained from the IVW method is equivalent to a two-stage approach using individual-level data. This basic model assumes that any differences in the causal estimates derived from multiple IVs can be explained by their variances, as these are assumed to represent the same underlying quantity (homogeneity assumption). This assumption can be tested using the classical Cohran's Q heterogeneity statistic.

Both the likelihood-based and the IVW methods assume that gene-gene interactions among the selected IVs are negligible and that the IVs are not in LD. Extensive simulation studies reveal that gene-gene interactions have little impact on the estimates obtained using summarized data MR methods [43]. On the other hand, when correlated variants are used as IVs the standard errors are underestimated, which may result in invalid statistical inferences. This warrants the need of statistical approaches that account for the correlation structure of the IVs [16]. Overall, the estimates obtained from the likelihood-based approach including robustly associated variants that are not in LD are unbiased and precise when compared against those derived by employing two-stage methods using individual-level data. The IVW approach also gives similar point estimates to two-stage methods [43].

The IVW and likelihood-based approaches are based on the idea to synthesize separate causal effects derived from multiple IVs in order to derive an overall causal estimate. Another perspective could be to combine multiple IVs and construct an allele score [46]. Unweighted or weighted scores can be constructed, and it has been shown that both approaches give unbiased results [46]. Formulas for the calculation of allele score based methods using summarized data have been presented and bias can be avoided if weights from an external population are used [47]. Allele scores accounting for variants in LD have been recently described allowing for the inclusion of multiple correlated IVs that further increase power of the causal estimates [47]. However, caution on the interpretation of the findings is necessary if the allele score is composed of invalid IVs. We conclude that synthesizing evidence using summarized data is a good compromise if individual-level data are not available.

5.3 Assessing IV Assumptions

We have discussed MR methods for estimating causal effects using summary association data. Here, we discuss methods that are used for assessing the validity of IV assumptions and present robust estimation methods that account for pleiotropy. Assessing IV assumptions is particularly challenging when individual level data are not available. To secure the non-violation of the first assumption of MR, genetic variants are selected that are robustly associated with the exposure of interest in GWAS. The strength of an instrument can be evaluated using the F statistic in the regression of the exposure on the IV [48]. In the case of summary data, $F = \frac{N-K-1}{K}\frac{R^2}{1-R^2}$, with R^2 approximately equal to $2\widehat{\beta}_{Xk} \times MAF\times (1 - MAF)$, where N is the sample size, K is the number of genetic variants, R^2 the proportion of the variance of the exposure explained by the IV and MAF the minor allele frequency. Thus, the F-statistic depends on the sample size, the number of IVs, MAF and the proportion of the variance explained by the IVs. If F is less than 10, this is an indication of weak instrument(s) [49]. However, this value is arbitrary and is valid only for two-stage methods [50]; it fluctuates according to the sample size and is calculated post-hoc [51]. Alternatively, the instrument strength could be quantified by a modification of the classical I^2 statistic [52], which is termed ${I_{GX}}^2$ [53] attributing the excess of variability of gene-exposure associations to measurement error. This statistic fluctuates from

0 to 1, and a value of 0.9 is equivalent to an F statistic of 10. The second assumption is testable only for known confounders. If summarized data are available, this assumption could be at least partially tested acquiring information from the literature or from checking for possible associations between the selected IVs and known confounders in the GWAS Catalogue [42].

Although the inclusion of multiple IVs derived from published GWAS can increase power to detect causal effects, it is more likely to introduce bias due to violation of the third MR assumption [46]. If the distinct causal estimates derived from each genetic variant differ, this may be an indication of pleiotropic effects. Formal statistical tests exist to test for those discrepancies including the classical Cohran's Q statistic, the I^2 statistic [54] or likelihood ratio tests. Heterogenous effects could also be detected by plotting causal estimates from the each included IV.

Moreover, pleiotropy could be tested applying the MR-Egger regression method [55]. We move back to the IVW estimate of Eq. (2), which is equivalent to fitting a weighted linear regression of the associations of the IVs with the outcome on the IVs with the exposure with no intercept term. This analysis assumes that all IVs are valid and no pleiotropic effects exist. The classical IVW method is a good fit only if pleiotropy is balanced. In order to account for directional pleiotropic effects, one could reformulate the aforementioned regression model with no constraint on the intercept term resulting in the so-called MR-Egger regression method [55]. This intercept term captures the average pleiotropic effects of the IVs and values away from zero are an indication of directional pleiotropy. The slope of the MR-Egger regression is a robust estimate of the causal effect. This approach assumes that the pleiotropic effects of the IVs on the outcome are distributed independently of the associations of the IVs with the exposure (InSIDE assumption). The InSIDE assumption is more likely to be satisfied if IVs are not associated with a confounder of the exposure-outcome association. An additional assumption that is required to hold is the so-called "NO Measurement Error" (NOME) where the variance of the IV-exposure association is negligible [43, 56]. In a two-sample MR design, violation of the NOME assumption results in underestimated causal effects and other approaches have been proposed [53], such as the simulation extrapolation approach (SIMEX) [57]. A limitation of the MR-Egger regression is the lack of power and poor performance when few instruments are used. MR-Egger regression is also more sensitive to the InSIDE assumption violation than IVW. Besides, the confidence intervals when the causal effect is not null are not precisely estimated and over-interpretation should be avoided.

Another robust method to account for directional pleiotropy is based on the simple idea to order the ratio estimates of the *k* genetic variants and report the median [58], which assumes that at least 50% of the variants are valid. The InSIDE assumption is not necessary. Violations of the second and the third assumptions are also allowed. One could also derive a weighted median estimate assigning weights proportionally to the precision of the causal estimate derived from each IV [59]. This approach requires at least 50% of the weights to originate from valid IVs. Simulation studies reveal that the weighted median approach results in more precise estimates, when compared against the MR-Egger regression method [59]. Extensions of the classical additive or multiplicative random effects models used in meta-analysis can accommodate both balanced and directional pleiotropy [60].

Statistical tests for assessing pleiotropy could be further enriched graphically. A typical graph presented in MR studies is to plot the gene-outcome against the gene-exposure associations. If pleiotropy is absent, we expect that a variant's association with outcome is proportional to its association with exposure, and therefore the plotted points fall along a line that passes through the origin and has a slope equal to the MR estimate. Additionally, one could create a funnel plot of the reciprocal of the standard error versus the MR causal estimate and check for any asymmetry.

Another aspect in an MR setting is that estimation methods of the causal effects assume linearity of the exposure-outcome association. This is important and most MR investigations do not check this, but future MR studies should check first if exposure-outcome relationships derived from multi-SNP scores are linear before using the suggested estimation methods.

5.4 MR in Practice

In this section we will describe step by step how one can perform an MR study using publicly available summary data. We will focus on the two most popular options, the MR-base platform (http://www.mrbase.org/) [21] and the MendelianRandomization package in R. MR-base is a database and an online platform that allows the user to run a two-sample MR analysis. Currently, it is a collective repertoire of 'complete summary data' from 1094 GWAS analyses from 44 consortia with approximately 4 billion associations between SNPs and phenotypes (i.e., diseases, risk factors, metabolites and immune system traits). This database populates information not only from the GWAS Catalog [42], but also gene expression quantitative trait loci (QTLs) [61], methylation level QTLs [62], metabolite level QTLs [63] and protein level QTLs [64]. In the first step, one has to select the exposure of interest from the appropriate source (GWAS catalog, gene expression QTLs, etc.), and robustly associated IVs (with the exposure) are extracted with respect to a p-value threshold for inclusion and/or LD threshold for pruning IVs that can be modified by the user. Alternatively, the user can upload a specific list of IVs manually with pre-calculated effect sizes and standard errors. In a second step, the user chooses the outcome of interest. For instance, if we were interested in testing the causal association of body mass index (exposure) and lung cancer (outcome), originally published by Carreras-Torres and coworkers [8], we would select IVs for the exposure from the Genetic Investigation of ANthropometric Traits (GIANT) consortium and for the outcome from the International Lung Cancer Consortium (ILCCO) by clicking on the respective GWAS [65, 66]. The platform also offers the functionality to use proxies if a particular IV is not present, harmonise gene-exposure and gene-outcome effect alleles to ensure a common effect allele is used in both associations, and correct for palindromic SNPs. The user then selects the method of analysis (e.g., IVW, maximum likelihood, etc.) and is navigated to the results window. One can retrieve summary information on the studies used for the exposure and outcome associations, the number of variants extracted, and the MR causal estimates from each predefined method. The presence of pleiotropy can be evaluated using the reported heterogeneity statistics and the p-value of the intercept from the MR-Egger regression method. Using the example of body mass index and risk of lung cancer, we retrieved a total of 79 IVs using default settings (i.e., p-value threshold for including IVs at 5×10^{-8}, LD R^2 values for pruning IVs at 0.001, clumping distance at 10.000, LD R^2 values for proxies at 0.8 and a MAF threshold for aligning palindromes at 0.3). None of the IVW, MR-Egger or weighted median approaches yielded statistically significant causal estimates. There was some evidence for heterogeneity, but evidence for directional pleiotropy was not present. We urge investigators to check for associations of the selected IVs with known confounders such as smoking in the particular example, and re-evaluate MR estimates after excluding those variants. Four plots are also available (i.e., causal effects calculated from each IV, IV-outcome associations against IV-exposure, causal effects derived removing one IV sequentially and a funnel plot of the reciprocal of the standard error versus the MR causal estimate). MR results and associated plots can also be converted in an HTML format. An interested researcher can alternatively use the TwoSampleMR package in R to perform the analysis (Box 1).

Box 1. Estimating causal association of body mass index with lung cancer using TwoSampleMR R package.

```
# Load TwoSampleMR R package:
. library(TwoSampleMR)
# Obtain data from MR Base GWAS database:
. ao<- available_outcomes()
# Extract IVs for an exposure, for example to obtain IVs for body mass index
using Locke et al. 2015 GIANT study, specifying the study ID:
. exposure_dat<- extract_instruments(ao$id[c(2)])
*Options are also available:
p1 = P-value threshold for keeping a SNP (default=5e-08)
clump = Whether or not to return independent SNPs only (default=TRUE)
r2 = The maximum LD R-square allowed between returned SNPs (default=0.001)
kb = The distance in which to search for LD R-square values (default=10.000)
# Extract IVs for an outcome, for example to obtain IVs for lung cancer
using Wang et al. 2014 ILCCO study, specifying the study ID, LD Rsq values
for proxies at 0.8 and a MAF threshold for aligning palindromes at 0.3:
. outcome_dat<- extract_outcome_data(exposure_dat$SNP, c(966), proxies = 1,
rsq = 0.8, align_alleles = 1, palindromes = 1, maf_threshold = 0.3)
# Harmonise exposure-outcome data to match the same reference allele,
inferring forward strand using allele frequency:
. dat<- harmonise_data(exposure_dat, outcome_dat, action = 2)
# Perform an MR analysis:
. mr_results<- mr(dat)
## Sensitivity analyses:
# Obtain heterogeneity statistics:
. mr_heterogeneity<- mr_heterogeneity(dat)
# Test for directional pleiotropy:
. mr_pleiotropy_test<- mr_pleiotropy_test(dat)
# Obtain MR estimates for each of the selected IVs:
```

```
. res_single<- mr_singlesnp(dat)

# Obtain MR estimates excluding one IV at a time:

. res_loo<- mr_leaveoneout(dat)

## Creating plots:

# Create scatter plot of IV-outcome associations against IV-exposure:

. p1<- mr_scatter_plot(mr_result, dat)

# Create forest plot of causal effects calculated from each IV:

. p2<- mr_forest_plot(res_single)

# Create plot of causal effects derived removing one IV sequentially:

. p3<- mr_leaveoneout_plot(res_loo)

# Create funnel plot of of the reciprocal of the standard error versus the

MR causal estimate:

. p4<- mr_funnel_plot(res_single)
```

Another option is to use the MendelianRandomization package in R. This package offers the extra functionality to model the correlation of IVs that are in LD which is not feasible via the TwoSampleMR package. Moreover, overlapping samples for estimating IV-exposure and IV-outcome associations can be accounted for. The I_{GX}^2 statistic [53] can be also calculated in order to measure the instrument strength. The user has to specify appropriately vectors including IV-exposure and IV-outcome beta estimates along with their standard errors and this information is not automatically retrieved as in MR-base. However, the authors are willing to directly import information from genetic association studies available in PhenoScanner (http://phenoscanner.medschl.cam.ac.uk) in the package in the near future. Optionally, names of the genetic variants, effect or non-effect alleles and effect allele frequencies can be provided by the user. For demonstration purposes, we reanalysed the harmonised data extracted from the MR Base for estimating the potential causal association of body mass index with lung cancer risk assuming that IVs are independent (Box 2).

Box 2.Estimating causal association of body mass index with lung cancer using MendelianRandomization R package.

```
# Load MendelianRandomzation R package:
. library(MendelianRandomization)
# Create MRInput object from the harmonised body mass index using Locke et
al. 2015 GIANT study and lung cancer using Wang et al. 2014 ILCCO study
obtained from MR Base GWAS database:
. MRInputObject <- mr_input(bx = dat$beta.exposure, bxse = dat$se.exposure,
by = dat$beta.outcome, byse = dat$se.outcome,exposure = "Body mass index",
outcome = "Lung cancer", snps = dat$SNP)
# Run IVW MR method:
. IVW<- mr_ivw(MRInputObject,
model = "default",
robust = FALSE,
penalized = FALSE,
weights = "simple",
distribution = "normal",
alpha = 0.05)
*Options for IVW method:
model = "default", "random" or "fixed" (default=fixed-effect with 3 IVs or
fewer)
robust = robust instead of standard regression can be performed
(default=FALSE)
penalized = penalty can be applied to downweight the contribution of genetic
variants with outlying ratio estimates (default=FALSE)
weights = "simple" or "delta", the latter option uses the delta method to
calculate the variance of the ratio estimates (default=simple)
distribution = "normal" or "t-dist" (default=normal)
# Run MR Egger method:
. Egger<- mr_egger(MRInputObject,
```

```
                          robust = FALSE,
                          penalized = FALSE,
                          distribution = "normal",
                          alpha = 0.05)
*Options as in IVW method
# Run ML method:
. MaxLik<- mr_maxlik(MRInputObject,
                            model = "default",
                            distribution = "normal",
                            alpha = 0.05)
*Options as in IVW method
# Run Median based method:
. Median<- mr_median(MRInputObject,
                                    weighting = "weighted",
                                    distribution = "normal",
                                    alpha = 0.05,
                                    iterations = 10000,
                                    seed = 314159265)
*Options for median based methods:
weighting = "simple", "weighted" or "penalized" (default=weighted)
distribution = "normal" or "t-dist" (default=normal)
iterations = bootstrap samples for calculating standard errors
(default=10000)
seed = seed to use when generating bootstrap samples (default=314159265)
# Run all methods:
. MR_all<- mr_allmethods(MRInputObject, method = "all")
## Creating plots:
# Create scatter plot of IV-outcome associations against IV-exposure:
. p<- mr_plot(MRInputObject,
error = TRUE,
orientate = FALSE,
```

```
interactive = TRUE,

labels = TRUE,

line = "ivw")

*Options for scatter plot:

error = include error bars (default=TRUE)

orientate = convert negative gene-exposure associations to positive (default=FALSE)

interactive = produces interactive plots (default=TRUE)

labels = displays IV labels (default=FALSE)

line = "ivw" or "egger" (default=ivw)
```

6 Discussion

MR is a powerful approach for deriving causal inferences about the effect of an exposure on an outcome overcoming limitations of observational epidemiology (i.e., confounding and reverse causation). As the sharing of summary data from consortia becomes common practice, numerous genetic variants can be utilized as possible IVs resulting in greater efficiency and more powerful causal estimates. We described the methods for conducting an MR study using summary association data and provided practical guidance using available software.

The MR methodology has great promise for advancing biomedical research, but is also subject to assumptions and limitations caused by unsuitable IVs, population stratification, LD and pleiotropy. We showed that MR assumptions are difficult to be evaluated when individual level data are available, which becomes even more difficult when only summary association data are available. MR is a relatively new field, and additional methodology is warranted to increase the sensitivity and power to detect potential violation of IV assumptions. For instance, MR methods that allow for automatic identification of specific genetic variants with pleiotropic effects that could be excluded from subsequent analysis could strengthen the MR approach. Moreover, selected genetic variants usually explain a small proportion of the variance in the different exposures. Given that many of these environmental exposures/traits are highly heritable, further work using additional genetic variants as instruments, when they become available from future GWAS, will increase power of MR studies and will allow investigations in subgroups. As in all science, replication of results from MR studies is vital.

Acknowledgements

NLD was supported by the IKY scholarship programme, which is co-financed by the European Union (European Social Fund - ESF) and Greek national funds through the action entitled "Reinforcement of Postdoctoral Researchers" in the framework of the Operational Programme "Human Resources Development Program, Education and Lifelong Learning" of the National Strategic Reference Framework (NSRF) 2014 – 2020. KKT was supported by the World Cancer Research Fund International Regular Grant Programme (WCRF 2014/1180).

References

1. Thomas DC, Conti DV (2004) Commentary: the concept of 'Mendelian Randomization'. Int J Epidemiol 33(1):21–25. https://doi.org/10.1093/ije/dyh048
2. Smith GD, Ebrahim S (2003) Mendelian randomization': can genetic epidemiology contribute to understanding environmental determinants of disease? Int J Epidemiol 32 (1):1–22
3. Lawlor DA, Harbord RM, Sterne JA et al (2008) Mendelian randomization: using genes as instruments for making causal inferences in epidemiology. Stat Med 27 (8):1133–1163. https://doi.org/10.1002/sim.3034
4. Bochud M, Rousson V (2010) Usefulness of Mendelian randomization in observational epidemiology. Int J Environ Res Public Health 7 (3):711–728. https://doi.org/10.3390/ijerph7030711
5. Burgess S, Butterworth A, Malarstig A et al (2012) Use of Mendelian randomisation to assess potential benefit of clinical intervention. BMJ 345:e7325. https://doi.org/10.1136/bmj.e7325
6. Kivimaki M, Smith GD, Timpson NJ et al (2008) Lifetime body mass index and later atherosclerosis risk in young adults: examining causal links using Mendelian randomization in the cardiovascular risk in young finns study. Eur Heart J 29(20):2552–2560. https://doi.org/10.1093/eurheartj/ehn252
7. Voight BF, Peloso GM, Orho-Melander M et al (2012) Plasma HDL cholesterol and risk of myocardial infarction: a mendelian randomisation study. Lancet 380(9841):572–580. https://doi.org/10.1016/S0140-6736(12)60312-2
8. Carreras-Torres R, Haycock PC, Relton CL et al (2016) The causal relevance of body mass index in different histological types of lung cancer: a Mendelian randomization study. Sci Rep 6:31121. https://doi.org/10.1038/srep31121
9. Dixon SC, Nagle CM, Thrift AP et al (2016) Adult body mass index and risk of ovarian cancer by subtype: a Mendelian randomization study. Int J Epidemiol 45(3):884–895. https://doi.org/10.1093/ije/dyw158
10. Gao C, Patel CJ, Michailidou K et al (2016) Genetically predicted body mass index and breast cancer risk: mendelian randomization analyses of data from 145,000 women of European descent. PLoS Med 13(8): e1002105. https://doi.org/10.1371/journal.pmed.1002105
11. Guo Y, Warren Andersen S, Shu XO et al (2016) Genetically predicted body mass index and breast cancer risk: mendelian randomization analyses of data from 145,000 women of European descent. PLoS Med 13(8): e1002105. https://doi.org/10.1371/journal.pmed.1002105
12. Didelez V, Sheehan N (2007) Mendelian randomization as an instrumental variable approach to causal inference. Stat Methods Med Res 16(4):309–330. https://doi.org/10.1177/0962280206077743
13. Glymour MM, Tchetgen Tchetgen EJ, Robins JM (2012) Credible Mendelian randomization studies: approaches for evaluating the instrumental variable assumptions. Am J Epidemiol 175(4):332–339. https://doi.org/10.1093/aje/kwr323
14. Hernan MA, Robins JM (2006) Instruments for causal inference: an epidemiologist's dream? Epidemiology 17(4):360–372. https://doi.org/10.1097/01.ede.0000222409.00878.37

15. Lawlor DA (2016) Commentary: two-sample Mendelian randomization: opportunities and challenges. Int J Epidemiol 45(3):908–915. https://doi.org/10.1093/ije/dyw127
16. Burgess S, Scott RA, Timpson NJ et al (2015) Using published data in Mendelian randomization: a blueprint for efficient identification of causal risk factors. Eur J Epidemiol 30 (7):543–552. https://doi.org/10.1007/s10654-015-0011-z
17. Burgess S, Small DS, Thompson SG (2015) A review of instrumental variable estimators for Mendelian randomization. Stat Methods Med Res. https://doi.org/10.1177/0962280215597579
18. Boef AG, Dekkers OM, le Cessie S (2015) Mendelian randomization studies: a review of the approaches used and the quality of reporting. Int J Epidemiol 44(2):496–511. https://doi.org/10.1093/ije/dyv071
19. Davies NM, Smith GD, Windmeijer F et al (2013) Issues in the reporting and conduct of instrumental variable studies: a systematic review. Epidemiology 24(3):363–369. https://doi.org/10.1097/EDE.0b013e31828abafb
20. Haycock PC, Burgess S, Wade KH et al (2016) Best (but oft-forgotten) practices: the design, analysis, and interpretation of Mendelian randomization studies. Am J Clin Nutr 103 (4):965–978. https://doi.org/10.3945/ajcn.115.118216
21. Hemani G, Zheng J, Wade KH et al (2016) MR-base: a platform for systematic causal inference across the phenome using billions of genetic associations. bioRxivr. https://doi.org/10.1101/078972
22. Greenland S (2000) An introduction to instrumental variables for epidemiologists. Int J Epidemiol 29(4):722–729
23. Martens EP, Pestman WR, de Boer A et al (2006) Instrumental variables: application and limitations. Epidemiology 17(3):260–267. https://doi.org/10.1097/01.ede.0000215160.88317.cb
24. Wald A (1940) The fitting of straight lines if both variables are subject to error. Ann Math Stat 11(3):284–300
25. Fieller E (1954) Some problems in interval estimation. J R Stat Soc Series B Stat Methodology 16(2):175–185
26. Efron B, Tibshirani R (1993) An introduction to the bootstrap. Chapman & Hall/CRC Press, Boca Raton, Florida
27. Anderson T, Rubin H (1949) Estimators of the parameters of a single equation in a complete set of stochastic equations. Ann Mathe Stat 21 (1):570–582
28. Moreira M (2003) A conditional likelihood ratio test for structural models. Econometrica 71(4):1027–1048
29. Ebrahim S, Davey Smith G (2008) Mendelian randomization: can genetic epidemiology help redress the failures of observational epidemiology? Hum Genet 123(1):15–33. https://doi.org/10.1007/s00439-007-0448-6
30. Angrist J, Pischke J (2009) Mostly harmless econometrics: an empiricist's companion. Chapter 4: instrumental variables in action: sometimes you get what you need. Princeton University Press, Princeton, New Jersey
31. Nagelkerke N, Fidler V, Bernsen R et al (2000) Estimating treatment effects in randomized clinical trials in the presence of non-compliance. Stat Med 19(14):1849–1864
32. Davidson R, MacKinnon J (1993) Estimation and inference in econometrics. Chapter 18: simultaneous equation models. Oxford University Press, Oxford
33. Kleibergen F, Zivot E (2003) Bayesian and classical approaches to instrumental variable regression. J Econom 114:29–72
34. Foster E (1997) Instrumental variables for logistic regression: an illustration. Soc Sci Res 26(4):487–504
35. Johnston KM, Gustafson P, Levy AR et al (2008) Use of instrumental variables in the analysis of generalized linear models in the presence of unmeasured confounding with applications to epidemiological research. Stat Med 27(9):1539–1556. https://doi.org/10.1002/sim.3036
36. Hansen LP, Heaton J, Yaron A (1996) Finite-sample properties of some alternative GMM estimators. J Bus Econ Stat 14(3):262–280
37. Bowden J, Vansteelandt S (2011) Mendelian randomization analysis of case-control data using structural mean models. Stat Med 30 (6):678–694. https://doi.org/10.1002/sim.4138
38. Greenland S, Lanes S, Jara M (2008) Estimating effects from randomized trials with discontinuations: the need for intent-to-treat design and G-estimation. Clin Trials 5(1):5–13. https://doi.org/10.1177/1740774507087703
39. Robins J (1986) A new approach to causal inference in mortality studies with a sustained exposure period–application to control of the healthy worker survivor effect. Math Model 7 (9–12):1393–1512
40. Pierce BL, Burgess S (2013) Efficient design for Mendelian randomization studies:

subsample and 2-sample instrumental variable estimators. Am J Epidemiol 178 (7):1177–1184. https://doi.org/10.1093/aje/kwt084

41. Pierce BL, Ahsan H, Vanderweele TJ (2011) Power and instrument strength requirements for Mendelian randomization studies using multiple genetic variants. Int J Epidemiol 40 (3):740–752. https://doi.org/10.1093/ije/dyq151
42. Welter D, MacArthur J, Morales J et al (2014) The NHGRI GWAS catalog, a curated resource of SNP-trait associations. Nucleic Acids Res 42 (Database issue):D1001–D1006. https://doi.org/10.1093/nar/gkt1229
43. Burgess S, Butterworth A, Thompson SG (2013) Mendelian randomization analysis with multiple genetic variants using summarized data. Genet Epidemiol 37(7):658–665. https://doi.org/10.1002/gepi.21758
44. Johnson T (2011) Conditional and joint multiple-SNP analysis of GWAS summary statistics identifies additional variants influencing complex traits. Technical report, Queen Mary University of London
45. Thomas DC, Lawlor DA, Thompson JR (2007) Re: estimation of bias in nongenetic observational studies using "Mendelian triangulation" by Bautista et al. Ann Epidemiol 17 (7):511–513. https://doi.org/10.1016/j.annepidem.2006.12.005
46. Burgess S, Thompson SG (2013) Use of allele scores as instrumental variables for Mendelian randomization. Int J Epidemiol 42 (4):1134–1144. https://doi.org/10.1093/ije/dyt093
47. Burgess S, Dudbridge F, Thompson SG (2016) Combining information on multiple instrumental variables in Mendelian randomization: comparison of allele score and summarized data methods. Stat Med 35 (11):1880–1906. https://doi.org/10.1002/sim.6835
48. Stock J, Wright J, Yogo M (2002) A survey of weak instruments and weak identification in generalized method of moments. J Bus Econ Stat 20(4):518–529
49. Staiger D, Stock J (1997) Instrumental variables regression with weak instruments. Econometrica 65(3):557–586
50. Burgess S, Granell R, Palmer TM et al (2014) Lack of identification in semiparametric instrumental variable models with binary outcomes. Am J Epidemiol 180(1):111–119. https://doi.org/10.1093/aje/kwu107
51. Burgess S, Thompson SG, CRP CHD Genetics Collaboration (2011) Avoiding bias from weak instruments in Mendelian randomization studies. Int J Epidemiol 40(3):755–764. https://doi.org/10.1093/ije/dyr036
52. Higgins JP, Thompson SG, Deeks JJ et al (2003) Measuring inconsistency in meta-analyses. BMJ 327(7414):557–560. https://doi.org/10.1136/bmj.327.7414.557
53. Bowden J, Del Greco MF, Minelli C et al (2016) Assessing the suitability of summary data for two-sample Mendelian randomization analyses using MR-egger regression: the role of the I2 statistic. Int J Epidemiol 45 (6):1961–1974. https://doi.org/10.1093/ije/dyw220
54. Greco MF, Minelli C, Sheehan NA et al (2015) Detecting pleiotropy in Mendelian randomisation studies with summary data and a continuous outcome. Stat Med 34(21):2926–2940. https://doi.org/10.1002/sim.6522
55. Bowden J, Davey Smith G, Burgess S (2015) Mendelian randomization with invalid instruments: effect estimation and bias detection through egger regression. Int J Epidemiol 44 (2):512–525. https://doi.org/10.1093/ije/dyv080
56. Brion MJ, Shakhbazov K, Visscher PM (2013) Calculating statistical power in Mendelian randomization studies. Int J Epidemiol 42 (5):1497–1501. https://doi.org/10.1093/ije/dyt179
57. Cook JR, Stefanski LA (1994) Simulation-extrapolation estimation in parametric measurement error models. J Am Stat Assoc 89 (428):1314–1328. https://doi.org/10.2307/2290994
58. Han C (2008) Detecting invalid instruments using L1-GMM. Econ Lett 101(3):285–287
59. Bowden J, Davey Smith G, Haycock PC et al (2016) Consistent estimation in mendelian randomization with some invalid instruments using a weighted median estimator. Genet Epidemiol 40(4):304–314. https://doi.org/10.1002/gepi.21965
60. Bowden J, Del Greco MF, Minelli C et al (2017) A framework for the investigation of pleiotropy in two-sample summary data Mendelian randomization. Stat Med. https://doi.org/10.1002/sim.7221
61. GTEx Consortium (2015) Human genomics. The genotype-tissue expression (GTEx) pilot analysis: multitissue gene regulation in humans. Science 348(6235):648–660. https://doi.org/10.1126/science.1262110
62. Gaunt TR, Shihab HA, Hemani G et al (2016) Systematic identification of genetic influences on methylation across the human life course.

Genome Biol 17:61. https://doi.org/10.1186/s13059-016-0926-z

63. Kettunen J, Demirkan A, Wurtz P et al (2016) Genome-wide study for circulating metabolites identifies 62 loci and reveals novel systemic effects of LPA. Nat Commun 7:11122. https://doi.org/10.1038/ncomms11122
64. Deming Y, Xia J, Cai Y et al (2016) Genetic studies of plasma analytes identify novel potential biomarkers for several complex traits. Sci Rep 6:18092. https://doi.org/10.1038/srep18092
65. Locke AE, Kahali B, Berndt SI et al (2015) Genetic studies of body mass index yield new insights for obesity biology. Nature 518 (7538):197–206. https://doi.org/10.1038/nature14177
66. Wang Y, McKay JD, Rafnar T et al (2014) Rare variants of large effect in BRCA2 and CHEK2 affect risk of lung cancer. Nat Genet 46 (7):736–741. https://doi.org/10.1038/ng.3002

Chapter 14

Copy Number Variation

Aurélien Macé, Zoltán Kutalik, and Armand Valsesia

Abstract

Differences between genomes can be due to single nucleotide variants (SNPs), translocations, inversions and copy number variants (CNVs, gain or loss of DNA). The latter can range from sub-microscopic events to complete chromosomal aneuploidies. Small CNVs are often benign but those larger than 250 kb are strongly associated with morbid consequences such as developmental disorders and cancer. Detecting CNVs within and between populations is essential to better understand the plasticity of our genome and to elucidate its possible contribution to disease or phenotypic traits.

While the link between SNPs and disease susceptibility has been well studied, to date there are still very few published CNV genome-wide association studies; probably owing to the fact that CNV analysis remains a slightly more complex task than SNP analysis (both in term of bioinformatics workflow and uncertainty in the CNV calling leading to high false positive rates and unknown false negative rates). This chapter aims at explaining computational methods for the analysis of CNVs, ranging from study design, data processing and quality control, up to genome-wide association study with clinical traits.

Key words Copy number variation, DNA, Duplication, Deletion, Structural variation, Genome-wide association studies, Human genetics, Human disease

1 Introduction

Genetic variations in the human genome take many forms ranging from large chromosomal anomalies (segmental aneuploidy) to single nucleotide variant (SNVs) [1]. Deletion, insertion and duplication events which give rise to copy number variations (CNVs) have been found genome-wide in humans [2–11] and other species [12–17]. CNVs can be observed both as simple bi-allelic events or more complex multi-allelic events (Fig. 1). CNVs are classically defined as events longer than 1 kb [3]; smaller events are referred to as indels. With the advent of next generation sequencing (NGS), CNVs as small as 500 bp can be identified. CNVs can occur at different frequencies in a given population. When this frequency is greater than 1%, the CNV is referred to as a copy number polymorphism (CNP) [3]. This contrasts with SNPs whose frequencies are by definition greater than 1%.

Evangelos Evangelou (ed.), *Genetic Epidemiology: Methods and Protocols*, Methods in Molecular Biology, vol. 1793, https://doi.org/10.1007/978-1-4939-7868-7_14, © Springer Science+Business Media, LLC, part of Springer Nature 2018

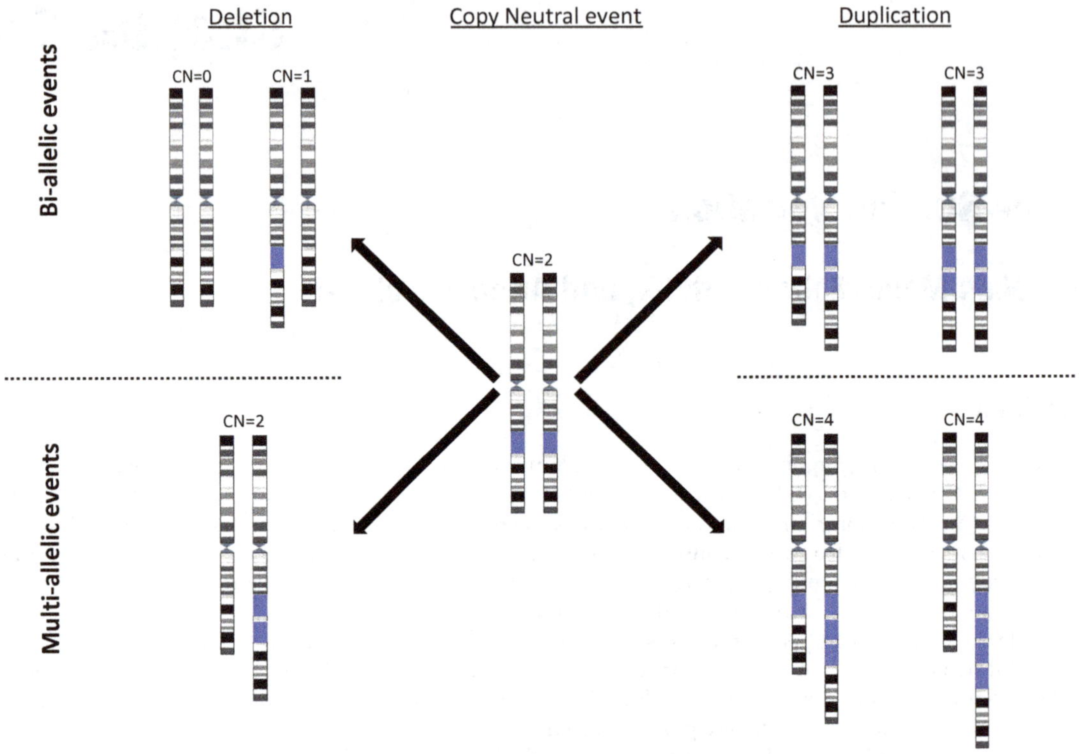

Fig. 1 Illustration of Copy Number Variants

The observation that CNVs and CNPs (here collectively referred to as CNVs) could occur both in normal [2–10, 18, 19] and disease [20–25] populations has opened a new chapter in human genomics. CNVs have been explored in European [9, 18, 19, 26, 27], African [28, 29], and several Asian populations: Chinese [30], Japanese [31], Korean [32, 33]. Comparisons have been performed between human populations [2, 34, 35] and across apes [7, 36, 37]. CNVs constitute a non-negligible part of the genetic diversity, with consequences in term of evolution and disease susceptibility [36]. Consequently, their detection and association with quantitative traits and clinical phenotype constitute an important step toward a better understanding of disease aetiology. However, their detection remains challenging. There are numerous factors in the data generation and computational analyses that can lead to spurious associations. Finally, the sheer amount of data that can be generated already for a single subject imposes severe challenges in terms of data interpretation.

In the following sections, we discuss on how to achieve a good design for a CNV study; explain how to process and quality-control the data obtained from the main high-throughput technologies (microarrays and sequencing); and finally how to conduct a genome-wide association study.

2 Materials

All methods described below make use of data generated following standard recommendations from the respective manufacturers.

3 Methods

3.1 Designing a CNV Study and Avoiding Batch Effects

3.1.1 Batch Effect Consequences

Batch effects have dramatic consequences in scientific studies, of any size and for any type of omics [38]. Any high-throughput experiment depends on a number of factors such as reagents, equipment, experimenters, time of experiment, sample handling etc. When conditions change during the course of the same study, it would introduce a bias in the data generation and subsequent quality. When the data displays different behavior according to experimental conditions and independently of the underlying biology, this is considered as a batch effect. For example, in case-control study, processing cases and controls with distinct set of experimental conditions creates a batch effect. De facto, any significant difference between the two groups is likely due to differences in experimental setup as opposed to the underlying biological and clinical differences.

Data normalization can help correcting for batch effects [39–42]. Yet, batch effect correction reduces statistical power, i.e., can mask true biological signal. Also, in the most pernicious scenario, the correction can introduce new confounders [43–45].

Batch effects have been identified in CNV studies [18, 38, 46]. CNV studies tend to be more sensitive to batch effect than genotyping studies owing to a stronger sensitivity to technological artifacts and to processing steps [47].

3.1.2 Detecting Batch Effects

Several approaches have been proposed for batch effect detection [38, 46, 48, 49] and can be used in an agnostic fashion. Those approaches rely on principal component analyses or unsupervised clustering. Those techniques allow to visually inspecting whether the data variance or sub-groups are observed with respect to plausible batch surrogates (such as date of processing, plate id, sample storage condition) or also clinical variables (case/control status, gender, age, study center etc.). Illustrations are given in Figs. 2–3, *see* also **Note 1** for recommendations for PCA-based analyses. Figure 2 shows hierarchical clustering for a real omics dataset using patients recruited in three distinct centers. Panel A displays a colored label according to the center and panel B displays a label according the subject's gender (M/F). A center effect can be seen (subjects tend to group according to the study center). The gender effect is less clear. Results with a principal component analysis (PCA) can be seen in Fig. 3 and provides clearer visualization.

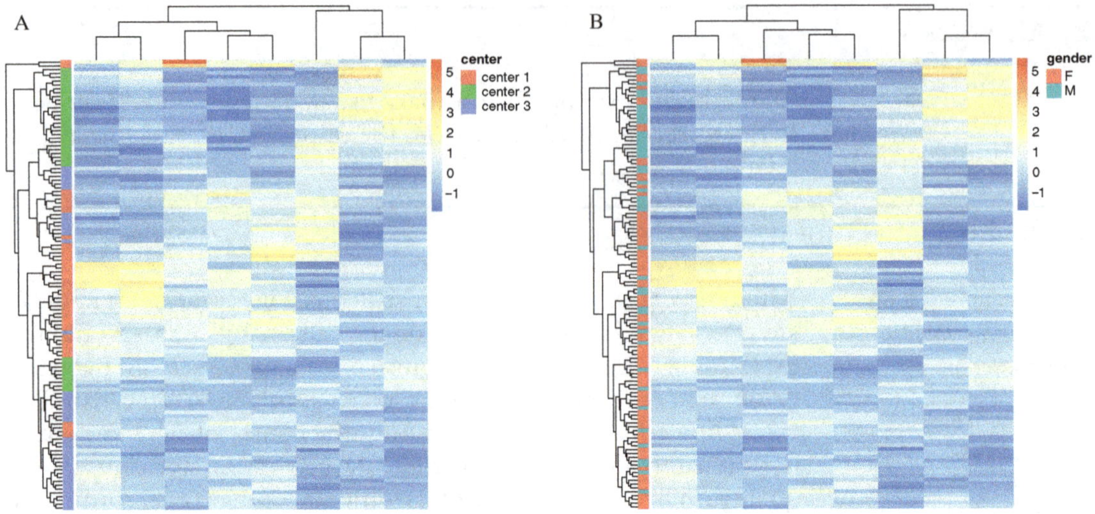

Fig. 2 Hierarchical clustering of a real omics dataset for patients recruited in three different centers. (**a**) The left dendrogram provides labels colored according to the patient's center and shows that patients from the same center tend to cluster together. (**b**) Labels are colored according to gender and no clear pattern can be seen (e.g., gender enrichment in the hierarchical clustering)

Another approach to detect batch effect would consist in doing exploratory analyses (*see* **Note 2**). For example, an analyst could summarize the data with PCA and then assess whether there is a significant association with one or several batch surrogates or clinical outcomes. Figure 3 illustrates this approach with a non-parametric approach (ranksum tests).

3.1.3 Accounting for Population Stratification

In genetic studies (SNP, CNV), analysts should also pay attention to population stratification. Genetic structure can be seen in PCA plots [50] and can induce a bias in genome-wide association studies. Fig. 4 shows data from another study that included participants having different genetic background and whose samples had been processed in two distinct labs. Although no obvious lab effect is observed, subjects cluster according to their genetic background. When such effects are detected, one may choose to discard subjects in order to keep a more homogeneous population (in term of genetic ancestry) and/or account for these differences in the analysis [51].

3.1.4 Preventing Batch Effects

Preventing batch effect is not always possible in large studies, simply because it is not possible to process the samples at the same time, within the same facility and by the same experimenter. Yet, studies should be designed upfront, in such a way that prevents or at least minimizes the possible batch effects. Unfortunately, it is common practice that data generation will start as soon as some samples are received and while the study (patient recruitment/sample collection) is still ongoing. This is often justified by the

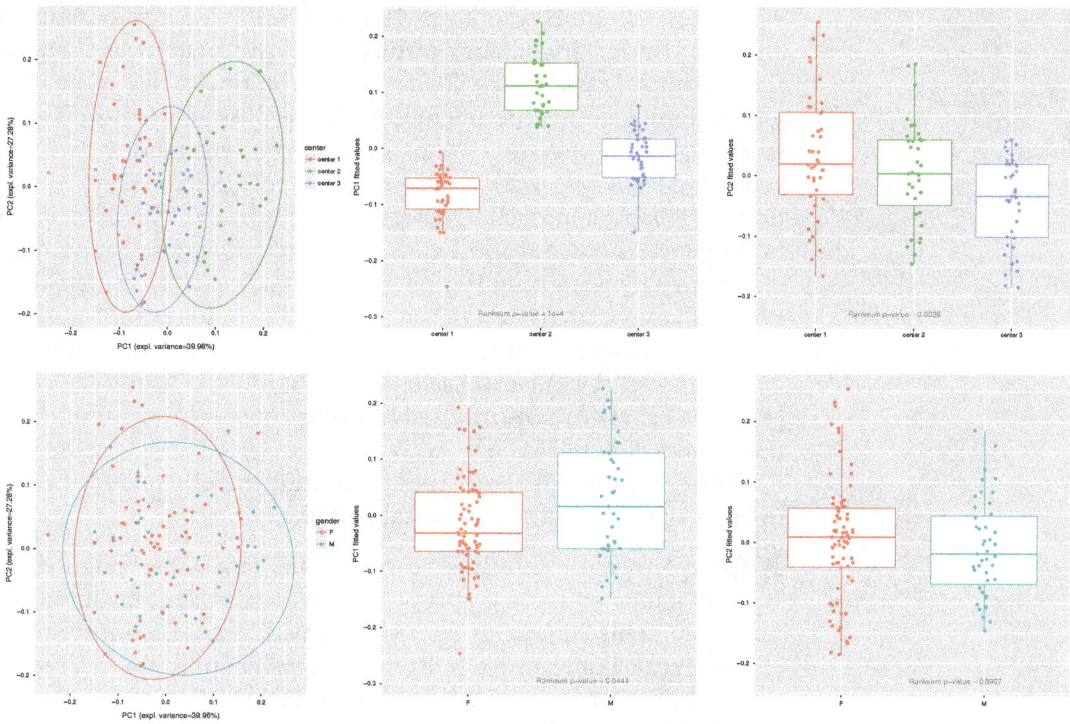

Fig. 3 Principal component analysis of a real omics dataset for patients recruited in three different centers. The top plots display principal component scores colored according to the patient's center. The bottom plots display the scores colored according to the patient's gender. The boxplots enable visualization of a single principal component grouped by a given confounding factor. The ranksum test *p*-value, as indicated in the boxplot, confirm the batch effect due to the center and highlight a slight effect due to gender

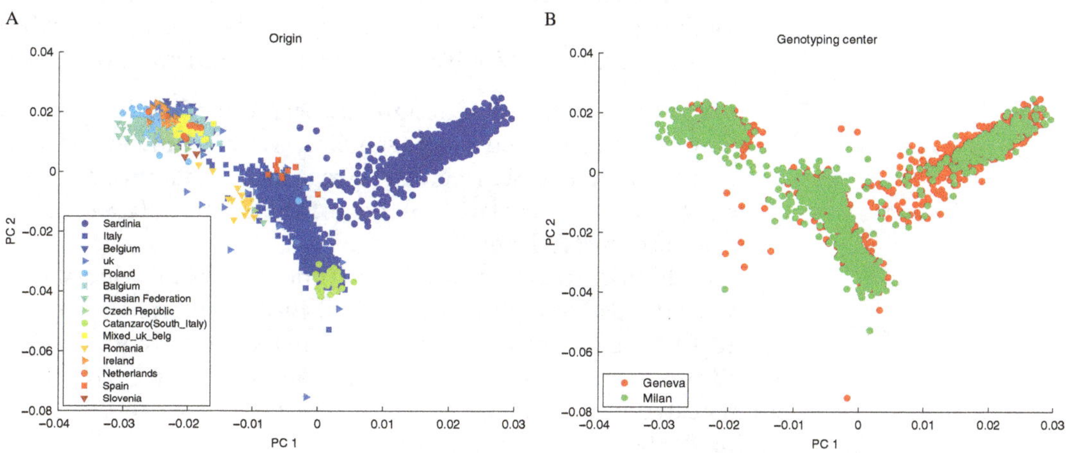

Fig. 4 Principal component analysis of a genetic dataset reveals population stratification. (**a**) PCA score plot showing a slight stratification according to the genetic background; (**b**) the same PCA showing that there was no strong effect on PC1 or PC2, linked with the processing lab

willingness to quickly obtain data and start the computational analyses (to get preliminary results). Yet, this practice is a recipe for potential disaster and will introduce profound biases in the data generation. A clear experimental design will make the results of a study stronger; limit the risk of spurious findings; and ultimately save significant resources (both in time and money). Randomization is a reliable approach to design an omics study; it helps creating homogeneous batches and limiting the risks of biases or judgment errors. In a randomized experimental design, the samples would be randomly attributed to a given processing unit (facility, experimenter, experiment date etc.). Experimental design and randomization have been extensively discussed for clinical trials [52–54]. There are also numerous references that are useful for designing studies [55–58].

Here, we describe two types of randomization (*see* **Note 3** for instructions using the R statistical language):

1. Complete randomization: samples are randomly assigned to processing units (e.g., samples are randomly attributed to plates). This can easily be achieved with any random number generator. For example in R, the *sample* function can be used to randomly attribute a processing plate ID to each biological sample. Complete randomization is often enough for observational studies (e.g., CNV analyses in the general population).
2. Block randomization: if specific differences are known prior doing the study (e.g., gender differences that may influence response to a given intervention/treatment), then subjects could be first divided into two homogeneous blocks (e.g., male/female) and then within each block subjects would be randomly assigned to the intervention (as in a complete randomization scheme). This setting might be appropriate when investigating CNV biomarkers in a clinical/intervention study.

Once the experimental design has been established, e.g., plate IDs have been attributed to the samples, we recommend checking with exploratory analyses (e.g., PCA, regression) that the attributed plate ID does not correlate with any of the existing data or metadata (*see* also **Notes 1** and **2**).

In addition to randomized experimental design, one should consider the use of replicates [58, 59]. Biological replicates correspond to parallel measurements of distinct subjects (e.g., drawing blood twice for different subjects). By contrast, technical replicates are repeated measurements of the same sample (e.g., several genotyping of the same DNA sample).

Technical replicates allow evaluating the experimental noise and its impact on the data. It can be useful to detect which plates had significantly lower quality and make decision whether such plates should be redone or discarded. Potentially, technical replicates might help renormalizing the data to account for the experimental variability. The use of biological replicates is strongly recommended as it allows checking the validity of the analyses (i.e. ensure that statistical assumptions of the methods are fulfilled and results reproduced).

3.2 CNV Detection with High-Throughput Technologies

Gross copy number alterations were initially detected with karyotyping in the early days of cytogenetics. Several large-scale aberrations [37, 60, 61] were identified before the development of higher resolution techniques. Fluorescence in situ hybridization (FISH) has increased this resolution, enabling the detection of *sub-microscopic* copy number variations that could not be detected with karyotyping. Today, the most widely used techniques can be classified as amplification-based (polymerase chain reaction), hybridization-based (FISH, CGH and SNP arrays) or sequencing-based. These techniques differ in precision, throughput and resolution.

3.2.1 Microarray-Based Methods

Single nucleotide polymorphism genotyping arrays

The Hapmap project [62] has played a major role in the discovery and characterization of single nucleotide polymorphisms (SNP). Investigation of genotype data from trios played a major role in the identification of CNVs from SNP genotyping arrays. Indeed CNVs have been detected from the following patterns: (1) SNPs violating Mendelian inheritance principle [63], (2) clusters of genotyping errors and (3) regions not in Hardy-Weinberg equilibrium [64]. Both Mc Carroll et al. [64] and Conrad et al. [63] showed that these events corresponded to deletions. This prompted the need to re-analyse SNP genotyping arrays for CNVs. Although these arrays were not primarily designed for CNV analysis, it is possible to obtain a copy number (CN) ratio by combining the intensities of the two alleles and normalizing this quantity with respect to reference. CNV can then be detected by identifying significant deviations from the baseline CN ratio. Some publicly available software combines CN and allelic ratio (the ratio of the allele intensities) to improve CNV detection (Table 1). Such strategy can be applied both for tumor analysis [65, 66] (Fig. 5) and diploid sample analysis [67–69]. Now, genotyping arrays include both SNP probes and copy number probes to cover previously established copy number variant regions. The choice of a method will depend on several factors: (1) which platform is to be analysed (Illumina or Affymetrix), (2) the desired output (discrete or continuous copy number prediction) and (3) the type of DNA to be analysed (germline or somatic CNV analysis). In addition, one should be aware that CNV software can lead to very distinct predictions, e.g., 70%–80% of the CNVs called by PennCNV [69] are not detected by both QuantiSNP [68] and CNVpartition [70]. Thus, it is often necessary to investigate the reliability of

Table 1
Algorithms for CNV detection from array data

Software	Affymetrix		Illumina						
	6.0	500 k	1 M	610 k	550 k	CGH	Method	Use Allelic Intensities	Copy number output
CRLMM [47]	X		X	X	X		Corrected robust linear model with maximum likelihood distance	X	Allele-specific copy number (CN)
ASCAT [106]	X	X	X	X	X		Allele-specific piecewise constant fitting	X	Allele-specific copy number (CN)
GMM [18]	X	X	X	X	X	X	Gaussian mixture model		Continuous CN
PICNIC [105]	X						Hidden-Markov model (HMM)	X	Continuous CN + CN genotypes
GLAD [125]	X	X	X	X	X	X	Adaptive weight smoothing		Discrete CN
PennCNV [69]	X*	X*	X	X	X		HMM	X	Discrete CN + CN genotypes
Birdsuite [104]	X						HMM	X	Discrete CN + CN genotypes
QuantiSNP [68]	X*	X*	X	X	X		HMM	X	Discrete CN + CN genotypes
Affymetrix. Aroma [126]	X	X					Robust multichip analysis (CRMA)		Unclassified segments
Cn.Farms [118]	X	X					Probabilistic latent variable model		Unclassified segments
GADA [127]	X	X	X	X	X	X	Sparse Bayesian learning		Unclassified segments
CBS [128]	X	X	X	X	X	X	Binary segmentation assessed by permutations		Unclassified segments

X* indicates a software not initially designed for such analysis, but that might be used providing upon additional pre-processing steps

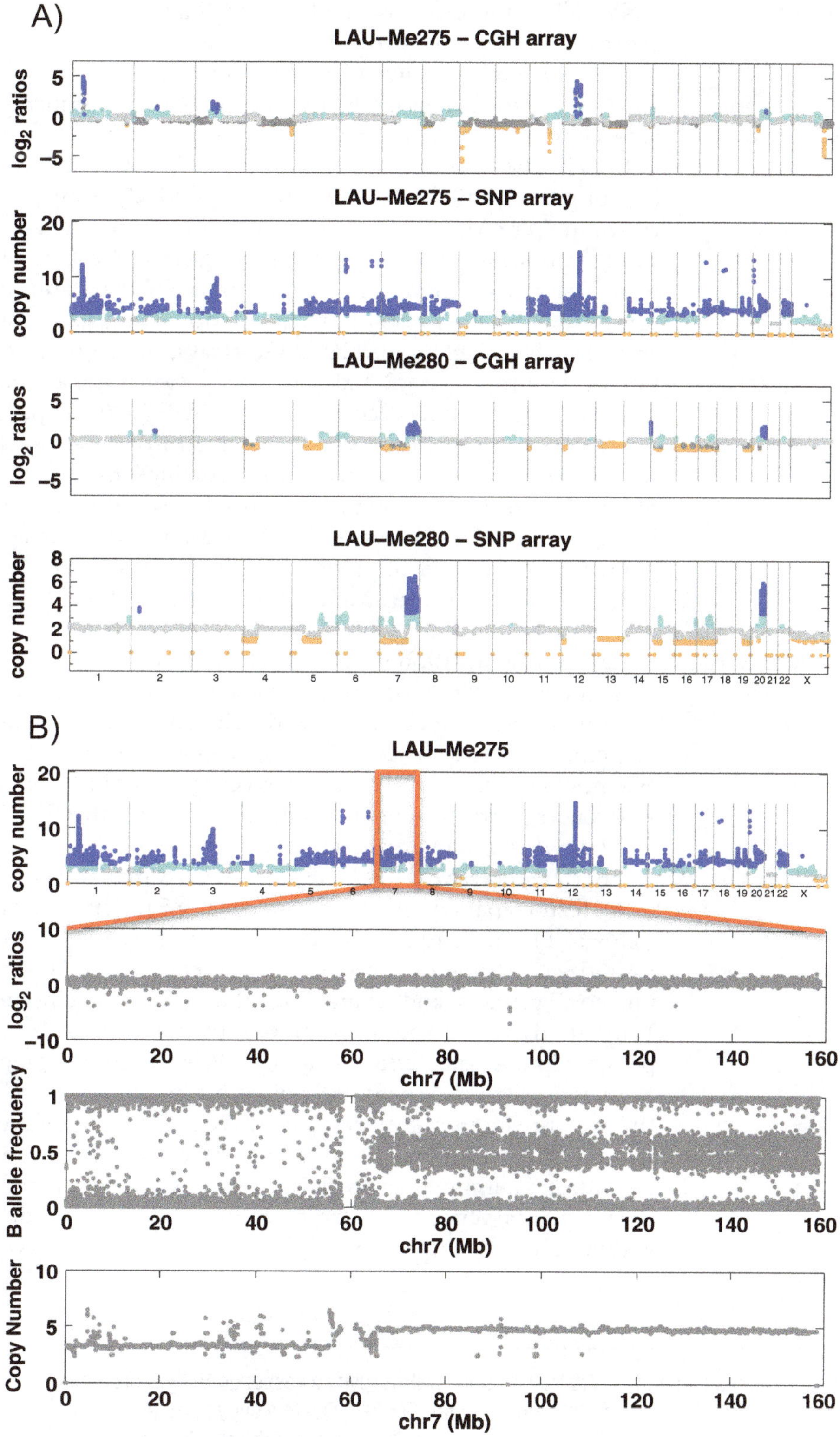

Fig. 5 SNP and CGH array analyses. (**a**) Analyses with SNP and CGH arrays of two melanoma samples (Me275 a tetraploid sample and Me280 with large deletions). Probe/SNP are plotted as a function of their genomic

CNV calls using different methods, technical replicates and post-processing filters (*see* **Note 4**).

Comparative Genome Hybridization arrays

Comparative Genome Hybridization (CGH) compares the relative copy number of a test DNA with respect to a reference DNA [71–74]. The two DNA samples are labelled with different dyes (red or green), and then hybridized competitively. A ratio of relative copy number changes can then be measured; significant deviations from the baseline indicate copy number gains or losses with respect to the reference genome (Fig. 5). Initial CNV detection was made using arrays having a resolution close to 50 kb [4, 9]. Current CGH arrays, such as Agilent SurePrint G3 arrays, have a median resolution of one probe every 2.1 kb. Such resolution is not as good as the one obtained from recent SNP arrays (~370 bp, Ilumina HumanOmni5-4) but the signals obtained from few CGH probes tend to be more reliable than those obtained from few adjacent SNPs [75, 76] and although allele-specific copy number cannot be inferred from CGH (as opposed to SNP arrays), these arrays remain popular for the detection of CNV both in somatic (tumours) [72, 77, 78] and in constitutional diagnostics [79–82].

3.2.2 Sequencing-Based Methods

Today, next generation sequencing (NGS) technologies allow one to sequence millions of reads in parallel [83]. Methods [84] for structural variant analysis were developed including paired-end mapping, read-depth analysis, split-read strategies and sequence assembly comparisons and more recently combinations of these. References to freely available tools are given in Table 2.

Paired-end mapping approaches

Before the advent of NGS, structural variants were detected from fosmid paired-end sequencing [7, 85]. The principle is as follow: (1) the genomic sequence is fragmented and cloned into fosmids. (2) Ends of the cloned fragments are sequenced using universal primers and aligned to the reference genome. (3) -Paired-ends, discordant in length or direction, indicate respectively possible indels or inversion (Fig. 6a). Paired-end mapping (PEM) enables precise breakpoint determination and performs well even in the presence of repetitive elements (LINE, SINE). However, it fails when both paired-ends map within repeats. Also the detection resolution is limited to the distance between pairs; therefore, neither large nor very small rearrangements can be detected, with the exception of large deletions.

Fig. 5 (continued) position on the *X* axis. *Y* axis for CGH arrays corresponds to hybridization ratios. *Y* axis for SNP arrays corresponds to the predicted copy number. Colors indicate a copy number state (orange$<$2 copies; gray = 2 copies; cyan = 3 copies; dark blue$>$3 copies). (**b**) Analysis of the Me275 sample with SNP array. The top panel shows genome-wide copy number. Subsequent panels show chromosome 7 with, from top to bottom: Hybridization log2 ratio, B allele frequency and copy number prediction

Table 2
Algorithms for CNV detection from NGS data

Strategy	Approach	References
Paired-end mapping	Detection of discordant end pairs Clustering of end-pairs	[85, 129–131] [7, 130, 132–134]
Read-depth analysis	Detection of local change points Detection of outliers compared to the read-depth baseline Event-wise testing Segmentation-based approach, adjusted across populations and copy number classification refined with mixture models	[119, 135–138] [139] [140] [141]
Split-read analysis	Identification of breakpoints with a pattern growth algorithm	[86, 142–146]
Sequence assembly analysis	De novo assembly and comparison to reference genome Burrows-wheeler transform Simultaneously assembly of multiple eukaryotic genomes Detection of small indels through local reassembly	[87, 88, 90] [90, 147] [82, 87, 89] [148]
Mixed strategies	Paired-end mapping and read-depth analysis Split-read and read depth / paired end Paired end and sequence assembly	[149] [145, 150, 151] [152, 153]
Whole-exome sequencing	Read-depth based	[154–160]

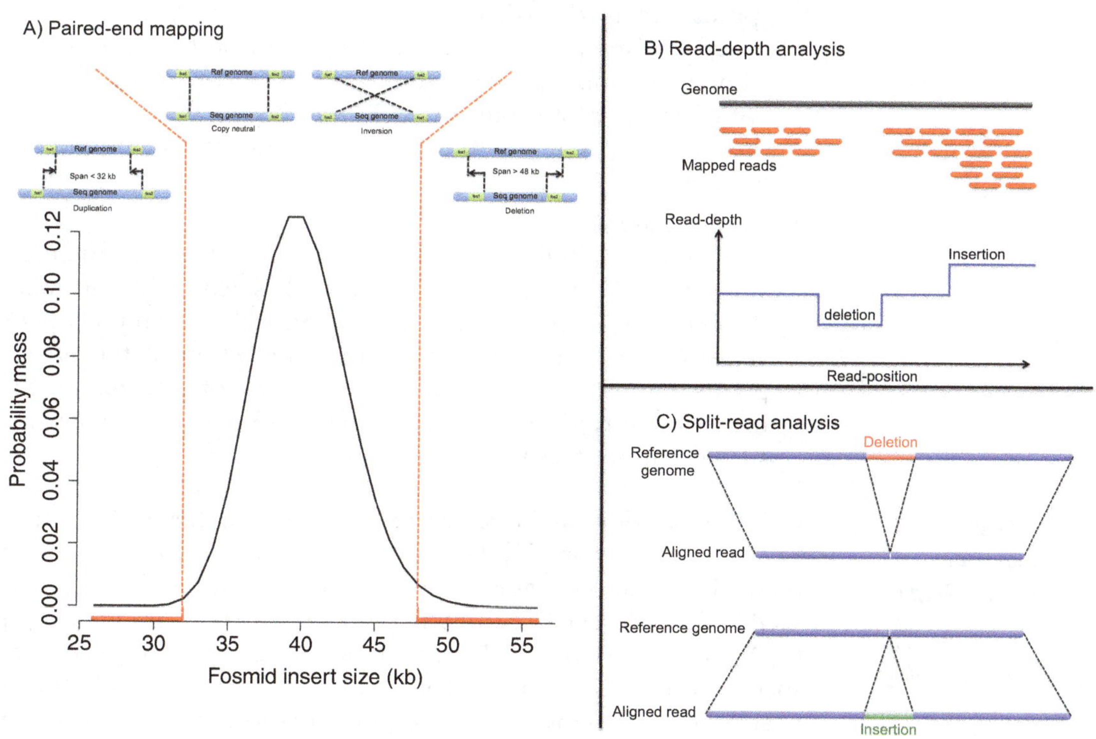

Fig. 6 Illustration of Next-Generation Sequencing (NGS) approaches. Analytical strategy to detect CNV from NGS data: (**a**) pair-end mapping approached, (**b**) read-depth approach and (**c**) split-read approach

1. Read-depth approach
   The read-depth analysis investigates changes in read coverage compared to an expected depth distribution (Fig. 6b). Mutual information about paired-reads is used to improve the mapping quality and to detect complex and large rearrangements. However, read-depth analysis is challenging in repeat-rich regions (due to mapping issues).
2. Split-read approach
   The split-read strategy entails in gapped-alignment of reads onto candidate breakpoints (Fig. 6c). The strategy is to detect paired-reads where only one end is uniquely mapped onto a reference genome [86]. The assumption is that the second paired-read could not be mapped, even with few mismatches allowed, because it corresponds to a deletion or insertion breakpoint. The mapped-read is used as an anchor and knowing both a maximum event length and the direction to search for the unmapped-read; alignment of the unmapped-read can be performed either by splitting it into two or three fragments whereby the former indicates a deletion event and the latter indicates an insertion event (Fig. 6c).
3. Sequence assembly comparison
   Provided a high sequencing depth, de novo assembly can be attempted [87–90] such that a sequence comparison can be made with the reference genome to identify deletions and insertions. The advantage of de novo assembling over PEM approaches is that deletions or insertions smaller than the paired-end insert size can be detected. But on the other hand, de novo assembling is very difficult for repeat-rich regions and until 2012 [89] was only possible with high read-depth. When this criterion is not met, several experiments can be pooled together [91].
4. Mixed strategies
   The above techniques present different and complementary advantages. Combining several approaches definitely empowers the detection of structural variations [92]. Paired-end mapping approach performs well for the exact detection of the breakpoints however the results are limited in case of large rearrangements while read-depth analysis attains good performances for such event but fails to accurately detect breakpoints.

3.3 Carrying Genome-Wide Association Studies

3.3.1 Input CNV Data for Association Studies

CNVs association can be run at different levels, either at the probe- or CNV- level. Probe-level corresponds to using the copy number prediction positioned at each probe from the micro-array (SNP or CGH). CNV-level correspond to working with a locus enriched in CNVs sharing essentially the same boundaries across subjects. Irrespectively of the input data (probe- or CNV- level), some additional post-processing steps are needed prior performing the association tests (*see* **Note 4**).

Performing association at the probe-level is rather straightforward, as a single matrix probe by individuals (with each element equals to the copy number state) can easily be derived and then analyzed with essentially the same tools as for SNP-based GWAs. The choice of the copy number representation can be either a continuous value (e.g., values ranging from 0 to 4 or higher), discrete (e.g., deletion, copy-neutral or duplication) or presence/absence of copy-neutral event (*see* **Note 5**). However when working at the probe-level, the statistical tests are not independent (the data would be highly redundant between adjacent probes) and thus appropriate multiple-testing correction must be performed (*see* **Note 6**).

By contrast, working at the CNV-level needs some additional processing. It requires to reconcile CNV regions from all individuals into a consensus region. Since CNV boundaries differ across individuals, defining a consensus region is a complex task [18]. This approach can be useful to identify clusters of CNVs with similar boundaries, to reduce the number of tests and help for the interpretation (Fig. 7). This can be done with the so-called merge-by-overlap approach [9, 63], where CNVs from different individuals are merged into the same CNV region if their reciprocal overlap satisfies a minimal cut-off (>50% is frequently used [9, 63]). It also exists an alternative approach based on principal component analysis and clustering [18].

3.3.2 Workflow of CNV-Based Genome Wide Association Studies (CNV-Based GWAs)

CNV-based GWAs can be made using similar tools than for SNP-based GWAs. For example, with case-control [20] designs, logistic regression, Fisher's exact test or Armitage-Cochrane trend test can be used to estimate whether CNV frequencies differ between the two groups. This approach has been successfully applied in the case of severe early-onset obesity [93]. For quantitative traits, linear regression approaches are applicable. More specialized CNV tools are described in Subheading 3.4.

As with SNP-based GWAs, it is important to properly adjust the analysis for potential confounding factors. Finally, specific imputation might be needed for meta-analysis of cohorts whose CNV detection was performed on slightly different chip versions (*see* **Note 7**).

Once association tests have been performed, critical attention should be paid to QQ plots and ensure that there is no massive p-value inflation (or deflation). Strong inflation is often linked with a serious confounding effect that is not adjusted (e.g., batch effect) or with low-quality CNV calling. While strong deflation may be linked with a lack of statistical power and/or a large number of inter-dependent tests. More details are provided in **Note 8** regarding QQ plot interpretations and possible solutions.

Association studies for CNV on chromosome X and Y needs special attention (*see* **Note 9**). By definition, males are expected to

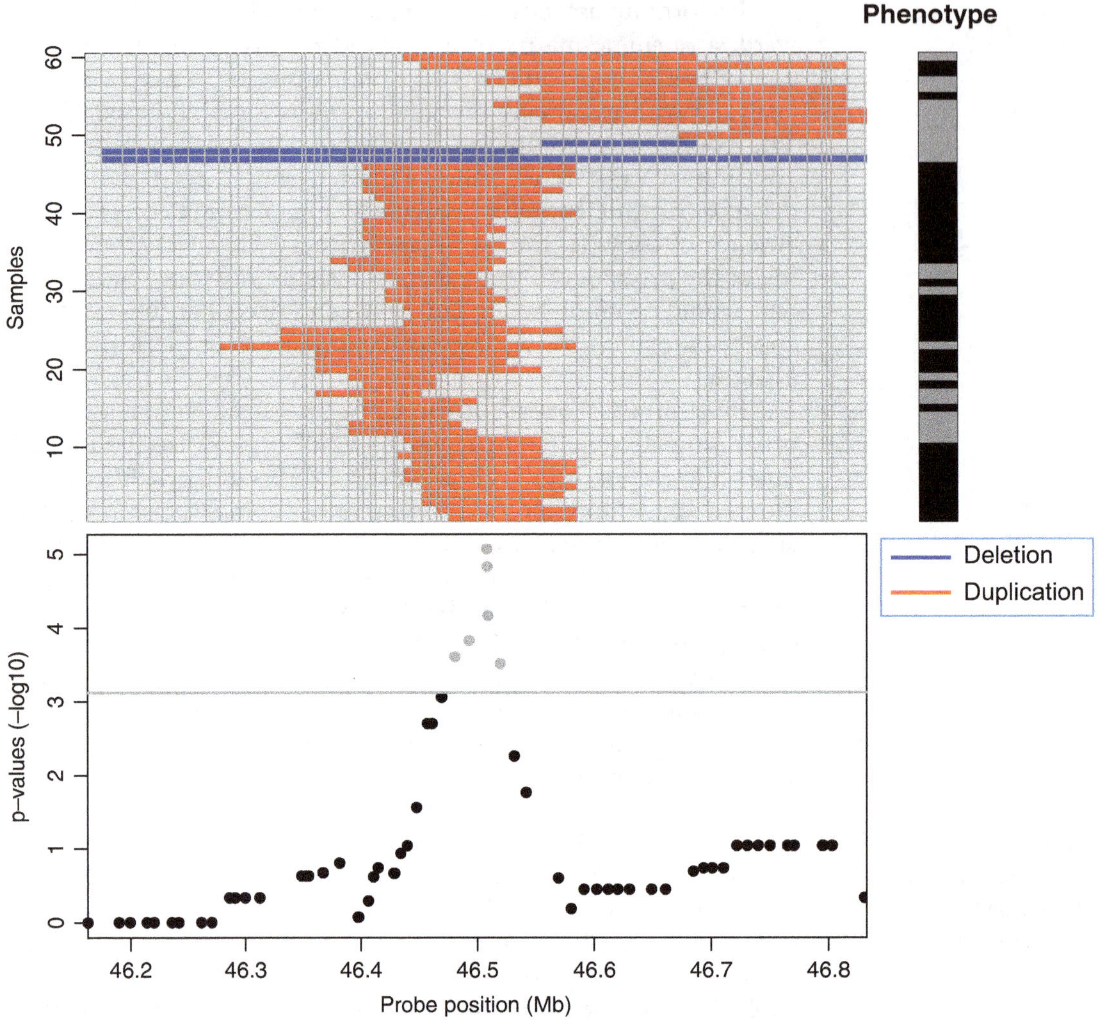

Fig. 7 Representation of CNV data and CNV-GWA analysis. The upper panel shows a matrix-based representation of the CNV along with the phenotype of the different subjects. Association results are presented in the bottom panel

have one copy of both chromosomes while females would be diploid for chromosome X and have no copy of the Y chromosome. This can affect data normalization, subsequent calling and potentially lead to spurious results on chromosome X and Y. Stratified analyses for sexual chromosomes are recommended. Furthermore, due to the highly repetitive nature of these chromosomes (in particular chromosome Y) stringent QC filters are recommended and/or validation of CNV calls using an independent technique [94].

3.4 Statistical Frameworks

In order to facilitate CNV-traits analysis, frameworks have been developed. Table 3 proposes a non-exhaustive list of freely available

Table 3
Frameworks for CNV analysis

Method	Approach	References
CNVtools	Likelihood ratio trend test	[95]
Birdsuite	Regression sum number copies each allele	[161]
Plink	Permutation-based test	[162]
CNVassoc	Latent class model	[96]
ParseCNV	Multi-step approach	[97]
CKAT	Kernel association test	[112]

software. CNVtools [95] is a popular framework for CNV association analyses. It is available as an R package and has been designed to perform both case-control and quantitative trait association tests. This method is platform-agnostic and can be applied when a (reference) diploid copy number is available. Other frameworks have been proposed like CNVassoc [96], and ParseCNV [97], both with functionalities for different types of design (case-control, cohort etc.). More recently, we proposed a complete pipeline [98] for SNP arrays that estimates the probability for a CNV call to be a true CNV. This CNV quality score can then be used for CNV-trait association. Using such probabilistic framework enables to increase statistical power while controlling the risk of spurious association [99]. All the steps ranging from the CNV call to the CNV-trait association including the quality score calculation are encapsulated in a single stand-alone pipeline (both code and documentation are available online http://goo.gl/T6yuFM).

Finally, a third type of association is possible and consists in testing CNV segregation in families or trios. The FBAT [100, 101] software remains a reference for family-based association studies from both SNP and CNV data. The method is based on the co-variance between the offspring trait and CNV data (hybridization intensities) while adjusting for parental CNV data. As advantage, this method does not require CNV intensity data to be clearly clustered in discrete copy number classes. The FBAT extensions (e.g., time-to-event or multivariate analyses) are also applicable for CNV-based association study. However, in presence of non-linear intensity—copy number relationship and departure from Hardy-Weinberg equilibrium, the FBAT CNV score statistics might be biased and lead to inflated type 1 error [102] and thus would require additional caution when evaluating association signals [103]. Such caution would apply for any CNV association study and stresses the need for replication using an independent technology and/or replication in an independent cohort (*see* **Note 10**).

3.5 Common/Rare CNVs Analyses

CNVs are usually divided into two groups depending on their frequency: CNVs with frequency higher than 1% will be considered as common and called Copy Number Polymorphisms (CNP) while the CNVs with frequency lower than 1% will be consider as rare. CNPs correspond mostly to ancestral events and segregate in the population with different allele frequencies (owing to the fact that many are multi-allelic [9, 104]). Studies from the WTCCC [20] found that only very few CNPs were likely to be associated with common diseases. It is likely that the effect size of CNPs is modest, and that lack of standardization between studies and small sample size challenge the identification of association signal. Instead of discrete CNV classification, (continuous) copy number genotypes are preferred for testing [104]. A number of software [69, 104–106] packages exist to compute copy number genotypes rendering such analyses possible.

For rare CNV association studies, a large sample size is needed to obtain the required statistical power. This can be achieved by pooling data from different cohorts [23, 24]. This task is challenging due to the differences between cohorts, platform vendors (and thus genomic content), analytical methods and even false discovery rate. Currently, the only reasonable approach is to re-analyze SNP arrays data used in previous GWAS [107, 108]. Large sample size studies based on sequencing or CGH arrays are not yet affordable. Ideally these cohorts should be genotyped on platforms as homogeneous as possible [109]. Although, it exists many different Illumina chips, the vast majority of them share the Illumina 1 M probe set, which can be a common set of probes to use.

Specific methods have been developed for the meta-analysis of rare variants like RAREMETAL [110]. More recently, the SKAT [111] method designed for rare variant association analysis has been adapted for rare CNVs in a method called CKAT [112]. In the case of rare CNVs and limited sample size, a classical approach is to perform CNV burden analysis [19]. This type of analysis does not investigate a specific CNV but instead a group of CNVs (e.g., deletions) and test for global differences (e.g., between cases and controls). This method has been successfully applied for the analysis of the effect of CNVs on cognitive traits in the general population. It has been shown, for example, that carriers of large (>250 kb) and rare (<0.05%) deletions will have a higher risk of intellectual disability and a lower educational level than the non-carriers.

4 Concluding Remarks

Copy number variation is widely spread within and between species. Numerous studies have documented CNVs among healthy subjects. Specific CNVs have been reported as risk factors for complex diseases; de novo events have also been documented in several genomic syndromes and somatic copy number aberrations are typical of cancer genomes. The contribution of CNVs to disease and the fraction of the genome that is potentially variable across individuals remain far less advanced than our understanding of the impact of SNVs. With the advent of very large cohorts, including large sequencing projects, and with the availability of massive datasets generated using very similar technologies studying the clinical impact of CNVs remains a fascinating research topic.

5 Notes

1. Using principal component analysis for batch effect detection
   Principal component analyses are widely used in genomic studies. Several functions in R can be used (*prcomp*, *svd* and several specialized R packages such as *FactoMiner* or *gPCA*). Fitting bivariate ellipses to each group in a PCA plot might help identifying outliers. The *ggbiplot* R package provides such functionality. Statistical methods for outlier detection can also be useful (see examples with the *outliers* R package). Once outliers (samples/subjects) have been identified and removed from the dataset, we recommend doing a second PCA to ensure that those previous outliers were not explaining a significant fraction of variance and hiding other outliers.
2. Checking an experimental design with exploratory analyses
   Once a plate ID has been (randomly) attributed to the samples to be processed (see additional details in **Note 3**), one could use exploratory analyses to ensure the attributed plate ID is not confounded with the subjects' age, gender, baseline clinical characteristics etc. By exploratory analyses, we mean to check the correlation/independence between a simple factor (e.g., gender) and the plate identifier. In such case, a simple proportion test (e.g., proportion of male per plates) or using a logistic regression would answer the question whether the gender repartition over the different plates is random. Similar tests can be conducted with continuous variable (e.g., weight, height, any important baseline variable). For e.g., a t-test, ranksum test, linear regression or simple correlation, would answer the question of having an independent relationship between plate ID and the continuous variable of interest.

   When the plate ID attrition has been made with random number generators, the analyses should not detect any significant association. If an association is found, then the investigator should consider whether the associated factor is important for the study and/or whether the design should be re-made, possibly using a different approach (e.g., block randomization).

3. Tools for randomization
   Complete randomization schemes can easily be implemented using the *sample* function in R. This function allows generating a sequence of number (e.g., 1–10) sorted in a random fashion, which can be useful to attribute to samples a randomly generated plate ID. In practice, complete randomization is suitable for most observational studies. For block-randomization, there are several tools that facilitate such design such as the ***blockrand*** R package. Yet, such design scheme is best discussed between the study investigator and a statistician/analyst, to ensure that pertinent blocking variable and blocking size are chosen.
4. CNV post-processing
   CNV post-processing is one of the key steps in CNV analysis. Many detected CNVs are small, located next to each other and therefore would need to be merged. PennCNV [69] proposes a filtering Perl script which merges two CNVs if the ratio between the total length of the CNVs and the distance between them is below a given threshold. Following CNV merging, additional checks are needed to remove potential false calls and/or samples with an aberrant number of CNVs. A recent study has shown that 70%–80% of the CNV calls by PennCNV are not detected by both QuantiSNP [68] and CNVpartition [70]. CNVs can be filtered based on several parameters listed in the Table 4. Unfortunately, there is no gold standard and there are almost as many QC thresholds as the number of studies. We recently proposed to combine the different criteria in a single score, which estimates the probability of a CNV called by PennCNV to be detected by the two other software. Finally, in the case of meta-analysis combining the results from several cohorts, one can decide to remove CNVs, which appear in too few cohorts, or with a too low frequency.
5. Copy number values for association studies
   One first approach for CNV-trait association is to consider the copy number value as continuous variables going from 0 to 4 and more. Or if the exact number of copies does not matter then one can just assign value −1 for deletion, 0 for copy neutral and 1 for duplication. These two approaches imply that there is a mirror effect from the CNV on the trait, or that only the deletions or the duplications have an impact. But these approaches will miss CNV-trait associations in the case the deletions and the duplications have effect going in the same direction (i.e., any departure from copy neutral state). A possible approach is to assign value 1 when there is a CNV (deletion or duplication) and 0 when it is copy neutral (i.e., presence/absence of copy-neutral event), and conduct the association test with such binary values.

Table 4
Metrics for CNV filtering

Metrics	Definition
CNV quality score	Statistical learning from a set of QC metrics to estimate the probability of false positive
Confidence	Likelihood of the most likely CN minus the 2nd most likely one
Length	CNV length in bp
N probes	Number of probes in the CNV
LRR mean	Mean LRR for a given sample
LRR sd	Standard deviation of the LRR
BAF mean	Mean BAF for a given sample
BAF sd	Standard deviation of the BAF
BAF drift	Summarize the proportion of BAF values falling out of the expected BAF (0, 0.5 and 1)
WF	Value measuring the strength of waviness in a given sample
N CNVs	Number of CNVs per sample
Call rate	Probes call rate from the SNP array

Different thresholds and combination of metrics have been used thorough CNV studies [69, 76, 97, 163, 164]. The CNV quality score [98] avoids using ad-hoc filters and provides a statistical framework for subsequent association studies

6. Multiple testing correction
   Similarly to the SNP GWAS, genome-wide CNV association studies are facing the issue of the multiple testing corrections. Since CNV regions are defined by stretch of SNPs/probes having the same predicted copy number, CNV data would exhibit stronger correlation patterns that SNP genotyping data. Thus the number of independent tests is not equal to the number of tested SNPs/probes and also depends on the study sample size. A naïve Bonferroni correction based on the number of tested markers would result in an overly conservative correction that would likely mask interesting loci. Instead, appropriate methods should be used to estimate the number of truly independent tests. A study [18] using the Colaus cohort (a population-based health survey with more than 5600 subjects genotyped on Affymetrix 500 k SNP arrays) showed that CN predictions obtained at 490 k autosomal SNPs could be compressed into about 8 k distinct CNV regions, including both rare and common CNVs. This number of regions gives a first approximation about the number of independent tests.

Using the simple *M* method [113], we estimated that the number of truly independent tests was 6643 corresponding to a 74-fold difference compared to the probe-level CN predictions. However, when the number of individuals included in the analysis increases, the CNV regions get more complex as the number of CNV increases, including an increase in the definition of CNV boundaries (breakpoints). Thus the number of independent probes, and then tests, will increase too. Number of effective tests calculation for a meta-analysis project (manuscript in preparation) based on ~191,161 samples with copy number information at the probe level from Illumina 1 M showed a number of independent tests equals to 399,665 corresponding at a 2.5-fold decrease compared to the number of probes on the Illumina 1 M platform and p-value threshold for significance equals to 1.7E-6.

7. Missing summary statistics for CNV meta-analysis
One issue with running a meta-analysis is the integration of data generated from different versions/formats of the same technology (e.g., Illumina 660-quad arrays, HumanCore, OmniExpress etc.) or a more complex scenario with data from different technologies (CGH-, SNP-arrays). For data from the same vendor, meta-analysis may be restricted to common probes (e.g., most of Illumina arrays tend to use a common base of markers). For data from different vendors/technologies, the data integration is more challenging. In which case, it may be necessary to work at the CNV region level (locus-level) [114] and to use random-effect modeling to account for cohort heterogeneity.

8. Interpretation and sanity checks of GWAs results
Non-Gaussian test statistic distributions can lead to spurious associations [99] and give rise to inflated p-values (as can be detected with QQ-plots). Although genomic control methods [115–117] allow correcting for inflated p-values in most cases, critical assessment of the CNV pipeline remains necessary both for sensitivity and specificity. Combining methods that estimate FDRs [118, 119] with technical replicates is essential to achieve a good sensitivity-specificity compromise.

Inflated *p*-values can be due to various violations of the model assumptions, e.g., non-normal trait distribution, dependence between tests, or confounding effects such as population stratification (including population admixture), cryptic- or familial relatedness. Careful covariate selection and diagnostic plots are needed to address the two first issues. For admixture and population stratification, many methods have been proposed to detect and adjust them [120, 121].

CNV-GWAs can also produce deflated QQ-plots owing to the fact the number of tested markers is much greater than the number of truly-independent tests. Methods used in multiple-testing adjustment in SNP-GWAs [113, 122, 123] can be useful to identify CN markers corresponding to independent tests and to produce the corresponding QQ plot using those markers only.

Controlling for false positives may in some cases require investigating subject-level data (profile of CN ratio and profile of allelic ratio), CNV frequencies and the genomic distance between the different signals. Correlated signals from probes adjacent to each other's would indicate a partially detected CNV (i.e., disrupted CNV prediction) while isolated signals located on different chromosome would more likely correspond to spurious associations. Increasing the stringency filter on very rare CNVs (e.g., removing CNVs with frequency smaller than 1/1000) might avoid the latter issue.

9. CNV detection on the X and Y chromosomes
Most of the studies focus on autosomes and do not consider the sex chromosomes. In fact, the X and Y chromosomes need to be treated specifically [94]. One approach is to consider males and females separately, in order to properly compare the copy number values on the X and Y chromosomes. Attention should be paid to the data normalization (prior CNV calling). Several methods [69, 119] include an option for CNV detection on sex chromosomes. Generally, the user needs to provide a file containing the sex information of all the subjects. Once CNVs have been called, association studies should also be conducted with caution, for example by carrying gender-stratified analyses.

10. Replication of CNV association signals
Since CNV detection methods remain prone to both false-positives and false-negatives, we strongly recommend any detected CNV association to be confirmed with an independent detection platform. With the cost reduction and throughput offered with in large-scale qPCR assays (e.g., Taqman, Multiplex Ligation-dependent Probe Amplification [124]) replicating the CNV using a subset (or integrality) of the cohort is now affordable. Replication with an independent cohort (if possible) should also remain a gold standard.

References

1. Valsesia A, Mace A, Jacquemont S et al (2013) The growing importance of CNVs: new insights for detection and clinical interpretation. Front Genet 4:92

2. Conrad DF, Pinto D, Redon R et al (2010) Origins and functional impact of copy number variation in the human genome. Nature 464(7289):704–712

3. Feuk L, Carson AR, Scherer SW (2006) Structural variation in the human genome. Nat Rev Genet 7(2):85–97
4. Fiegler H, Redon R, Andrews D et al (2006) Accurate and reliable high-throughput detection of copy number variation in the human genome. Genome Res 16(12):1566–1574
5. Freeman JL, Perry GH, Feuk L et al (2006) Copy number variation: new insights in genome diversity. Genome Res 16 (8):949–961
6. Iafrate AJ, Feuk L, Rivera MN et al (2004) Detection of large-scale variation in the human genome. Nat Genet 36(9):949–951
7. Kidd JM, Cooper GM, Donahue WF et al (2008) Mapping and sequencing of structural variation from eight human genomes. Nature 453(7191):56–64
8. Perry GH, Yang F, Marques-Bonet T et al (2008) Copy number variation and evolution in humans and chimpanzees. Genome Res 18 (11):1698–1710
9. Redon R, Ishikawa S, Fitch KR et al (2006) Global variation in copy number in the human genome. Nature 444(7118):444–454
10. Sharp AJ, Locke DP, McGrath SD et al (2005) Segmental duplications and copy-number variation in the human genome. Am J Hum Genet 77(1):78–88
11. Valsesia A, Rimoldi D, Martinet D et al (2011) Network-guided analysis of genes with altered somatic copy number and gene expression reveals pathways commonly perturbed in metastatic melanoma. PLoS One 6 (4):e18369
12. Dopman EB, Hartl DL (2007) A portrait of copy-number polymorphism in Drosophila melanogaster. Proc Natl Acad Sci U S A 104 (18056801):19920–19925
13. Fontanesi L, Martelli PL, Beretti F et al (2010) An initial comparative map of copy number variations in the goat (Capra hircus) genome. BMC Genomics 11(21083884):639
14. Graubert TA, Cahan P, Edwin D et al (2007) A high-resolution map of segmental DNA copy number variation in the mouse genome. PLoS Genet 3(1):e3
15. Guryev V, Saar K, Adamovic T et al (2008) Distribution and functional impact of DNA copy number variation in the rat. Nat Genet 40(5):538–545
16. Lee AS, Gutiérrez-Arcelus M, Perry GH et al (2008) Analysis of copy number variation in the rhesus macaque genome identifies candidate loci for evolutionary and human disease studies. Hum Mol Genet 17(8):1127–1136
17. Liu GE, Hou Y, Zhu B et al (2010) Analysis of copy number variations among diverse cattle breeds. Genome Res 20 (20212021):693–703
18. Valsesia A, Stevenson BJ, Waterworth D et al (2012) Identification and validation of copy number variants using SNP genotyping arrays from a large clinical cohort. BMC Genomics 13:241
19. Mannik K, Magi R, Mace A et al (2015) Copy number variations and cognitive phenotypes in unselected populations. JAMA 313 (20):2044–2054
20. Craddock N, Hurles ME, Cardin N et al (2010) Genome-wide association study of CNVs in 16,000 cases of eight common diseases and 3,000 shared controls. Nature 464 (7289):713–720
21. Firth HV, Richards SM, Bevan AP et al (2009) DECIPHER: database of chromosomal imbalance and phenotype in humans using ensembl resources. Am J Hum Genet 84(19344873):524–533
22. Grozeva D, Kirov G, Ivanov D et al (2010) Rare copy number variants: a point of rarity in genetic risk for bipolar disorder and schizophrenia. Arch Gen Psychiatry 67 (20368508):318–327
23. Jacquemont S, Reymond A, Zufferey F et al (2011) Mirror extreme BMI phenotypes associated with gene dosage at the chromosome 16p11.2 locus. Nature 478(7367):97–102
24. Walters RG, Jacquemont S, Valsesia A et al (2010) A new highly penetrant form of obesity due to deletions on chromosome 16p11.2. Nature 463(7281):671–675
25. Zhang F, Gu W, Hurles ME et al (2009) Copy number variation in human health, disease, and evolution. Annu Rev Genomics Hum Genet 10(19715442):451–481
26. Gayán J, Galan JJ, González-Pérez A et al (2010) Genetic structure of the Spanish population. BMC Genomics 11:326
27. Li J, Yang T, Wang L et al (2009) Whole genome distribution and ethnic differentiation of copy number variation in Caucasian and Asian populations. PLoS One 4(11):e7958
28. Matsuzaki H, Wang P-H, Hu J et al (2009) High resolution discovery and confirmation of copy number variants in 90 Yoruba Nigerians. Genome Biol 10(11):R125
29. McElroy JP, Nelson MR, Caillier SJ et al (2009) Copy number variation in African Americans. BMC Genet 10:15
30. Lin C-H, Li L-H, Ho S-F et al (2008) A large-scale survey of genetic copy number variations

among Han Chinese residing in Taiwan. BMC Genet 9:92

31. Takahashi N, Tsuyama N, Sasaki K et al (2008) Segmental copy-number variation observed in Japanese by array-CGH. Ann Hum Genet 72(Pt 2):193–204
32. Jeon JP, Shim SM, Jung JS et al (2009) A comprehensive profile of DNA copy number variations in a Korean population: identification of copy number invariant regions among Koreans. Exp Mol Med 41(9):618–628
33. Kang T-W, Jeon Y-J, Jang E et al (2008) Copy number variations (CNVs) identified in Korean individuals. BMC Genomics 9:492
34. Jakobsson M, Scholz SW, Scheet P et al (2008) Genotype, haplotype and copy-number variation in worldwide human populations. Nature 451(7181):998–1003
35. Kato M, Kawaguchi T, Ishikawa S et al (2010) Population-genetic nature of copy number variations in the human genome. Hum Mol Genet 19(5):761–773
36. Conrad DF, Hurles ME (2007) The population genetics of structural variation. Nat Genet 39(7 Suppl):S30–S36
37. Nistér M, Wedell B, Betsholtz C et al (1987) Evidence for progressional changes in the human malignant glioma line U-343 MGa: analysis of karyotype and expression of genes encoding the subunit chains of platelet-derived growth factor. Cancer Res 47 (18):4953–4960
38. Leek JT, Scharpf RB, Bravo HC et al (2010) Tackling the widespread and critical impact of batch effects in high-throughput data. Nat Rev Genet 11(10):733–739
39. Allison DB, Cui X, Page GP, Sabripour M (2006) Microarray data analysis: from disarray to consolidation and consensus. Nat Rev Genet 7(1):55–65
40. Benito M, Parker J, Du Q et al (2004) Adjustment of systematic microarray data biases. Bioinformatics 20(1):105–114
41. Irizarry RA, Hobbs B, Collin F et al (2003) Exploration, normalization, and summaries of high density oligonucleotide array probe level data. Biostatistics 4(2):249–264
42. Johnson WE, Li C, Rabinovic A (2007) Adjusting batch effects in microarray expression data using empirical Bayes methods. Biostatistics 8(1):118–127
43. Leek JT, Storey JD (2007) Capturing heterogeneity in gene expression studies by surrogate variable analysis. PLoS Genet 3 (9):1724–1735
44. Nygaard V, Rodland EA, Hovig E (2016) Methods that remove batch effects while retaining group differences may lead to exaggerated confidence in downstream analyses. Biostatistics 17(1):29–39
45. Oytam Y, Sobhanmanesh F, Duesing K et al (2016) Risk-conscious correction of batch effects: maximising information extraction from high-throughput genomic datasets. BMC Bioinformatics 17(1):332
46. Reese SE, Archer KJ, Therneau TM et al (2013) A new statistic for identifying batch effects in high-throughput genomic data that uses guided principal component analysis. Bioinformatics 29(22):2877–2883
47. Scharpf RB, Ruczinski I, Carvalho B et al (2011) A multilevel model to address batch effects in copy number estimation using SNP arrays. Biostatistics 12(1):33–50
48. Chung NC, Storey JD (2015) Statistical significance of variables driving systematic variation in high-dimensional data. Bioinformatics 31(4):545–554
49. Manimaran S, Selby HM, Okrah K et al (2016) BatchQC: interactive software for evaluating sample and batch effects in genomic data. Bioinformatics 32(24):3836–3838
50. Novembre J, Johnson T, Bryc K et al (2008) Genes mirror geography within Europe. Nature 456(7218):98–101
51. Yang J, Lee SH, Goddard ME et al (2011) GCTA: a tool for genome-wide complex trait analysis. Am J Hum Genet 88(1):76–82
52. Lachin JM, Matts JP, Wei LJ (1988) Randomization in clinical trials: conclusions and recommendations. Control Clin Trials 9 (4):365–374
53. Altman DG (1991) Randomisation. BMJ 302 (6791):1481–1482
54. Altman DG, Bland JM (1999) How to randomise. BMJ 319(7211):703–704
55. Box GEP, Hunter JS, Hunter WG (2005) Statistics for experimenters : design, innovation, and discovery, 2nd edn. Wiley-Interscience.; xvii, Hoboken, N.J, p 633
56. Fisher RA, Bennett JH, Fisher RA et al (1990) Statistical methods, experimental design, and scientific inference. Oxford University Press, Oxford England; New York
57. Maxwell SE, Delaney HD (2004) Designing experiments and analyzing data : a model comparison perspective, 2nd edn. Lawrence Erlbaum Associates, Mahwah, N.J

58. Montgomery DC (2008) Design and analysis of experiments, 7th edn. Wiley. xvii, Hoboken, NJ, p 656
59. Blainey P, Krzywinski M, Altman N (2014) Points of significance: replication. Nat Methods 11(9):879–880
60. Dowjat K, Włodarska I (1981) G-banding patterns in mouse lymphoblastic leukemia L1210. J Natl Cancer Inst 66(1):177–182
61. Pepler WJ, Smith M, van Niekerk WA (1968) An unusual karyotype in a patient with signs suggestive of Down's syndrome. J Med Genet 5(1):68–71
62. International HapMap Consortium (2003) The international HapMap project. Nature 426(6968):789–796
63. Conrad DF, Andrews TD, Carter NP et al (2006) A high-resolution survey of deletion polymorphism in the human genome. Nat Genet 38(1):75–81
64. McCarroll SA, Hadnott TN, Perry GH et al (2006) Common deletion polymorphisms in the human genome. Nat Genet 38(1):86–92
65. Attiyeh EF, Diskin SJ, Attiyeh MA et al (2009) Genomic copy number determination in cancer cells from single nucleotide polymorphism microarrays based on quantitative genotyping corrected for aneuploidy. Genome Res 19(2):276–283
66. LaFramboise T, Weir BA, Zhao X et al (2005) Allele-specific amplification in cancer revealed by SNP array analysis. PLoS Comput Biol 1 (6):e65
67. Coin LJM, Asher JE, Walters RG et al (2010) cnvHap: an integrative population and haplotype-based multiplatform model of SNPs and CNVs. Nat Methods 7(7):541–546
68. Colella S, Yau C, Taylor JM et al (2007) QuantiSNP: an objective Bayes hidden-Markov model to detect and accurately map copy number variation using SNP genotyping data. Nucleic Acids Res 35(6):2013–2025
69. Wang K, Li M, Hadley D, Liu R et al (2007) PennCNV: an integrated hidden Markov model designed for high-resolution copy number variation detection in whole-genome SNP genotyping data. Genome Res 17 (11):1665–1674
70. Illumina. CNVpartition. http://wwwillumi-nacom/documents/products/technotes/technote_cnv_algorithmspdf
71. Carter NP (2007) Methods and strategies for analyzing copy number variation using DNA microarrays. Nat Genet 39(7 Suppl):S16–S21
72. Kallioniemi A, Kallioniemi OP et al (1992) Comparative genomic hybridization for molecular cytogenetic analysis of solid tumors. Science 258(5083):818–821
73. Redon R, Rigler D, Carter NP (2009) Comparative genomic hybridization: DNA preparation for microarray fabrication. Methods Mol Biol 529:259–266
74. Ylstra B, van den Ijssel P, Carvalho B et al (2006) BAC to the future! Or oligonucleotides: a perspective for micro array comparative genomic hybridization (array CGH). Nucleic Acids Res 34(2):445–450
75. Curtis C, Lynch AG, Dunning MJ et al (2009) The pitfalls of platform comparison: DNA copy number array technologies assessed. BMC Genomics 10:588
76. Pinto D, Darvishi K, Shi X et al (2011) Comprehensive assessment of array-based platforms and calling algorithms for detection of copy number variants. Nat Biotechnol 29 (6):512–520
77. Bignell GR, Santarius T, Pole JCM et al (2007) Architectures of somatic genomic rearrangement in human cancer amplicons at sequence-level resolution. Genome Res 17 (9):1296–1303
78. Pinkel D, Albertson DG (2005) Array comparative genomic hybridization and its applications in cancer. Nat Genet 37(Suppl): S11–S17
79. Oostlander AE, Meijer GA, Ylstra B (2004) Microarray-based comparative genomic hybridization and its applications in human genetics. Clin Genet 66(6):488–495
80. Shaffer LG, Bejjani BA (2006) Medical applications of array CGH and the transformation of clinical cytogenetics. Cytogenet Genome Res 115(3–4):303–309
81. Edelmann L, Hirschhorn K (2009) Clinical utility of array CGH for the detection of chromosomal imbalances associated with mental retardation and multiple congenital anomalies. Ann N Y Acad Sci 1151:157–166
82. Boone PM, Bacino CA, Shaw CA et al (2010) Detection of clinically relevant exonic copy-number changes by array CGH. Hum Mutat 31(12):1326–1342
83. Goodwin S, McPherson JD, McCombie WR (2016) Coming of age: ten years of next-generation sequencing technologies. Nat Rev Genet 17(6):333–351
84. Pirooznia M, Goes FS, Zandi PP (2005) Whole-genome CNV analysis: advances in computational approaches. Front Genet 6:138
85. Tuzun E, Sharp AJ, Bailey JA et al (2005) Fine-scale structural variation of the human genome. Nat Genet 37(7):727–732

86. Ye K, Schulz MH, Long Q et al (2009) Pindel: a pattern growth approach to detect break points of large deletions and medium sized insertions from paired-end short reads. Bioinformatics 25(21):2865–2871
87. Simpson JT, Wong K, Jackman SD et al (2009) ABySS: a parallel assembler for short read sequence data. Genome Res 19 (6):1117–1123
88. Li R, Zhu H, Ruan J et al (2010) De novo assembly of human genomes with massively parallel short read sequencing. Genome Res 20(2):265–272
89. Iqbal Z, Caccamo M, Turner I et al (2012) De novo assembly and genotyping of variants using colored de Bruijn graphs. Nat Genet 44(2):226–232
90. Simpson JT, Durbin R (2012) Efficient de novo assembly of large genomes using compressed data structures. Genome Res 22 (3):549–556
91. Abecasis GR, Altshuler D, 1000 Genomes Project Consortium et al (2010) A map of human genome variation from population-scale sequencing. Nature 467 (7319):1061–1073
92. Mills RE, Walter K, Stewart C et al (2011) Mapping copy number variation by population-scale genome sequencing. Nature 470(7332):59–65
93. Wheeler E, Huang N, Bochukova EG et al (2013) Genome-wide SNP and CNV analysis identifies common and low-frequency variants associated with severe early-onset obesity. Nat Genet 45(5):513–517
94. Johansson MM, Van Geystelen A, Larmuseau MH et al (2015) Microarray analysis of copy number variants on the human Y chromosome reveals novel and frequent duplications overrepresented in specific haplogroups. PLoS One 10(8):e0137223
95. Barnes C, Plagnol V, Fitzgerald T et al (2008) A robust statistical method for case-control association testing with copy number variation. Nat Genet 40(10):1245–1252
96. Subirana I, Diaz-Uriarte R, Lucas G, Gonzalez JR (2011) CNVassoc: association analysis of CNV data using R. BMC Med Genet 4:47
97. Glessner JT, Li J, Hakonarson H (2013) ParseCNV integrative copy number variation association software with quality tracking. Nucleic Acids Res 41(5):e64
98. Mace A, Tuke MA, Beckmann JS et al (2016) New quality measure for SNP array based CNV detection. Bioinformatics 32 (21):3298–3305
99. Kutalik Z, Johnson T, Bochud M et al (2011) Methods for testing association between uncertain genotypes and quantitative traits. Biostatistics 12(1):1–17
100. Ionita-Laza I, Perry GH, Raby BA et al (2008) On the analysis of copy-number variations in genome-wide association studies: a translation of the family-based association test. Genet Epidemiol 32(3):273–284
101. Murphy A, Won S, Rogers A et al (2010) On the genome-wide analysis of copy number variants in family-based designs: methods for combining family-based and population-based information for testing dichotomous or quantitative traits, or completely ascertained samples. Genet Epidemiol 34 (6):582–590
102. Zanda M, Onengut S, Walker N et al (2012) Validity of the family-based association test for copy number variant data in the case of non-linear intensity-genotype relationship. Genet Epidemiol 36(8):895–898
103. Zanda M, Onengut-Gumuscu S, Walker N et al (2014) A genome-wide assessment of the role of untagged copy number variants in type 1 diabetes. PLoS Genet 10(5): e1004367
104. McCarroll SA, Kuruvilla FG, Korn JM et al (2008) Integrated detection and population-genetic analysis of SNPs and copy number variation. Nat Genet 40(10):1166–1174
105. Greenman CD, Bignell G, Butler A et al (2010) PICNIC: an algorithm to predict absolute allelic copy number variation with microarray cancer data. Biostatistics 11 (1):164–175
106. Van Loo P, Nordgard SH, Lingjærde OC et al (2010) Allele-specific copy number analysis of tumors. Proc Natl Acad Sci U S A 107 (39):16910–16915
107. Locke AE, Kahali B, Berndt SI et al (2015) Genetic studies of body mass index yield new insights for obesity biology. Nature 518 (7538):197–206
108. Wood AR, Esko T, Yang J et al (2014) Defining the role of common variation in the genomic and biological architecture of adult human height. Nat Genet 46 (11):1173–1186
109. Voight BF, Kang HM, Ding J et al (2012) The Metabochip, a custom genotyping array for genetic studies of metabolic, cardiovascular, and anthropometric traits. PLoS Genet 8 (8):e1002793
110. Feng S, Liu D, Zhan X et al (2014) RAREMETAL: fast and powerful meta-analysis for

rare variants. Bioinformatics 30 (19):2828–2829

111. Wu MC, Lee S, Cai T et al (2011) Rare-variant association testing for sequencing data with the sequence kernel association test. Am J Hum Genet 89(1):82–93

112. Zhan X, Girirajan S, Zhao N et al (2016) A novel copy number variants kernel association test with application to autism spectrum disorders studies. Bioinformatics 32 (23):3603–3610

113. Gao X, Starmer J, Martin ER (2008) A multiple testing correction method for genetic association studies using correlated single nucleotide polymorphisms. Genet Epidemiol 32(4):361–369

114. Walters RG, Jacquemont S, Valsesia A et al (2010) A new highly penetrant form of obesity due to deletions on chromosome 16p11.2. Nature 463(20130649):671–675

115. Devlin B, Roeder K (1999) Genomic control for association studies. Biometrics 55 (4):997–1004

116. Kang HM, Sul JH, Service SK et al (2010) Variance component model to account for sample structure in genome-wide association studies. Nat Genet 42(4):348–354

117. Loh PR, Tucker G, Bulik-Sullivan BK et al (2015) Efficient Bayesian mixed-model analysis increases association power in large cohorts. Nat Genet 47(3):284–290

118. Clevert DA, Mitterecker A, Mayr A et al (2011) Cn.FARMS: a latent variable model to detect copy number variations in microarray data with a low false discovery rate. Nucleic Acids Res 39(12):e79

119. Klambauer G, Schwarzbauer K, Mayr A et al (2012) Cn.MOPS: mixture of Poissons for discovering copy number variations in next-generation sequencing data with a low false discovery rate. Nucleic Acids Res 40(9):e69

120. Cardon LR, Palmer LJ (2003) Population stratification and spurious allelic association. Lancet 361(9357):598–604

121. Rosenberg NA, Huang L, Jewett EM et al (2010) Genome-wide association studies in diverse populations. Nat Rev Genet 11 (5):356–366

122. Cheverud JM (2001) A simple correction for multiple comparisons in interval mapping genome scans. Heredity (Edinb) 87 (Pt 1):52–58

123. Nyholt DR (2004) A simple correction for multiple testing for single-nucleotide polymorphisms in linkage disequilibrium with each other. Am J Hum Genet 74(4):765–769

124. Stuppia L, Antonucci I, Palka G et al (2012) Use of the MLPA assay in the molecular diagnosis of gene copy number alterations in human genetic diseases. Int J Mol Sci 13 (3):3245–3276

125. Hupe P, Stransky N, Thiery JP et al (2004) Analysis of array CGH data: from signal ratio to gain and loss of DNA regions. Bioinformatics 20(18):3413–3422

126. Bengtsson H, Irizarry R, Carvalho B et al (2008) Estimation and assessment of raw copy numbers at the single locus level. Bioinformatics 24(6):759–767

127. Pique-Regi R, Monso-Varona J, Ortega A et al (2008) Sparse representation and Bayesian detection of genome copy number alterations from microarray data. Bioinformatics 24 (3):309–318

128. Olshen AB, Venkatraman ES, Lucito R et al (2004) Circular binary segmentation for the analysis of array-based DNA copy number data. Biostatistics 5(4):557–572

129. Chen K, Wallis JW, McLellan MD, Larson DE, Kalicki JM, Pohl CS et al (2009) BreakDancer: an algorithm for high-resolution mapping of genomic structural variation. Nat Methods 6(9):677–681

130. Korbel JO, Abyzov A, Mu XJ, Carriero N, Cayting P, Zhang Z et al (2009) PEMer: a computational framework with simulation-based error models for inferring genomic structural variants from massive paired-end sequencing data. Genome Biol 10(2):R23

131. Lee WP, Stromberg MP, Ward A et al (2014) MOSAIK: a hash-based algorithm for accurate next-generation sequencing short-read mapping. PLoS One 9(3):e90581

132. Hormozdiari F, Alkan C, Eichler EE et al (2009) Combinatorial algorithms for structural variation detection in high-throughput sequenced genomes. Genome Res 19 (7):1270–1278

133. Korbel JO, Urban AE, Affourtit JP et al (2007) Paired-end mapping reveals extensive structural variation in the human genome. Science 318(5849):420–426

134. Lee S, Hormozdiari F, Alkan C et al (2009) Detecting small indels from clone-end sequencing with mixtures of distributions. Nat Methods 6(7):473–474

135. Campbell PJ, Stephens PJ, Pleasance ED et al (2008) Identification of somatically acquired rearrangements in cancer using genome-wide massively parallel paired-end sequencing. Nat Genet 40(6):722–729

136. Chiang DY, Getz G, Jaffe DB et al (2009) High-resolution mapping of copy-number

alterations with massively parallel sequencing. Nat Methods 6(1):99–103

137. Li X, Chen S, Xie W et al (2014) PSCC: sensitive and reliable population-scale copy number variation detection method based on low coverage sequencing. PLoS One 9 (1):e85096

138. Wang H, Nettleton D, Ying K (2014) Copy number variation detection using next generation sequencing read counts. BMC Bioinformatics 15:109

139. Alkan C, Kidd JM, Marques-Bonet T et al (2009) Personalized copy number and segmental duplication maps using next-generation sequencing. Nat Genet 41 (10):1061–1067

140. Yoon S, Xuan Z, Makarov V et al (2009) Sensitive and accurate detection of copy number variants using read depth of coverage. Genome Res 19(9):1586–1592

141. Nguyen HT, Merriman TR, Black MA (2014) The CNVrd2 package: measurement of copy number at complex loci using high-throughput sequencing data. Front Genet 5:248

142. Lin K, Smit S, Bonnema G et al (2015) Making the difference: integrating structural variation detection tools. Brief Bioinform 16 (5):852–864

143. Schroder J, Hsu A, Boyle SE et al (2014) Socrates: identification of genomic rearrangements in tumour genomes by re-aligning soft clipped reads. Bioinformatics 30 (8):1064–1072

144. Trappe K, Emde AK, Ehrlich HC et al (2014) Detecting and correctly classifying SVs in the NGS twilight zone. Bioinformatics 30 (24):3484–3490

145. Jiang Y, Wang Y, Brudno M (2012) PRISM: pair-read informed split-read mapping for base-pair level detection of insertion, deletion and structural variants. Bioinformatics 28 (20):2576–2583

146. Zhang ZD, Du J, Lam H et al (2011) Identification of genomic indels and structural variations using split reads. BMC Genomics 12:375

147. Simpson JT, Durbin R (2010) Efficient construction of an assembly string graph using the FM-index. Bioinformatics 26(12): i367–i373

148. Massouras A, Hens K, Gubelmann C et al (2010) Primer-initiated sequence synthesis to detect and assemble structural variants. Nat Methods 7(7):485–486

149. Medvedev P, Fiume M, Dzamba M et al (2010) Detecting copy number variation with mated short reads. Genome Res 20 (11):1613–1622

150. Marschall T, Hajirasouliha I, Schonhuth A (2013) MATE-CLEVER: Mendelian-inheritance-aware discovery and genotyping of midsize and long indels. Bioinformatics 29(24):3143–3150

151. Zhang J, Wu Y (2011) SVseq: an approach for detecting exact breakpoints of deletions with low-coverage sequence data. Bioinformatics 27(23):3228–3234

152. Quinlan AR, Clark RA, Sokolova S et al (2010) Genome-wide mapping and assembly of structural variant breakpoints in the mouse genome. Genome Res 20(5):623–635

153. Hajirasouliha I, Hormozdiari F, Alkan C et al (2010) Detection and characterization of novel sequence insertions using paired-end next-generation sequencing. Bioinformatics 26(10):1277–1283

154. Jiang Y, Oldridge DA, Diskin SJ et al (2015) CODEX: a normalization and copy number variation detection method for whole exome sequencing. Nucleic Acids Res 43(6):e39

155. Bansal V, Dorn C, Grunert M et al (2014) Outlier-based identification of copy number variations using targeted resequencing in a small cohort of patients with tetralogy of Fallot. PLoS One 9(1):e85375

156. Magi A, Tattini L, Cifola I et al (2013) EXCAVATOR: detecting copy number variants from whole-exome sequencing data. Genome Biol 14(10):R120

157. Coin LJ, Cao D, Ren J et al (2012) An exome sequencing pipeline for identifying and genotyping common CNVs associated with disease with application to psoriasis. Bioinformatics 28(18):i370–i3i4

158. Fromer M, Moran JL, Chambert K et al (2012) Discovery and statistical genotyping of copy-number variation from whole-exome sequencing depth. Am J Hum Genet 91 (4):597–607

159. Krumm N, Sudmant PH, Ko A et al (2012) Copy number variation detection and genotyping from exome sequence data. Genome Res 22(8):1525–1532

160. Plagnol V, Curtis J, Epstein M et al (2012) A robust model for read count data in exome sequencing experiments and implications for copy number variant calling. Bioinformatics 28(21):2747–2754

161. Korn JM, Kuruvilla FG, McCarroll SA et al (2008) Integrated genotype calling and association analysis of SNPs, common copy number polymorphisms and rare CNVs. Nat Genet 40(10):1253–1260

162. Purcell S, Neale B, Todd-Brown K et al (2007) PLINK: a tool set for whole-genome association and population-based linkage analyses. Am J Hum Genet 81(3):559–575

163. Palta P, Kaplinski L, Nagirnaja L et al (2015) Haplotype phasing and inheritance of copy number variants in nuclear families. PLoS One 10(4):e0122713

164. Chettier R, Ward K, Albertsen HM (2014) Endometriosis is associated with rare copy number variants. PLoS One 9(8):e103968

Chapter 15

From Identification to Function: Current Strategies to Prioritise and Follow-Up GWAS Results

Antonio J. Berlanga-Taylor

Abstract

Along with family-based studies, dozens of genome-wide association studies (GWAS) have clearly identified the genetic basis of common diseases and complex traits. There are currently hundreds of single nucleotide polymorphisms (SNP) associated with human disease as well as biochemical and physiological phenotypes. Although this is only the tip of the iceberg, we are now confronted with a general lack of understanding of how these trait-associated variants act. How do these genetic changes lead to overt clinical phenotypes? What are the molecular mechanisms? Can we harness this information to develop better preventive and curative strategies? Current efforts are shifting to focus on these questions as we move from identifying variants to understanding their effects. Here I provide a broad overview of the main technical concerns and current bottlenecks as we approach this new phase.

Key words Functional genomics, GWAS, Human disease, Variant function, Genotype, Phenotype, Complex traits, Fine-mapping

1 Introduction

The study of complex traits, typically those which are polygenic with many presumed gene–gene and gene–environment interactions, has accelerated since the publication of the human genome. Genome-wide association studies (GWAS) have yielded thousands of associations between genotypes and phenotypes and have become a cornerstone of complex trait research methods. GWAS observations are critical in our understanding since they are mostly germline variants and thus likely causal. GWAS observations do not tell us about the mechanisms through which these variants act however and biomedical translation is unlikely to occur at greater pace without this knowledge. Functional genomics came into existence with the advent of next-generation sequencing, adaptation of molecular methods that probe genetic function and increasingly powerful statistical and computational methods. It is the marriage of molecular biology with quantitative genetics and aims to answer

Evangelos Evangelou (ed.), *Genetic Epidemiology: Methods and Protocols*, Methods in Molecular Biology, vol. 1793, https://doi.org/10.1007/978-1-4939-7868-7_15,

a fundamental question: what are the effects and functional consequences of genetic variation? Functional genomics has thus recently grown in importance as the post-GWAS focus shifts towards gaining this understanding. Excitingly, further advances in molecular biology, namely in genome editing, promise greater expansion with experimental manipulation at unprecedented resolution.

Important limitations exist however, both philosophical and technical. What does causality mean in this context? How do we define functionality? What constitutes a (relevant) phenotype? How to make reliable observations directly in humans? How to translate findings from model organisms? How to increase high-throughput methods? Some of these questions are pertinent to other related fields but have become acutely important in disease genomics in the post-GWAS era. In this review I cover some of the main methods as well as technical and experimental issues that we currently face. The aim is to provide an overview of the current challenges in understanding what the effects of genetic variation are. Although I do not cover important aspects such as how to define causality, function and phenotype in genomics in any detail, these are fundamental issues that will guide future research.

2 The Success and Limitations of GWAS

The genetic basis to complex disease has been clearly established based on replicable and robust methodology [1]. Many key observations have been made over the last decade including that genetic risk is polygenic, pleotropic, both shared and private to populations, families and individuals and that risk variants occur at different allele frequencies and are not only rare [2, 3]. These issues remain under scrutiny and vary between traits however.

Perhaps most importantly, genetic association studies have repeatedly observed that the seat of complex traits is in regulatory regions, namely in non-coding sequences such as enhancers. This key observation is rapidly shifting the efforts of methodological development towards genetic dissection at scale and systems-level approaches. Many questions have been opened from this period of discovery, including missing or hidden heritability, the biological and clinical relevance of small effect sizes, and the realisation of the important limitations of GWAS.

Much more remains to be discovered, such as the degree of epistasis, largely unobserved so far [4] and robust study designs to capture gene–environment interactions. A point to remember is that so far we have largely focussed on single nucleotide polymorphisms (SNPs). Although copy number variants (CNVs) are unlikely to play a major role in common disease [5], other variants such as larger insertions and/or deletions (indels), complex architectures or the full spectrum of genetic variation across individuals and populations remain to be explored in greater depth.

Overall, the degree of complexity that we face remains as daunting as ever. After the large genome and variant mapping efforts and the success of association studies two of the most pressing questions are to determine which variants are causal and through which mechanisms they act.

3 Causality, Function and Phenotypes in Complex Trait Genetics

The use of the term "causal variant" to refer to significant results from association studies is somewhat of a misnomer. What is often meant by this is a variant, one (or a set) in high linkage disequilibrium, having an effect on disease (directly or indirectly). Variants in GWASs are unlikely to be somatic [6] and we can thus assume that they are germline and present before disease. GWAS results are also unlikely to be 'synthetic' (spurious) [7] except in a minority of cases such as non-coding variants in the NOD2 region [8].

Virtually anything that is not a genotype could be described as a phenotype. Traits which are organismal, systemic, tissue, cellular, biochemical, epigenetic, etc., can be used to make associations with genetic variation or probe functional genetic effects. Key questions are whether a given trait is actually relevant and if it can be accurately defined and measured, both for biomedical and statistical reasons [9].

At one end of the spectrum we can define functional genetic variation as that which has a biochemical effect [10]. An extreme example of this is that the whole genome, because it replicates, is functional, making it a contentious definition and less useful operationally [11]. At the other end is the evolutionary view that genetic variation is functional if selective pressure has acted on it (for a discussion see [12]). The former is overly simplistic and the latter only accounts for genetic variation on which particular environments have exerted an effect on over many generations. Thus, how to define functionality in genomics has important philosophical and practical implications. Here I refer to function as the evolutionary and causal mechanism of a genetic variant (the 'selected-effect', see [13]) and effect as the 'activity' of a variant (i.e., any biochemical or other read-out that can be assigned to DNA sequence) [14]. As biological, medical and other sciences interface it is critical that a common vocabulary is maintained. Ultimately, a combined approach will yield better answers [15].

4 Effects of Genetic Variation at the Molecular and Cellular Levels

In terms of impact on biochemical and other activity, variants can be divided according to effects on chromatin status, transcription, mRNA stability and translation, and protein function, stability or localisation. Variants in regulatory regions (but not exclusively), such as in promoters and enhancers, can prevent or modify transcript levels, timing of expression, cell specificity, DNA methylation levels and DNase regions for example [16–19].

In post-GWAS analysis, effects have been broadly categorised according to the location of the genetic variant as coding versus non-coding. Indeed, a key observation from complex trait genomics association studies has been that ~93% of trait-associated variants are non-coding [20] and that variants lying within regulatory elements (e.g., enhancers) account for a higher heritability than those in protein-coding sequences [21]. In autoimmune diseases (AID) for example, genomic analysis has provided deeper insight into how variants likely act in concert through common pathways [22]. Analysis of tens of GWAS in AID have shown that many susceptibility loci are shared but the relationship is complex, observing opposing direction of effects for different diseases, locus heterogeneity (different variants associated with different diseases nearby) and large effect loci which are more likely to be disease specific.

The simple and useful categorisation of coding versus non-coding can be misleading however, as overlap of effects where coding sequences act as non-coding and vice-versa have been documented [23, 24].

5 Strategies to Determine the Effect of Genetic Variants

As DNA sequencing has become standardised and accessible, genomics has transitioned from mapping to describing and probing function. Global experimentation based on high throughput approaches combining statistical and computational analysis with bio-medical interpretation (but also agricultural, paleontological and others) is the cornerstone of functional genomics [25, 26]. Classical molecular biology approaches, including the study of gene expression, DNA–protein interactions, non-coding and regulatory elements, 3D interactions and DNA methylation, amongst others, are now followed by microarray or sequencing measurements and are at the heart of functional genomics [27].

5.1 Genome Editing

Of particular note are genome editing techniques based on programmable nucleases such zinc-fingers, transcription activator-like effector nucleases and CRISPR (clustered regularly interspaced short palindromic repeat)-associated protein 9 (Cas9) RNA-guided engineered nucleases (reviewed in [28]). Of the various methods, CRISPR/Cas9, a prokaryotic immune system which can recognise and cleave foreign genetic material, has received the most attention in the last few years. Since its discovery it has been developed into a powerful editing technique [29], enabling targeted mutagenesis in eukaryotic cells. CRISPR/Cas9, consisting of a guide RNA and the Cas9 enzyme, causes DNA double-strand breaks followed by homology-directed repair. This allows targeted insertions, corrections, point mutagenesis and, through additional modifications, chromosomal rearrangements.

CRISPR based methods have been adapted in order to perform not only knockouts but also to carry out transcriptional modulation by harnessing catalytically inactive Cas9 (dCas9) with transcriptional activator, repressor and recruitment domains without causing irreversible genetic modifications [30, 31]. CRISPR-based techniques have very recently been adapted to allow genome-scale interrogation, achieving knockdowns >90% compared to controls with minimal off-target effects (as measured by negative control sgRNAs) as well as 100-fold activation range [31] (reviewed in [32, 33]). Novel methods such as Perturb-seq and barcoding combine single-cell RNA sequencing, CRISPR-based manipulation and sophisticated analytical methods in order to dissect cellular phenotypes at scale [34–36].

Genome editing methods now allow in vivo manipulation of whole organisms for disease treatment [37] and have been used in clinical trials [38]. The study by Suzuki et al. [37] partially restored MERTK function and showed physiological improvement in rats suffering retinitis pigmentosa using a homology-independent targeted integration (HITI) method. This method was based on CRISPR/Cas9 and permits DNA knock-in in dividing and non-dividing cells in vivo. Tebas et al. [38] showed in a clinical trial that an autologous $CD4^+$ T cell infusion with a zinc-finger nuclease inactivated *CCR5* was safe. Clinical trials using CRISPR-Cas9 systems have recently been approved [39]. Although tantalising, CRISPR-based approaches are still in their infancy and issues such as consistency, false-positive and negative rates, off-target effects, scaling and full adaptation to human cells need to be overcome. Most importantly, ethical implications and societal impact must be addressed.

5.2 Epigenomic and Transcriptomic Assays

The epigenome, a series of chemical modifications to DNA and its surrounding histones, contains crucial information for genomic regulation which is thought to be heritable, cell specific and modifiable by environmental factors [40]. Epigenomic methods can identify regulatory regions by analysing DNA methylation, open chromatin, chromatin immunoprecipitation (ChIP) and 3D chromatin capture, amongst others [41].

DNA methylation, addition of a methyl group to cytosines by DNA methyltransferases, regulates gene expression through generally repressive effects. It can be investigated using a variety of techniques from targeted methods to whole genome analysis [42]. Genome-wide methods such as DNase I hypersensitive sites sequencing (DNase-seq), formaldehyde-assisted identification of regulatory elements (FAIRE-seq) and assay for transposase-accessible chromatin (ATAC-seq) identify genetic regulatory elements such as enhancers and promoters by determining chromatin accessibility followed by high-through put sequencing [43–46].

Maps of transcription factor binding and post-translational histone modifications can be described using chromatin immunoprecipitation based techniques which make use of specific antibodies to isolate targeted DNA–protein interactions (binding events) and chemical modifications of histones [47]. ChIP, as well as many other related experimental techniques, can be followed by polymerase chain reaction (ChIP-PCR, ChIP-qPCR) based assays, microarray measurements (ChIP-chip) or next-generation DNA sequencing (ChIP-seq). Chromatin conformation capture (3C) based experiments can identify 3D chromatin interactions between bound proteins. Techniques such as 3C, 4C, 5C, 6C (reviewed in [48]) and Capture-C [49, 50] determine the 3D state of DNA (looping) for targeted regions. Techniques such as Hi-C [51] and chromatin interaction analysis with paired-end tag sequencing (ChIAPET) [52] can scale genome-wide albeit in a small number of samples per experiment.

Coding and non-coding RNA molecules can be investigated using specifically designed sample preparation methods to determine mRNA, long non-coding RNA, microRNA and several other RNA classes [53]. Single cell analysis has adapted many of these methods, revealing deep insights into how cells act within a population [54–56]. RNA molecules are not necessarily confined intracellularly, microRNAs circulate in plasma and can be used as disease biomarkers [57].

The spatiotemporal nuclear organisation of a cell is critical in transcriptional regulation. New methods combine DNA sequencing based functional assays with imaging techniques [58]. Chen et al. [58] developed ATAC-see, based on a combination with ATAC-seq, to understand how neutrophil extracellular traps, chromatin structures with antimicrobial molecules, are released. Such methods have the potential to reveal how DNA regulatory elements map within their native nuclear context through cell-specific direct imaging techniques followed by next-generation sequencing of transposase identified regions.

Experimental and technological progress now enable assays to be performed with limited input and cell numbers, allowing clinical samples and rare cell-types to be studied. Improved resolution, such as that afforded by ChIP-exo (ChIP treated with exonucleases followed by sequencing) can provide single base-pair precision mapping [59]. Many experimental and analytical challenges remain however, including data integration, robust differential analysis and scaling genome-wide methods to thousands of samples.

5.3 Linking Genetic Variation to Molecular Phenotypes

Similar to GWAS methods, molecular and cellular traits can be associated with genetic data. Statistical approaches such as quantitative trait locus (QTL) analysis aim to identify the genetic basis of complex phenotypes by determining their actions, interactions, quantity and location [60]. QTL mapping has a long history and has been used in many organisms, revealing condition, gender, environment and context specific effects which would otherwise remain obscure [61]. Loci are often found in non-coding regions as has been the case for GWAS identified variants [62].

Recent studies have investigated the effect of genetic variation on molecular phenotypes such as gene expression, transcription factor binding and chromatin landscape [63–66]. Genetic variation can alter DNA–protein interactions, affect binding specificity and contribute to inter-individual differences in transcriptional regulation and expression. These differences, such as for open chromatin accessibility, metabolomic, proteomic or transcriptomic variation, can be detected by allelic biases determined by high-throughput DNA sequencing coupled with quantitative measurements of the trait of interest.

One of the most widely used molecular phenotypes is gene expression. Lower costs and advances in transcriptomic methods allow measurements in thousands of individuals which can be associated with their genotype using QTL analysis [67] (also termed genetical genomics). These genome-wide methods, coupling DNA and RNA in a so-called unbiased way, allow high-throughput characterisation of the molecular effects of genetic variation. Methods are computationally intensive however and further advances in statistical techniques are needed in order to better understand these complex relationships.

5.4 Systems Analysis

So far, studies have mainly tested individual elements (gene expression or transcription factor binding for example) but organismal effects likely come from a combination of factors, including dynamic events, and as such should ideally be studied using system-level approaches (partly reviewed in [68]). These approaches study biological components as a whole with the aim of predicting behaviours which cannot be elucidated from their dissection alone. Systems sciences attempt to model complex biological phenomena using computational, mathematical and statistical tools based on new or existing biological knowledge in order to discover cell, tissue, organism or species properties [69]. Systems genetics studies the flow of biological information pertaining to complex phenotypes by measuring intermediate quantitative phenotypes. Such systems-level approaches can identify genetic variants, molecules (transcripts, non-coding RNAs, metabolites and proteins), pathways and networks underpinning complex traits [68].

QTL studies in human cohorts or cell lines now routinely combine genotype–phenotype results with external annotations (such as those from ENCODE [10]), in order to contextualise and interpret the meaning of the associations found (see for example [70, 71]). Studies in model organisms also integrate systems methods. Song et al. [72] used genome-wide differential transcription factor binding with differentially expressed genes to investigate environmental stress response networks for example. Although genetic variation was not part of the study it is straightforward to conceive how population level projects could scale to identify genetic determinants.

5.5 Metabolomics and Proteomics

Although gene expression and DNA methylation have had greater attention as intermediate phenotypes, other molecules of the 'omics type are maturing into robust and high-throughput technologies with hundreds to thousands of measurements being performed simultaneously. Regulatory region QTLs [18], metabolome QTLs [73–75], protein QTLs [76] and cytomics [74] have all gained traction in the past several years. The study by Wu et al. [76] for example measured the levels of 5953 proteins in the supernatant of human lymphoblastoid cell lines from the Hapmap Project [77] and assessed the effect of genetic variation on these. The authors used isobaric tag-based quantitative mass spectrometry to determine relative protein levels and found that, as with gene expression, protein levels are heritable with high inter-individual, gender and population variation. Protein expression is regulated by post-transcriptional processes and does not correlate perfectly with mRNA levels thus making it essential to understand genotype–protein abundance correlations. Earlier studies measuring transcriptomics [78] also took advantage of Hapmap resources that had been established for genetic variation mapping and have since been used to explore biological mechanisms using shared and accessible samples. More recently, Hapmap has been expanded and superseded by the 1000 Genomes project [79, 80].

6 Experimental and Analytical Challenges

The studies described above and many others are creating an increasingly rich catalogue of the effects of genetic variation. Large, consortium-led projects such as ENCODE [10], BLUEPRINT/IHEC [81, 82] FANTOM5 [83], Roadmap Epigenomics Mapping Consortium [84], International Cancer Genome Consortium (ICGC) [85] and GTEx [19] have performed hundreds of experiments assessing the biochemical effects of sequence variation. Primarily, they have provided an excellent source of external annotation. Among other results, these multi-country, multi-laboratory projects have helped standardise protocols. Importantly, they have strongly promoted open data, open source and open access, allowing the re-use of data and software tools by other researchers. As these and other projects have become community resources they have resulted in hundreds of additional independent publications.

Although great progress has been made, it is important to remind ourselves of the limitations that remain in characterising the effects of genomic and epigenomic mechanisms. These range from sample obtention and preparation (with minimal invasion and manipulation, in sufficient quantity and without introducing biases) to statistical methods development, computational tractability and interpretation bottlenecks. An extended discussion is beyond the scope of this review however. As an example of an experimental challenge, an important disadvantage in methods which investigate DNA-protein interactions is that many rely on formaldehyde crosslinking (termed X-ChIP, such as in ChIP based assays, FAIRE-seq and others). Although largely reliable, formaldehyde crosslinking can induce important artefacts as it preferentially produces protein–protein crosslinks which can appear as artefactual DNA binding events [86]. Less frequently used alternatives are ultraviolet crosslinking, which bypasses protein–protein artefacts as it only generates protein–nucleic acid crosslinks [87] and is used successfully to analyse RNA–protein interactions [88], and native ChIP (N-ChIP) [89, 90].

ChIP-seq and ChIP-exo methods often show many low-occupancy peaks with degenerate motifs which are thought to be more likely artefacts than true positive signals [91]. Tests with reporter assays in Drosophila showed that these low occupancy sites do not induce expression [92]. Biases towards open chromatin are also important to note and may show different patterns according to the enzyme used. Perhaps most importantly, the lack of input controls severely limits wider interpretation of assays such as ChIP-exo and ATAC-seq. New alternatives to nucleosome determination such as chemical histone mapping [93] could provide higher accuracy and consistency compared to MNase-seq methods but remain to be fully tested. In fields such as metabolomics, target molecule identification is a high priority and solutions require an integrated approach between bioinformatics and experimental methods. Handling, processing, analysis and integration of high-density molecular data require specialised statistical and bioinformatics tools. Data analysis challenges mostly relate to scale, heterogeneity and the lack of individuals with the appropriate mix of computational, statistical and biological skills. Efforts towards data standardisation and accessibility, development of multivariate methods (simultaneous analysis of more than two variables), multiple testing and p-value correction, testing of multiple phenotypes, applications in machine learning, development of tools for visualisation, and efficient computational algorithms and data structures are areas of intense investigation. The increased availability of computational power and rapid development of experimental and analytical methods have considerably broadened the horizon. Many limitations can be overcome with appropriate study design, careful choice of statistical analysis and orthogonal observations. Important challenges for future research include improving our understanding of aetiology and molecular mechanisms, increasing the predictive ability of genomics and translating research findings into clinical benefit across the diversity of individuals and populations.

7 Examples of Functional Follow-Up in Disease

7.1 Rare Variants

Until recently the extent to which rare (minor allele frequency (MAF) $\leq 1\%$) and low-frequency (MAF 1–5%) variants contributed to complex trait variance had been relatively understudied. The UK10K Consortium, composed of population based and disease cohorts, undertook whole genome and exome sequencing of almost 10,000 individuals [94]. It generated community resources of sequence and phenotype data, methodological advancements in single-marker and rare variant aggregation tests and described novel biomedical insights.

In one example, UK10K investigated the contribution of rare non-coding genetic variants to bone mineral density (BMD), a heritable predictor of osteoporotic fractures with known associations to both common non-coding and rare coding DNA changes [95]. The study identified variants with comparatively large effect sizes associated with increased BMD ($n = 53{,}236$) and decreased risk of fracture ($n = 508{,}253$) using a combination of whole-genome ($n = 2882$), whole-exome ($n = 3549$) and genotype imputation ($n = 26{,}534$) followed by de novo replication (genotyping, $n = 20{,}271$). To understand the effects of the genetic variants, the researchers performed functional genomics, cellular and mouse studies on *EN1*, a novel locus encoding a homeobox gene known to be critical to limb formation in mice. Zheng et al. [95] carried out conditional loss of *En1* experiments in En1(cre/-flox) mice to test activity in adult bones observing lower bone mass by computed tomography in mutants as compared to littermate controls. Together with other observations, they concluded that low bone mass is secondary to increased osteoclastic activity derived from *En1* null osteogenic cells. Overall, UK10K researchers found more associations in deleterious coding and conserved non-coding variants than in other categories and advocate for larger sequencing studies in both healthy and disease populations [95]. Such studies should be followed by functional experiments to better understand possible physiological and disease mechanisms.

7.2 Common Variants and Systems-Level Approaches

Hundreds of common genetic variants have been associated with complex traits but we generally lack an understanding of the mechanisms through which they act. An example where researchers combined biochemical observations with evolutionary analysis to understand how non-coding *cis*-regulatory variation modulates disease risk is the study by Claussnitzer et al. [96]. The authors developed a method, phylogenetic module complexity analysis, which analyses conserved co-occurring transcription factor binding sites (TFBS) to identify functional regulatory variants and applied it to type 2 diabetes. The computational based strategy fine-maps GWAS loci by harnessing cross-species data of conserved motif clusters. In other words, previously associated GWAS identified SNPs are analysed for co-localisation with known enhancer regions (or TFBS, as defined by ENCODE for instance) in a relevant human cell type in order to prioritise candidate disease variants for functional follow-up experiments (see for example the analysis performed by Trynka et al. [97] for relevant tissue identification). Results from Claussnitzer et al. [96] identified paired related homeobox 1 (PRRX1), a nuclear homeobox DNA-associated protein usually acting as a transcription coactivator, as a repressor of PPARG2 expression in adipose cells. PPARG2, peroxisome proliferator-activated receptor gamma (PPAR-γ, glitazone receptor, NR1C3 or PPARG2) is an adipose tissue regulator of fatty acid storage and glucose metabolism. Further analysis showed that the rs4684847 risk allele, which alters PRRX1 binding, modulates negative effects on lipid metabolism and insulin sensitivity [96]. This and other studies show how transcription factor binding differences may affect disease risk [98]. Other studies have investigated the effect of a single locus using statistical and experimental fine-mapping of GWAS results with functional laboratory follow-up in human and animal models [99]. Small et al. [99] investigate the effects of type 2 diabetes associated risk alleles near *KLF14*, a transcription factor and master regulator of gene expression in adipose tissue. The authors show that *KLF14* risk alleles act in adipose tissue, reduce KLF14 expression and modulate the expression of 385 distant genes. Remarkably, effects are sex specific to both the subject and parent of origin.

8 Future Outlook: Beyond GWAS

Beyond GWAS it is very likely that there will be more GWAS which integrate functional genomics analyses in order to elucidate mechanisms behind genetic susceptibility and protection in complex traits. Efforts to understand genetic risk have moved in various directions but overall aim to answer questions surrounding causality, functionality and determining effects which can inform strategies for disease diagnosis, prognosis, prevention and treatment.

Understanding the genetic basis of complex traits has undoubtedly already contributed to our biological understanding of disease [100, 101] and has served to aid the understanding and discovery of current and novel drugs [102, 103].

Further integration of evolutionary, experimental and statistical approaches together with experimental and technical advances will allow scaling to larger sample sizes and multiple tissues in clinical cohorts. Although I do not discuss in any detail, a crucial aspect that will underpin future development is increased computational power and efficiency coupled with more sophisticated statistical methods such as mixed models and Bayesian approaches. Biological and statistical fine-mapping techniques are rapidly developing in order to aid the prioritisation of candidate genetic variants that could inform clinical strategies. These methods can still yield tens to hundreds of candidate SNPs however and techniques such as scaled CRISPR-based methods and massively parallel reporter assays will be necessary to further dissect candidates.

Increasing availability of DNA sequencing and genotyping data in studies with larger samples sizes, deep molecular phenotyping and standardised procedures [10, 104] together with open source tools and data will yield unique biomedical insights with reproducible and replicable results.

As more cell types, tissues, populations and environmental and other factors are studied in relation to genetic variation and effects we will gain a deeper understanding of possible causal relationships, particularly of gene–gene and gene–environment interactions across time. The exposome, the sum of all environmental exposures in an individual [105] quantitated in human bio-samples (as opposed to questionnaires) using hi-plex (hundreds to thousands of simultaneous measurements) methods [106] may become a routine concept and practice.

Systems approaches which integrate evolutionary methods with genetic, molecular and organismal phenotypes in human observational studies are becoming more common practice. Randomised, placebo-controlled clinical trials in humans are now utilising eQTL methods to investigate genetic determinants of drug response [107, 108]. Similarly, large-scale efforts are underway using prospective cohorts coupled to biobanking with sample sizes in the tens of thousands [109, 110]. These studies combine gold-standard epidemiological designs in interventional and observational studies with high-throughput molecular methods and provide detailed insights associating genomics with molecular and clinical events. Finally, further advances in genome editing techniques and personal 'omics will increase our capacity to tailor treatments and modify what previously were unmodifiable factors with the aim of preventing or treating disease.

Acknowledgements

I am funded by a Medical Research Council Intermediate Fellowship through the UK MED-BIO Programme (MR/L01632X/1).

References

1. WTCCC (2007) Genome-wide association study of 14,000 cases of seven common diseases and 3,000 shared controls. Nature 447 (7145):661–678. https://doi.org/10.1038/nature05911
2. Visscher PM, Brown MA, McCarthy MI et al (2012) Five years of GWAS discovery. Am J Hum Genet 90(1):7–24. https://doi.org/10.1016/j.ajhg.2011.11.029
3. Gibson G (2012) Rare and common variants: twenty arguments. Nat Rev Genet 13 (2):135–145. https://doi.org/10.1038/nrg3118
4. Strange A, Capon F, Spencer CC et al (2010) A genome-wide association study identifies new psoriasis susceptibility loci and an interaction between HLA-C and ERAP1. Nat Genet 42(11):985–990. https://doi.org/10.1038/ng.694
5. Craddock N, Hurles ME, Cardin N et al (2010) Genome-wide association study of CNVs in 16,000 cases of eight common diseases and 3,000 shared controls. Nature 464 (7289):713–720. https://doi.org/10.1038/nature08979
6. Abecasis GR, Altshuler D, Auton A et al (2010) A map of human genome variation from population-scale sequencing. Nature 467(7319):1061–1073. https://doi.org/10.1038/nature09534
7. Dickson SP, Wang K, Krantz I et al (2010) Rare variants create synthetic genome-wide associations. PLoS Biol 8(1):e1000294. https://doi.org/10.1371/journal.pbio.1000294
8. Anderson CA, Soranzo N, Zeggini E et al (2011) Synthetic associations are unlikely to account for many common disease genome-wide association signals. PLoS Biol 9(1): e1000580. https://doi.org/10.1371/journal.pbio.1000580
9. Wojczynski MK, Tiwari HK (2008) Definition of phenotype. Adv Genet 60:75–105. https://doi.org/10.1016/s0065-2660(07)00404-x
10. Dunham I, Kundaje A, Aldred SF et al (2012) An integrated encyclopedia of DNA elements in the human genome. Nature 489 (7414):57–74. https://doi.org/10.1038/nature11247
11. Graur D, Zheng Y, Price N et al (2013) On the immortality of television sets: "function" in the human genome according to the evolution-free gospel of ENCODE. Genome Biol Evol 5(3):578–590. https://doi.org/10.1093/gbe/evt028
12. Doolittle WF (2013) Is junk DNA bunk? A critique of ENCODE. Proc Natl Acad Sci U S A 110(14):5294–5300. https://doi.org/10.1073/pnas.1221376110
13. Millikan RG (1984) Language, thought, and other biological categories: new foundations for realism. In: Bradford book. MIT Press, Cambridge
14. Doolittle WF, Brunet TD, Linquist S et al (2014) Distinguishing between "function" and "effect" in genome biology. Genome Biol Evol 6(5):1234–1237. https://doi.org/10.1093/gbe/evu098
15. Kellis M, Wold B, Snyder MP et al (2014) Defining functional DNA elements in the human genome. Proc Natl Acad Sci U S A 111(17):6131–6138. https://doi.org/10.1073/pnas.1318948111
16. Fairfax BP, Makino S, Radhakrishnan J et al (2012) Genetics of gene expression in primary immune cells identifies cell type-specific master regulators and roles of HLA alleles. Nat Genet 44(5):502–510. https://doi.org/10.1038/ng.2205. [doi]. ng.2205 [pii]
17. Fairfax BP, Humburg P, Makino S et al (2014) Innate immune activity conditions the effect of regulatory variants upon monocyte gene expression. Science 343 (6175):1246949. https://doi.org/10.1126/science.1246949
18. Degner JF, Pai AA, Pique-Regi R et al (2012) DNase I sensitivity QTLs are a major determinant of human expression variation. Nature 482(7385):390–394. https://doi.org/10.1038/nature10808
19. GTex Consortium (2013) The genotype-tissue expression (GTEx) project. Nat Genet 45(6):580–585. https://doi.org/10.1038/ng.2653

20. Maurano MT, Humbert R, Rynes E et al (2012) Systematic localization of common disease-associated variation in regulatory DNA. Science 337(6099):1190–1195. https://doi.org/10.1126/science.1222794. [doi]. science.1222794 [pii]
21. Gusev A, Lee SH, Trynka G et al (2014) Partitioning heritability of regulatory and cell-type-specific variants across 11 common diseases. Am J Hum Genet 95(5):535–552. https://doi.org/10.1016/j.ajhg.2014.10.004
22. Parkes M, Cortes A, van Heel DA et al (2013) Genetic insights into common pathways and complex relationships among immune-mediated diseases. Nat Rev Genet 14 (9):661–673. https://doi.org/10.1038/nrg3502
23. Stergachis AB, Haugen E, Shafer A et al (2013) Exonic transcription factor binding directs codon choice and affects protein evolution. Science 342(6164):1367–1372. https://doi.org/10.1126/science.1243490
24. Birnbaum RY, Clowney EJ, Agamy O et al (2012) Coding exons function as tissue-specific enhancers of nearby genes. Genome Res 22(6):1059–1068. https://doi.org/10.1101/gr.133546.111
25. Hieter P, Boguski M (1997) Functional genomics: it's all how you read it. Science 278 (5338):601–602
26. Weinstein JN (1998) Fishing expeditions. Science 282(5389):628–629
27. Green MR, Sambrook J (2012) Molecular cloning: a laboratory manual, 4th edn. Cold Spring Harbor Laboratory Press, Cold Spring Harbor, N.Y
28. Kim H, Kim JS (2014) A guide to genome engineering with programmable nucleases. Nat Rev Genet 15(5):321–334. https://doi.org/10.1038/nrg3686
29. Jinek M, Chylinski K, Fonfara I et al (2012) A programmable dual-RNA-guided DNA endonuclease in adaptive bacterial immunity. Science 337(6096):816–821. https://doi.org/10.1126/science.1225829
30. Konermann S, Brigham MD, Trevino AE et al (2015) Genome-scale transcriptional activation by an engineered CRISPR-Cas9 complex. Nature 517(7536):583–588. https://doi.org/10.1038/nature14136
31. Gilbert LA, Horlbeck MA, Adamson B et al (2014) Genome-scale CRISPR-mediated control of gene repression and activation. Cell 159(3):647–661. https://doi.org/10.1016/j.cell.2014.09.029
32. Shalem O, Sanjana NE, Zhang F (2015) High-throughput functional genomics using CRISPR-Cas9. Nat Rev Genet 16 (5):299–311. https://doi.org/10.1038/nrg3899
33. Komor AC, Badran AH, Liu DR (2016) CRISPR-based technologies for the manipulation of eukaryotic genomes. Cell 168 (1–2):20–36. https://doi.org/10.1016/j.cell.2016.10.044
34. Dixit A, Parnas O, Li B et al (2016) Perturb-seq: dissecting molecular circuits with scalable single-cell RNA profiling of pooled genetic screens. Cell 167(7):1853–1866.e1817. https://doi.org/10.1016/j.cell.2016.11.038
35. Adamson B, Norman TM, Jost M et al (2016) A multiplexed single-cell CRISPR screening platform enables systematic dissection of the unfolded protein response. Cell 167 (7):1867–1882.e1821. https://doi.org/10.1016/j.cell.2016.11.048
36. Jaitin DA, Weiner A, Yofe I et al (2016) Dissecting immune circuits by linking CRISPR-pooled screens with single-cell RNA-Seq. Cell 167(7):1883–1896.e1815. https://doi.org/10.1016/j.cell.2016.11.039
37. Suzuki K, Tsunekawa Y, Hernandez-Benitez R et al (2016) In vivo genome editing via CRISPR/Cas9 mediated homology-independent targeted integration. Nature 540(7631):144–149. https://doi.org/10.1038/nature20565
38. Tebas P, Stein D, Tang WW et al (2014) Gene editing of CCR5 in autologous CD4 T cells of persons infected with HIV. N Engl J Med 370 (10):901–910. https://doi.org/10.1056/NEJMoa1300662
39. Cyranoski D (2016) Chinese scientists to pioneer first human CRISPR trial. Nature 535 (7613):476–477. https://doi.org/10.1038/nature.2016.20302
40. Heard E, Martienssen RA (2014) Transgenerational epigenetic inheritance: myths and mechanisms. Cell 157(1):95–109. https://doi.org/10.1016/j.cell.2014.02.045
41. Rivera CM, Ren B (2013) Mapping human epigenomes. Cell 155(1):39–55. https://doi.org/10.1016/j.cell.2013.09.011
42. Krueger F, Kreck B, Franke A et al (2012) DNA methylome analysis using short bisulfite sequencing data. Nat Methods 9 (2):145–151. https://doi.org/10.1038/nmeth.1828
43. Boyle AP, Davis S, Shulha HP, Meltzer P et al (2008) High-resolution mapping and characterization of open chromatin across the

genome. Cell 132(2):311–322. https://doi.org/10.1016/j.cell.2007.12.014

44. Birney E, Stamatoyannopoulos JA, Dutta A et al (2007) Identification and analysis of functional elements in 1% of the human genome by the ENCODE pilot project. Nature 447(7146):799–816. https://doi.org/10.1038/nature05874
45. Thurman RE, Rynes E, Humbert R et al (2012) The accessible chromatin landscape of the human genome. Nature 489 (7414):75–82. https://doi.org/10.1038/nature11232
46. Buenrostro JD, Giresi PG, Zaba LC et al (2013) Transposition of native chromatin for fast and sensitive epigenomic profiling of open chromatin, DNA-binding proteins and nucleosome position. Nat Methods 10 (12):1213–1218. https://doi.org/10.1038/nmeth.2688
47. Furey TS (2012) ChIP-seq and beyond: new and improved methodologies to detect and characterize protein-DNA interactions. Nat Rev Genet 13(12):840–852. https://doi.org/10.1038/nrg3306
48. Dekker J, Marti-Renom MA, Mirny LA (2013) Exploring the three-dimensional organization of genomes: interpreting chromatin interaction data. Nat Rev Genet 14 (6):390–403. https://doi.org/10.1038/nrg3454
49. Davies JO, Telenius JM, McGowan SJ et al (2016) Multiplexed analysis of chromosome conformation at vastly improved sensitivity. Nat Methods 13(1):74–80. https://doi.org/10.1038/nmeth.3664
50. Hughes JR, Roberts N, McGowan S et al (2014) Analysis of hundreds of cis-regulatory landscapes at high resolution in a single, high-throughput experiment. Nat Genet 46(2):205–212. https://doi.org/10.1038/ng.2871
51. Lieberman-Aiden E, van Berkum NL, Williams L et al (2009) Comprehensive mapping of long-range interactions reveals folding principles of the human genome. Science 326(5950):289–293. https://doi.org/10.1126/science.1181369
52. Fullwood MJ, Liu MH, Pan YF et al (2009) An oestrogen-receptor-alpha-bound human chromatin interactome. Nature 462 (7269):58–64. https://doi.org/10.1038/nature08497. [doi]. nature08497 [pii]
53. Djebali S, Davis CA, Merkel A et al (2012) Landscape of transcription in human cells. Nature 489(7414):101–108. https://doi.org/10.1038/nature11233
54. Schwartzman O, Tanay A (2015) Single-cell epigenomics: techniques and emerging applications. Nat Rev Genet 16(12):716–726. https://doi.org/10.1038/nrg3980
55. Buenrostro JD, Wu B, Litzenburger UM et al (2015) Single-cell chromatin accessibility reveals principles of regulatory variation. Nature 523(7561):486–490. https://doi.org/10.1038/nature14590
56. Nagano T, Lubling Y, Stevens TJ et al (2013) Single-cell hi-C reveals cell-to-cell variability in chromosome structure. Nature 502 (7469):59–64. https://doi.org/10.1038/nature12593
57. Gilad S, Meiri E, Yogev Y et al (2008) Serum microRNAs are promising novel biomarkers. PLoS One 3(9):e3148. https://doi.org/10.1371/journal.pone.0003148
58. Chen X, Shen Y, Draper W et al (2016) ATAC-see reveals the accessible genome by transposase-mediated imaging and sequencing. Nat Methods 13(12):1013–1020. https://doi.org/10.1038/nmeth.4031
59. Rhee HS, Pugh BF (2011) Comprehensive genome-wide protein-DNA interactions detected at single-nucleotide resolution. Cell 147(6):1408–1419. https://doi.org/10.1016/j.cell.2011.11.013
60. Falconer DSDS, Mackay TFC, Falconer D et al (1996) Introduction to quantitative genetics, 4th ed edn. Pearson, Prentice Hall, Harlow
61. Mackay TF (2001) Quantitative trait loci in Drosophila. Nat Rev Genet 2(1):11–20. https://doi.org/10.1038/35047544
62. Welter D, MacArthur J, Morales J et al (2014) The NHGRI GWAS Catalog, a curated resource of SNP-trait associations. Nucleic Acids Res 42(Database issue): D1001–D1006. https://doi.org/10.1093/nar/gkt1229
63. Gallone G, Haerty W, Disanto G et al (2016) Identification of genetic variants affecting vitamin D receptor binding and associations with autoimmune disease. Hum Mol Genet 26(11):2164–2176
64. Kilpinen H, Waszak SM, Gschwind AR et al (2013) Coordinated effects of sequence variation on DNA binding, chromatin structure, and transcription. Science 342 (6159):744–747. https://doi.org/10.1126/science.1242463
65. Kasowski M, Kyriazopoulou-Panagiotopoulou S, Grubert F et al (2013) Extensive variation in chromatin states across humans. Science 342(6159):750–752. https://doi.org/10.1126/science.1242510

66. McVicker G, van de Geijn B, Degner JF et al (2013) Identification of genetic variants that affect histone modifications in human cells. Science 342(6159):747–749. https://doi.org/10.1126/science.1242429
67. Westra HJ, Peters MJ, Esko T et al (2013) Systematic identification of trans eQTLs as putative drivers of known disease associations. Nat Genet 45(10):1238–1243. https://doi.org/10.1038/ng.2756
68. Civelek M, Lusis AJ (2014) Systems genetics approaches to understand complex traits. Nat Rev Genet 15(1):34–48. https://doi.org/10.1038/nrg3575
69. Kitano H (2002) Systems biology: a brief overview. Science 295(5560):1662–1664. https://doi.org/10.1126/science.1069492
70. Gaffney DJ, Veyrieras JB, Degner JF et al (2012) Dissecting the regulatory architecture of gene expression QTLs. Genome Biol 13 (1):R7. https://doi.org/10.1186/gb-2012-13-1-r7
71. Lee MN, Ye C, Villani AC et al (2014) Common genetic variants modulate pathogen-sensing responses in human dendritic cells. Science 343(6175):1246980. https://doi.org/10.1126/science.1246980
72. Song L, Huang SC, Wise A et al (2016) A transcription factor hierarchy defines an environmental stress response network. Science 354(6312). https://doi.org/10.1126/science.aag1550
73. Rhee EP, Ho JE, Chen MH et al (2013) A genome-wide association study of the human metabolome in a community-based cohort. Cell Metab 18(1):130–143. https://doi.org/10.1016/j.cmet.2013.06.013
74. Kettunen J, Tukiainen T, Sarin AP et al (2012) Genome-wide association study identifies multiple loci influencing human serum metabolite levels. Nat Genet 44(3):269–276. https://doi.org/10.1038/ng.1073
75. Shin SY, Fauman EB, Petersen AK et al (2014) An atlas of genetic influences on human blood metabolites. Nat Genet 46 (6):543–550. https://doi.org/10.1038/ng.2982
76. Wu L, Candille SI, Choi Y et al (2013) Variation and genetic control of protein abundance in humans. Nature 499(7456):79–82. https://doi.org/10.1038/nature12223
77. Altshuler DM, Gibbs RA, Peltonen L et al (2007) Population genomics of human gene expression. Nat Genet 39(10):1217–1224. https://doi.org/10.1038/ng2142
78. Stranger BE, Nica AC, Forrest MS, Dimas A, Bird CP, Beazley C, Ingle CE, Dunning M, Flicek P, Koller D, Montgomery S, Tavare S, Deloukas P, Dermitzakis ET (2007) Population genomics of human gene expression. Nat Genet 39(10):1217–1224. https://doi.org/10.1038/ng2142
79. Auton A, Brooks LD, Durbin RM et al (2015) A global reference for human genetic variation. Nature 526(7571):68–74. https://doi.org/10.1038/nature15393
80. Sudmant PH, Rausch T, Gardner EJ et al (2015) An integrated map of structural variation in 2,504 human genomes. Nature 526 (7571):75–81. https://doi.org/10.1038/nature15394
81. Stunnenberg HG, Hirst M (2016) The international human epigenome consortium: a blueprint for scientific collaboration and discovery. Cell 167(5):1145–1149. https://doi.org/10.1016/j.cell.2016.11.007
82. Kundaje A, Meuleman W, Ernst J et al (2015) Integrative analysis of 111 reference human epigenomes. Nature 518(7539):317–330. https://doi.org/10.1038/nature14248
83. Andersson R, Gebhard C, Miguel-Escalada I et al (2014) An atlas of active enhancers across human cell types and tissues. Nature 507 (7493):455–461. https://doi.org/10.1038/nature12787
84. Bernstein BE, Stamatoyannopoulos JA, Costello JF et al (2010) The NIH roadmap epigenomics mapping consortium. Nat Biotechnol 28(10):1045–1048. https://doi.org/10.1038/nbt1010-1045
85. Hudson TJ, Anderson W, Artez A et al (2010) International network of cancer genome projects. Nature 464(7291):993–998. https://doi.org/10.1038/nature08987. [doi]. nature08987 [pii]
86. Teytelman L, Thurtle DM, Rine J et al (2013) Highly expressed loci are vulnerable to misleading ChIP localization of multiple unrelated proteins. Proc Natl Acad Sci U S A 110 (46):18602–18607. https://doi.org/10.1073/pnas.1316064110
87. Zhang L, Zhang K, Prandl R et al (2004) Detecting DNA-binding of proteins in vivo by UV-crosslinking and immunoprecipitation. Biochem Biophys Res Commun 322 (3):705–711. https://doi.org/10.1016/j.bbrc.2004.07.202
88. Licatalosi DD, Mele A, Fak JJ et al (2008) HITS-CLIP yields genome-wide insights into brain alternative RNA processing. Nature 456(7221):464–469. https://doi.org/10.1038/nature07488
89. O'Neill LP, Turner BM (2003) Immunoprecipitation of native chromatin: NChIP. Methods 31(1):76–82

90. Kasinathan S, Orsi GA, Zentner GE et al (2014) High-resolution mapping of transcription factor binding sites on native chromatin. Nat Methods 11(2):203–209. https://doi.org/10.1038/nmeth.2766
91. Fisher WW, Li JJ, Hammonds AS et al (2012) DNA regions bound at low occupancy by transcription factors do not drive patterned reporter gene expression in drosophila. Proc Natl Acad Sci U S A 109(52):21330–21335. https://doi.org/10.1073/pnas.1209589110
92. Chen J, Zhang Z, Li L et al (2014) Single-molecule dynamics of enhanceosome assembly in embryonic stem cells. Cell 156 (6):1274–1285. https://doi.org/10.1016/j.cell.2014.01.062
93. Voong LN, Xi L, Sebeson AC et al (2016) Insights into nucleosome organization in mouse embryonic stem cells through chemical mapping. Cell 167(6):1555–1570.e1515. https://doi.org/10.1016/j.cell.2016.10.049
94. Walter K, Min JL, Huang J et al (2015) The UK10K project identifies rare variants in health and disease. Nature 526 (7571):82–90. https://doi.org/10.1038/nature14962
95. Zheng HF, Forgetta V, Hsu YH et al (2015) Whole-genome sequencing identifies EN1 as a determinant of bone density and fracture. Nature 526(7571):112–117. https://doi.org/10.1038/nature14878
96. Claussnitzer M, Dankel SN, Klocke B et al (2014) Leveraging cross-species transcription factor binding site patterns: from diabetes risk loci to disease mechanisms. Cell 156 (1–2):343–358. https://doi.org/10.1016/j.cell.2013.10.058
97. Trynka G, Sandor C, Han B et al (2013) Chromatin marks identify critical cell types for fine mapping complex trait variants. Nat Genet 45(2):124–130. https://doi.org/10.1038/ng.2504
98. Tehranchi AK, Myrthil M, Martin T et al (2016) Pooled ChIP-Seq links variation in transcription factor binding to complex disease risk. Cell 165(3):730–741. https://doi.org/10.1016/j.cell.2016.03.041
99. Small KS, Todorcevic M, Civelek M et al (2018) Regulatory variants at KLF14 influence type 2 diabetes risk via a female-specific effect on adipocyte size and body composition. Nat Genet. 50(4):572-80. doi:10.1038/s41588-018-0088-x
100. Billings LK, Florez JC (2010) The genetics of type 2 diabetes: what have we learned from GWAS? Ann N Y Acad Sci 1212:59–77. https://doi.org/10.1111/j.1749-6632.2010.05838.x
101. Locke AE, Kahali B, Berndt SI et al (2015) Genetic studies of body mass index yield new insights for obesity biology. Nature 518 (7538):197–206. https://doi.org/10.1038/nature14177
102. Nelson MR, Wegmann D, Ehm MG et al (2012) An abundance of rare functional variants in 202 drug target genes sequenced in 14,002 people. Science 337(6090):100–104. https://doi.org/10.1126/science.1217876
103. Harper AR, Topol EJ (2012) Pharmacogenomics in clinical practice and drug development. Nat Biotechnol 30(11):1117–1124. https://doi.org/10.1038/nbt.2424
104. Lappalainen T, Sammeth M, Friedlander MR et al (2013) Transcriptome and genome sequencing uncovers functional variation in humans. Nature 501(7468):506–511. https://doi.org/10.1038/nature12531
105. Wild CP (2005) Complementing the genome with an "exposome": the outstanding challenge of environmental exposure measurement in molecular epidemiology. Cancer Epidemiol Biomark Prev 14(8):1847–1850. https://doi.org/10.1158/1055-9965.epi-05-0456
106. Holmes E, Loo RL, Stamler J et al (2008) Human metabolic phenotype diversity and its association with diet and blood pressure. Nature 453(7193):396–400. https://doi.org/10.1038/nature06882
107. Gibson G, Powell JE, Marigorta UM (2015) Expression quantitative trait locus analysis for translational medicine. Genome Med 7 (1):60. https://doi.org/10.1186/s13073-015-0186-7
108. Berlanga-Taylor, A. J., Plant, Dahl, A. et al (2017) Effect of vitamin D supplementation on biomarkers of inflammation and immune function: functional genomics analysis of the BEST-D trial. bioRxiv. https://doi.org/10.1101/217612
109. Elliott P, Vergnaud AC, Singh D et al (2014) The airwave health monitoring study of police officers and staff in great Britain: rationale, design and methods. Environ Res 134:280–285. https://doi.org/10.1016/j.envres.2014.07.025
110. Sudlow C, Gallacher J, Allen N et al (2015) UK biobank: an open access resource for identifying the causes of a wide range of complex diseases of middle and old age. PLoS Med 12(3):e1001779. https://doi.org/10.1371/journal.pmed.1001779

Chapter 16

Translating Human Genetics into Novel Drug Targets

Karol Estrada
Alzheimer's Disease Neuroimaging Initiative

Abstract

The most important promise of the human genome sequencing project is the identification of the genetic cause of devastating human diseases and the subsequent deliver of novel drug therapies to treat these diseases with high unmet medical need. In the last 10 years we have successfully identified hundreds of genetic loci associated with many traits and diseases. The translation of these findings into novel therapies is not straightforward and poses challenges that are usually overlooked in traditional gene mapping. This chapter describes some of the most common challenges and opportunities to use human genetics to identify and validate novel drug targets.

Key words Human genetics, Drug targets, Translation genomics

1 Introduction

The process of drug discovery starts with the generation of a hypothesis of a potential drug target to treat a human disease. There are several ways in which these hypotheses are generated, the most common are the exploration of proteins that have been reported to be part of a pathway of relevance, the repositioning of already in use drugs for new therapeutic areas, and the exploration of similar targets to those already in use or that have been previously proposed but lacked efficacy or failed safety. The major inherited disadvantage of all these strategies is the high risk of failure when they are finally ready to be tested for the first time in humans. It is easy to understand the main reason for this high failure rate, the generation of the hypothesis most of the time comes from

Data used in preparation of this article were obtained from the Alzheimer's Disease Neuroimaging Initiative (ADNI) database (adni.loni.usc.edu). As such, the investigators within the ADNI contributed to the design and implementation of ADNI and/or provided data but did not participate in analysis or writing of this report. A complete listing of ADNI investigators can be found at: http://adni.loni.usc.edu/wp-content/uploads/how_to_apply/ADNI_Acknowledgement_List.pdf

Evangelos Evangelou (ed.), *Genetic Epidemiology: Methods and Protocols*, Methods in Molecular Biology, vol. 1793, https://doi.org/10.1007/978-1-4939-7868-7_16, © Springer Science+Business Media, LLC, part of Springer Nature 2018

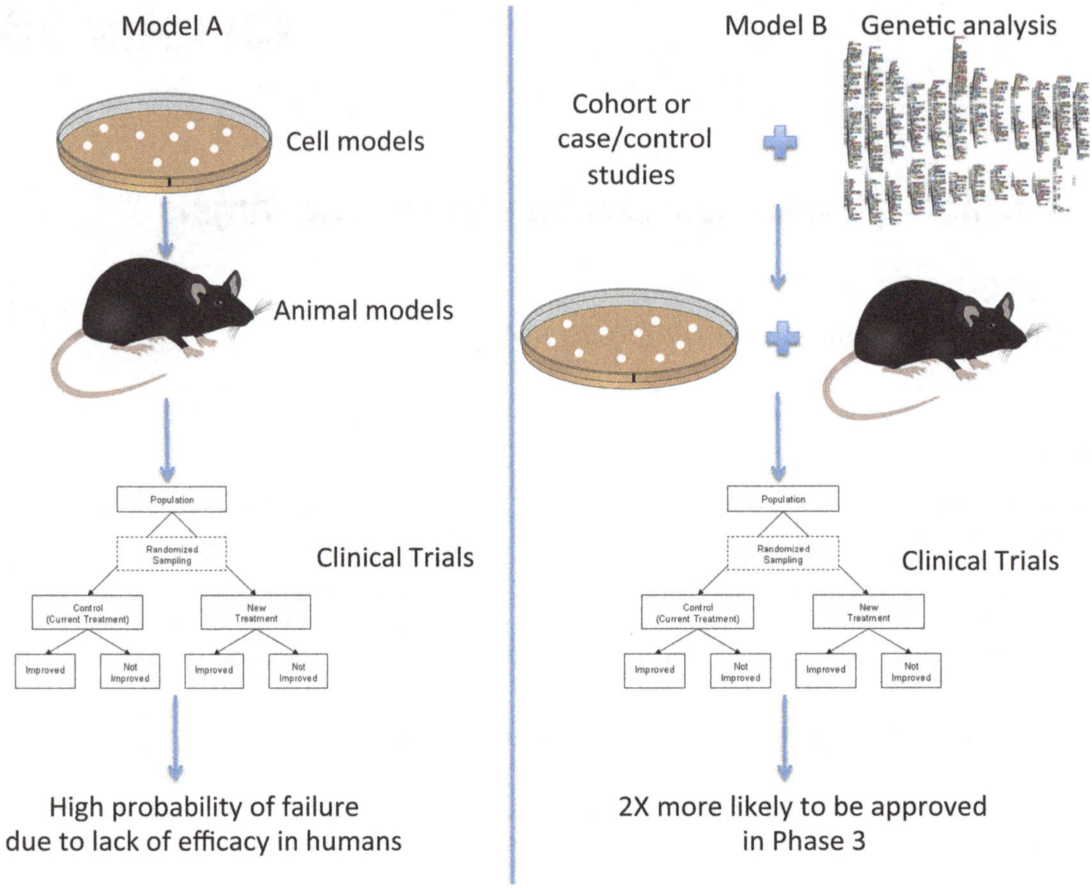

Fig. 1 Model A. Typical drug identification in pharma starting with an interesting observation in a cell model for a given disease. An observation on a cell model leads a scientist to believe that targeting gene X will be useful for targeting a human disease. After spending years and substantial lab work the target is approved for pre-clinical animal testing. The target then can show positive and/or conflicting results in animal models and therefore it is decided to test its effect for the first time in humans using the typical Phase I to III stages. Model A has a high probability of failure in clinical trials because it has never been observed/tested in humans. Model B. Similar scenario, as Model A, the main difference is that a novel gene Y has been observed to be mutated in humans in the disease of interest at statistically convincing levels. This gives us a sense of certainty that if our protein chemists are able to design a compound that mimics the naturally occurring variants, we have a high chance of success. Model B still has to go through cell and animal models because there is a need to understand the mechanism of action of the new target before being able to design and optimize a lead compound. It has been shown retrospectively that this model has two times more probability of being successful in phase III clinical trials

observations in cellular models, animal models or other systems that are several steps away from the complex biology involved in disease mechanism in humans (Fig. 1).

A more sensitive approach would be to start testing hypotheses directly generated from the same species (humans), but until recently little did we know about the biology of common diseases in humans. It has been shown that a drug target with support from human genetics is two times more likely to succeed from phase I all the way to phase III [1] (Fig. 1).

Genome-wide association studies (GWAS) have identified thousands of sites in the human genome that are consistently replicated across studies with an increased risk for most major diseases [2]. This plethora of novel biology does not automatically get translated into novel drug targets. This paper highlights some of the major challenges to overcome the translation of gene discovery into drug discovery.

2 Identifying Novel and Consistently Associated Risk Variants

Gene discovery for rare diseases has been in general successful using collections of families under the linkage approach. It was still a long-term process from finding a region with linkage to disease until an actual gene mutation could be determined. The linkage peaks on those studies could contain hundreds of genes, and testing variants on each of those was not as systematized as it is nowadays. This strategy however was not very successful for common complex diseases, the majority of the linkage peaks for common diseases, if any, were hard to replicate. A seminal paper from Risch and Merikangas, [3] titled "The future of genetic studies of complex human diseases", set the tone for what was set to be a revolution in the field. They correctly predicted that for complex diseases the linkage approach would require many more samples to identify without doubt a signal as compared to an association study.

The subsequent creation of the HapMap project, [4] the SNP microarray technology, combined with the ever larger collection of disease cohorts created a revolution in gene discovery of complex diseases. The Genome-Wide Association Study (GWAS) catalog lists to date (2016-08-25) a total of $n = 24{,}218$ unique SNP-trait associations [2].

The path from a successful GWAS of a common disease to the first wave of successful GWAS for neurological and psychiatric diseases was not straightforward. For many years without success of identifying genetic loci for schizophrenia, it was suggested that perhaps some of these common diseases had a majority of contribution from rare or de-novo type of genetic variation [5]. The reality was that these diseases are from nature more heterogeneous than other more quantitative and precise traits (such as adult height and bone mineral density) [6, 7]. Therefore, it required the hard work of coordinating several scientific groups in other to reach the sufficient sample size to be powered to find up to 108 genetic loci for schizophrenia at genome-wide significant levels [8]. This is explained by power estimations that show that even with 50,000 cases and 50,000 controls, there is limited power to identify common genetic variants (MAF > 0.05) of weak effects ($0.9 <$ OR <1.1) (Fig. 2).

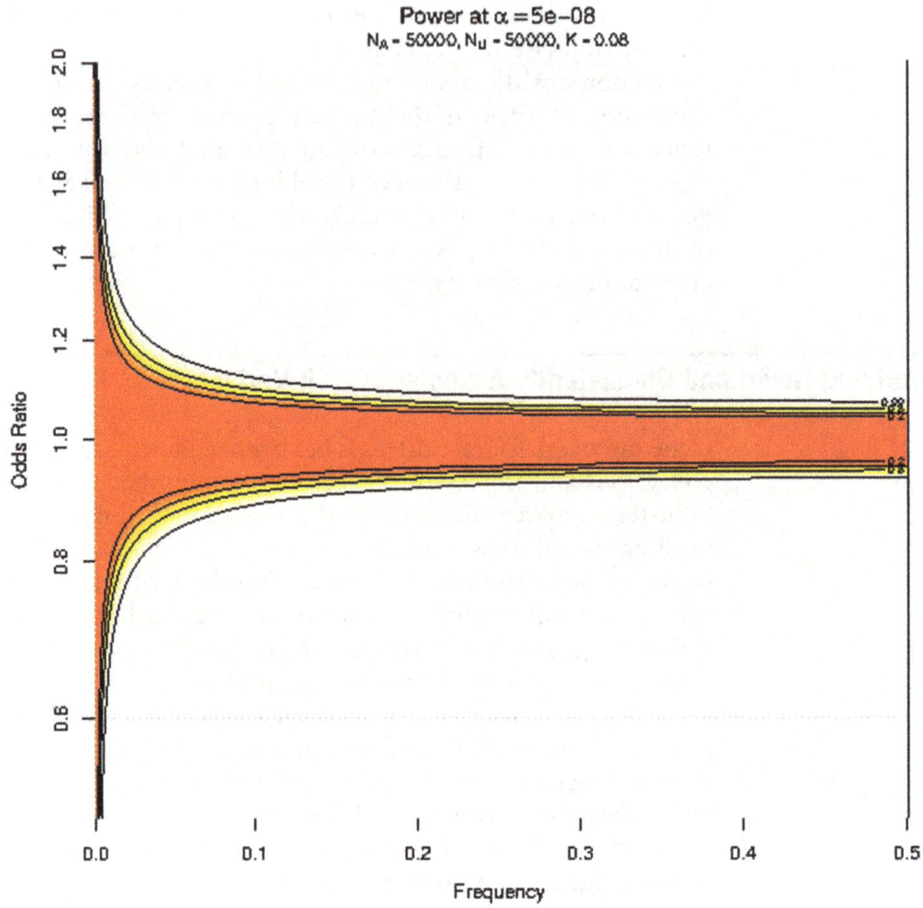

Fig. 2 Power estimations to identify a genetic variant associated under different scenarios. The model assumes a study with 50,000 cases and 50,000 controls of a disease with a prevalence of 8% and alpha $= 5 \times 10^{-8}$. The red zone identifies regions where power is less than 0.2, the different shades from red to white show where power starts increasing (white means power = 100%). Even with these samples sizes, variants of common frequency have limited power if their odds ratios are smaller than 1.10. This problem intensifies when we go down in the allele frequency expectrum

3 Identifying the Causal Genetic Variant

3.1 Linkage Disequilibrium, your Friend and Worst Enemy

As early as in 2002, it was found that the human genome is organized in haplotype blocks, these blocks vary in size depending on the location in the genome, but also on the ancestry of the population being studied [9]. The International HapMap project [4] was set to characterize at genome scale the diversity of these haplotypes and to understand the patterns of linkage disequilibrium across SNPs. It was observed that in individuals of European origin a common SNP is usually highly correlated ($r^2 >= 0.80$) to several other SNPs in a window that averages 500 kb but can be as large as 10,000 kb. This is in one way useful because most SNP arrays do not have a comprehensive coverage of all common SNPs on the human genome, and therefore without this feature we would easily miss a hit if by chance the array did not contain a causal variant. On the other hand, this feature is one of the worst enemies for the process of drug discovery. The fact that we are never sure that a variant is causal and acknowledging that it is more likely to be a correlated variant to the real causal one, indicates that extra work is needed.

3.2 Fine Mapping

In most circumstances we would like to know which causal variant is driving a genetic association. The preferred approach to do so is known as "fine mapping", it consists on designing a dense genotyping array targeting the regions where a genome-wide association has been found. In the past, these arrays were designed using data from sequencing projects such as the 1000 Genomes Project [10–12]. But for fine mapping to be successful, a study also requires to be powerful enough to find the original associations discovered in a typical GWAS. This strategy is required but not sufficient to find the casual variant, as we will see below, other statistical methods are required to deconvolute a GWAS signal.

3.3 Allelic Heterogeneity

Another interesting feature of the genetic architecture of human traits and diseases is the overwhelmingly common presence of multiple independent signals. Originally it was found that signals tended to be dispersed across all human chromosomes, but more recently it has been evident that even in the same locus there is persistent allelic heterogeneity that when a study is powered enough can be distinguished from linkage disequilibrium using either a statistical approach known as conditional analysis, or by using newer methods like the joint analysis [13].

3.4 Credible Set Analysis

When fine mapping data is available, a Bayes theorem application known as credible set analysis is preferred [14]. Using this method it is possible to determine a region (credible set) that have 95% posterior probability of containing a causal disease-associated SNP. Studies using this technique have found that around 20% of the loci can be mapped to a single SNP with 95% probability of being causal [14]. A recent implementation of this process has been published in a tool called FINEMAP [15].

4 Linking a Genetic Association to a Gene

4.1 Using Expression Quantitative Loci

When we read a typical GWAS paper describing a novel signal for a given disease it is commonly assigned to a gene symbol. This annotation however often relies on an imperfect method using proximity of the identified variant to a gene symbol. Knowing which gene is driving the association is one of the most challenging aspects of novel drug target identification. One method is to use data from expression quantitative trait locus (eQTL) to try to map a GWAS signal to a gene. Also, a recent paper reported that many GWAS signals could be explained by a different type of transcription modifier known as splicing factor or splicing QTL (sQTL) [16]. While this sounds straightforward given that an eQTL or sQTL has both an rsID and a Gene symbol associated, it has proven to be challenging for many reasons which are detailed below.

1. Incorrect tissue sample. The transcription of genes can be modulated in a tissue-dependent manner. Therefore if a gene is being controlled by a genetic variant ONLY in a certain tissue or cell type we might completely loose the eQTL signal. We have just started understanding these tissue expression challenges in recent efforts like the GTEX project [17] which characterized the transcriptome of 43 tissues from 175 individuals. Analyzed eQTLs are freely available from this project at http://gtexportal.org
2. Correct tissue, but incorrect timing. Another complication of gene expression data is the temporality of transcription events. Genes are not always turned on, there are certain genes that are active in certain development stages and after a particular time or event become inactive. This is a particularly challenging problem for eQTL analysis as there is little gene expression data generated from the same individuals but in different time points or conditions. One exception would be immune diseases where expression data of relevant cell types have been generated under different conditions that are known to be important for disease, this can however can be explained by the simplicity of the tissue of interest, which in most cases comes from access to blood samples. In neurological diseases this has been challenging as it is already hard to get access to brain human samples and would be literally impossible to get human samples at different time points (current available data comes from post-mortem samples).
3. Multiple eQTLS and/or multiple GWAS signals in the same locus. The preferred method to identify a causal gene via eQTL mapping is called co-localization analysis. It relies on a statistical model that assigns a probability that a given eQTL signal is the functional event driving a GWAS signal. Methods have been implemented using this approach [18]. This method however assumes that each GWAS locus contains a single causal variant. Novel methods to address this problem are being developed [16, 19].

4.2 Using Epigenetics

The ENCODE project [20] has identified and mapped thousands of regions that regulate transcription based on mapping of transcription factor binding sites, chromatin structures, DNase.

I hypersensitivity sites (DHS), and many other methods that collectively are called "epigenetics" or beyond genetics. One could use this data as an alternative of eQTL co-localization to identify the target gene. There are multiple ways to do this mapping, a recent manuscript has suggested to use DHS sites together with its effects on gene expression to map GWAS signals, the authors found that using this method they can prioritize a single gene in almost 80% across nine autoimmune and inflammatory diseases. These methods however has the same limitations as the use of eQTLs mentioned above.

5 The Beauty of Rare Protein Coding Variants

Ten years ago a new technology called "Next Generation Sequencing" came to the market and started a revolution in the way we do gene discovery. For the first time we were able to read the sequence of the human genome of multiple samples for prices several fold lower than the first human genome sequenced. This revolution allowed us to systematically sequence most protein coding variants independently of their allele frequencies (assuming same power, coding variant associated with disease tend to have lower allele frequencies but larger effect sizes) [21]. The main difference between the rare coding variants and the common non-coding variants is that the former are automatically linked to one single gene, while the later not. As we discussed above, mapping a non-coding variant to a gene is not straightforward. This step is particularly important in the context of target identification in drug discovery because a target is usually a gene product (protein) and not a genetic variant. The process of linking a common non-coding genetic variant to a gene can take several years and may not even be successful.

A rare protein coding variant or a collection therefore, associated with disease is particularly important when the variant confers a loss of protein function and at the same time is protective for a given disease [22]. The reason may not be immediately evident, until one thinks in the context of the typical drug target. Usually a drug is easier to design if three conditions are met: (1) the protein target is known and the drug is specific to that target, (2) the drug is an antagonist (meaning the drug that confers therapeutic value will somehow disrupt the function of the protein) and (3) there are not side-effects of targeting that protein. When a set of individuals have loss of protein function variants in a given gene that protects them from disease and are otherwise normal (in the sense that no other enrichment for other diseases), this is a perfect naturally occurring experiment in which we can say that a drug that targets that gene will have a higher probability of meeting the three points mentioned above.

The concept of using naturally occurring loss of protein function variants as a way to identify new drug targets is currently being tested. One of the best examples is the proprotein convertase subtilisin kexin 9 (PCSK9) gene. In 2005, it was found that rare loss of function variants in PCSK9 were associated with reduced levels of LDL cholesterol and reduced incidence of coronary heart disease [23]. In 2012, randomized control trials showed that following the logic explained above, a PCSK9-directed monoclonal antibody significantly reduced LDL cholesterol in humans [24, 25]. The first two PCSK9 inhibitors were approved by the FDA in 2015, exactly 10 years after the initial discovery of the relationship between PCSK9 and disease. This example shows that even after having a clear and perfect target validated by human genetic tools, the regular process to develop a new drug is still the main bottleneck to see all these discoveries translated into a clinically useful application.

6 Understanding the Mechanism of Action

6.1 Genetics of Endophenotypes

The majority of complex diseases have a heterogeneous etiology. For example, Type 2 diabetes is characterized by high glucose levels which is mostly derived by insulin resistance. Other example is Alzheimer's disease, which is characterized by two consistent observations on the brains of diseased individuals: accumulation of amyloid plaques and tau tangles (both different forms of abnormally aggregated proteins) [26]. If we believe in the mentioned hypotheses, then a genetic variant that has been associated with disease through one of these mechanisms would also show association with those characteristic endophenotypes. For Alzheimer's disease (AD) we can use GWAS for two biomarkers that are currently used in clinical trials to measure amyloid load and tau levels (Amyloid Beta measured with PET (positron emission tomography) AV45 from the Alzheimer's Disease Neuroimaging Initiative (ADNI, *see* Methods) and summary statistics from a GWAS for tau levels measured from Cerebrospinal fluid (CSF) [27]. By plotting the effect size of these two biomarkers on the 22 AD-associated loci [28] we can see that there is a clear correlation of AD-associated alleles with increasing levels of both amyloid beta and tau levels (Fig. 3). The strongest AD risk locus represented by the APOE e4 allele is a strong predictor of amyloid levels (rs429358, Beta = 0.12 for each C allele, $P = 9.9 \times 10^{-35}$) as well as for pTau (Beta = 0.11, $P = 0.024$), But more importantly, we observe that some AD genes have a nominal association with increasing levels of amyloid levels (ABCA7, represented by rs4147929, Beta = 0.044 SD per A allele,

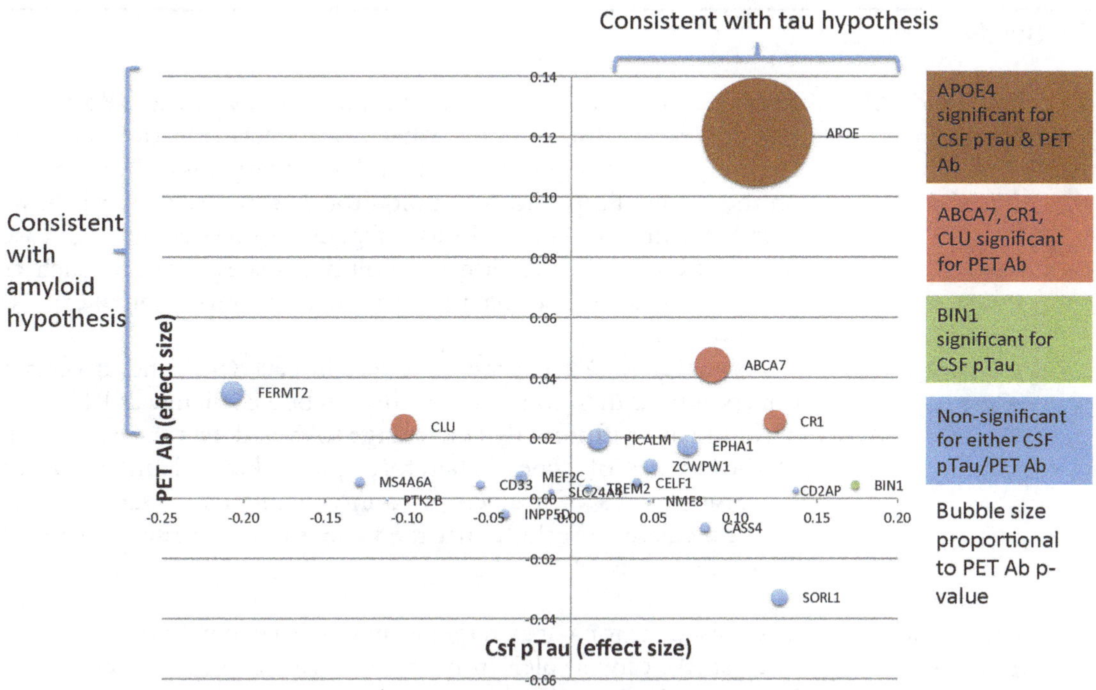

Fig. 3 Using endophenotypes to understand the mechanism of action of a target gene. Plotted are the 22 genome-wide significant loci for Alzheimer's disease. The allele represented in the diagram is always the one conferring risk for Alzheimer's disease. The *X*-axis represents the effect of the given allele in phosphorylated tau levels (in SDs from CSF). The *Y*-axis represents the effect of the same allele in amyloid beta levels (in SDs from PET). From this data we can conclude that there are some targets such as APOE and ABCA7 that have a clear role via amyloid beta metabolism while other targets such as BIN1 seem to be acting via modulation of pTau levels

$P = 3.6 \times 10^{-4}$) while BIN1 has a nominal association with tau levels but not amyloid (rs6733839, Beta = 0.17 SD for each T allele, $P = 0.04$). This information can provide insights into the potential mechanisms that these genes are acting to increase the risk for AD.

6.2 Pathways

Another method to gain insight into the mechanisms of action of genes of interest is to look into the known pathways that the gene is involved. For example, in our latest GEFOS meta-analysis of bone mineral density [6] we observed an enrichment of genes involved in three main pathways: Canonical Wnt signaling, RANK-RANKL-OPG, and the mesenchymal stem cell differentiation. While this information does not preclude that a gene may have another pleiotropic effect, the observation that many of the GWAS hits for BMD are enriched on each one of these pathways provides input into the potential way in which the novel genetic variants are modifying disease risk.

7 Safety

7.1 Tissue and Cell Type Expression Profile

Knowing in which tissues/cells of a human body a gene is expressed can be very useful to know what side effects one can cause by targeting that gene product. An ideal good target is only expressed on the tissue of interest, (not ubiquitously expressed), this is however uncommon. The majority of genes associated with disease show differential expression on multiple tissues. Projects such as GTEX are a useful resource for the rapid characterization of expression profiles.

Some genes are expressed at certain cell types, and at certain time points, as mentioned above this can be a challenge as RNA-seq may not have sufficient dynamic range to even detect the expression of these types of genes. Therefore, the lack of identification of expression levels of a given gene in a whole-tissue sample does not immediately preclude that the gene is not expressed in sub-set of cells.

7.2 Association with Other Traits and Diseases

The ideal gene for a drug target is only associated with the disease of interest. We can use pleiotropic effects as a measure of target safety. For example, imagine that we have found a gene where loss of function mutations are protective for Alzheimer's disease. However, we also find that other variation of unknown functional effect are associated with cardiovascular disease. While this observation does not preclude the gene being a good target, it does provide evidence that it is possible that targeting this gene may also have influence in unwanted side effects. Useful resources to identify these associations with disease are: the Online Mendelian Inheritance in Man (OMIM), ClinVar for rare diseases and the target validation platform of Open Targets (https://www.targetvalidation.org) for common diseases. When we know the exact SNP identifier and want to know if that marker is associated with other human disease or trait, a tool the Pheno Scanner is useful. (http://www.phenoscanner.medschl.cam.ac.uk/phenoscanner).

7.3 Constraint Scores and Human Knock-Outs

Imagine again a target where loss of function mutations are protective for disease. It would be ideal if we could know if the gene has a susceptibility for eliminating novel loss of function mutations from the gene pool via natural selection. This could be an indication that the same variation that protects for one disease may have also other unknown side effects. Using a large scale exome sequencing database such as ExAC, [29] http://exac.broadinstitute.org) and a method that compares the observed vs expected number of variants of three coding categories, [30] it is possible to estimate how likely it is that a gene is haploinsufficient (in ExAC, labeled as pLI). A gene with a pLI = 1 means that there is a significant depletion of loss of function mutations in the gene and therefore a very high chance that removing one copy of this gene will create a phenotypic effect. While we cannot tell exactly what that effect will be, it is a red flag that needs to be followed up more closely.

8 Conclusions

Target identification and further validation is an expensive and time consuming activity. It has been shown retrospectively that targets with strong evidence from human genetics could save up to 25% of the costs coming from failures in randomized clinical trials [31]. From 2005 to 2015 we were witness of a revolution in the identification of systematically replicated novel loci for multiple diseases. Most of these research lines stopped right after a *P*-value of association reached the threshold of genome-wide significance. The new phase of human genetics for drug identification and validation requires much more work than that. Understanding which causal variant, gene and mechanism drives that association is the next logical step. Joint academic and private initiatives such as the Open Targets and the Accelerating Medicines Partnerships are currently defining the processes, methods, tools and data sharing mechanisms that will facilitate how we use human genetics for the identification and validation of novel drug targets in the next 10 years.

9 Methods

9.1 Samples

Data used in the preparation of this article were obtained from the Alzheimer's Disease Neuroimaging Initiative (ADNI) database (http://adni.loni.usc.edu). The ADNI was launched in 2003 as a public-private partnership, led by Principal Investigator Michael W. Weiner, MD. The primary goal of ADNI has been to test whether serial magnetic resonance imaging (MRI), positron emission tomography (PET), other biological markers, and clinical and neuropsychological assessment can be combined to measure the progression of mild cognitive impairment (MCI) and early Alzheimer's disease (AD). For up-to-date information, *see* http://www.adni-info.org.

Merged datasets (ADNIMERGE) containing data from ADNI 1/GO/2 clinical data and numeric summaries were downloaded from the ADNI website. Composite SUVR values for amyloid beta measured with AV45 were obtained from the variable AV45, in total 1063 individuals were assessed. Detailed information on how the PET data was collected has been described elsewhere [32].

9.2 Genotypes & Quality Control

633 and 368 samples were genotyped with the Illumina Omni 2.5 and the Illumina Omni express arrays. Only samples clustering near the European group based on principal components were included. Individuals with first degree relatedness were removed. At the end 943 samples remained. A/T C/G SNPs were removed, and the remaining 674,143 variants where matched to the alleles represented in the Haplotype Reference Consortium (HRC) version 1.0 [33]. The Michigan Imputation Server was used to impute into HRC 1.0 which implements a pre-phasing and imputation pipeline using Shapeit and IMPUTE2.

After imputation, the following 22 SNPs taken from the list of genome-wide significant signals in the latest Alzheimer's Disease meta-analysis [28] were extracted and aligned for the increasing AD risk allele: APOE e4, rs429358; INPP5D, rs35349669; PICALM, rs10792832; TREM2, rs9381040; BIN1, rs6733839; FERMT2, rs17125944; CR1, rs6656401; CD2AP, rs10948363; NME8, rs2718058; ABCA7, rs4147929; ZCWPW1, rs1476679; MEF2C, rs190982; CLU, rs9331896; PTK2B, rs28834970; MS4A6A, rs983392; CASS4, rs7274581; SORL1, rs11218343; CELF1, rs10838725; CD33, rs3865444; EPHA1, rs11771145; SLC24A4, rs10498633; APOE e2, rs7412.

9.3 Association Analysis and Summary Statistics

The 22 SNPs were tested for association with amyloid levels (AV45) using a linear regression adjusted for the first four principal components, age, sex, and AD/MCI/normal status using dummy variables. The effect size (Beta) was aligned to match the AD-risk increasing allele previously reported [28].

Summary statistics GWAS for tau levels measured from Cerebrospinal fluid (CSF) were obtained from a previously published paper [27].

Acknowledgements

Data collection and sharing for this project was funded by the Alzheimer's Disease Neuroimaging Initiative (ADNI) (National Institutes of Health Grant U01 AG024904) and DOD ADNI (Department of Defense award number W81XWH-12-2-0012). ADNI is funded by the National Institute on Aging, the National Institute of Biomedical Imaging and Bioengineering, and through generous contributions from the following: AbbVie, Alzheimer's Association; Alzheimer's Drug Discovery Foundation; Araclon Biotech; BioClinica, Inc.; Biogen; Bristol-Myers Squibb Company; CereSpir, Inc.; Cogstate; Eisai Inc.; Elan Pharmaceuticals, Inc.; Eli Lilly and Company; EuroImmun; F. Hoffmann-La Roche Ltd. and its affiliated company Genentech, Inc.; Fujirebio; GE Healthcare; IXICO Ltd.; Janssen Alzheimer Immunotherapy Research & Development, LLC.; Johnson & Johnson Pharmaceutical Research

& Development LLC.; Lumosity; Lundbeck; Merck & Co., Inc.; Meso Scale Diagnostics, LLC.; NeuroRx Research; Neurotrack Technologies; Novartis Pharmaceuticals Corporation; Pfizer Inc.; Piramal Imaging; Servier; Takeda Pharmaceutical Company; and Transition Therapeutics. The Canadian Institutes of Health Research is providing funds to support ADNI clinical sites in Canada. Private sector contributions are facilitated by the Foundation for the National Institutes of Health (http://www.fnih.org). The grantee organization is the Northern California Institute for Research and Education, and the study is coordinated by the Alzheimer's Therapeutic Research Institute at the University of Southern California. ADNI data are disseminated by the Laboratory for Neuro Imaging at the University of Southern California.

References

1. Nelson MR, Tipney H, Painter JL et al (2015) The support of human genetic evidence for approved drug indications. Nat Genet 47 (8):856–860. https://doi.org/10.1038/ng.3314
2. Welter D, MacArthur J, Morales J et al (2014) The NHGRI GWAS Catalog, a curated resource of SNP-trait associations. Nucleic Acids Res 42(Database issue):D1001–D1006. https://doi.org/10.1093/nar/gkt1229
3. Risch N, Merikangas K (1996) The future of genetic studies of complex human diseases. Science 273(5281):1516–1517
4. International HapMap Consortium (2003) The international hapmap project. Nature 426(6968):789–796. https://doi.org/10.1038/nature02168
5. Goldstein DB (2009) Common genetic variation and human traits. N Engl J Med 360 (17):1696–1698. https://doi.org/10.1056/NEJMp0806284
6. Estrada K, Styrkarsdottir U, Evangelou E et al (2012) Genome-wide meta-analysis identifies 56 bone mineral density loci and reveals 14 loci associated with risk of fracture. Nat Genet 44(5):491–501. https://doi.org/10.1038/ng.2249
7. Lango Allen H, Estrada K, Lettre G et al (2010) Hundreds of variants clustered in genomic loci and biological pathways affect human height. Nature 467(7317):832–838. https://doi.org/10.1038/nature09410
8. Schizophrenia Working Group of the Psychiatric Genomics Consortium (2014) Biological insights from 108 schizophrenia-associated genetic loci. Nature 511(7510):421–427. https://doi.org/10.1038/nature13595
9. Gabriel SB, Schaffner SF, Nguyen H et al (2002) The structure of haplotype blocks in the human genome. Science 296 (5576):2225–2229. https://doi.org/10.1126/science.1069424
10. Cortes A, Brown MA (2011) Promise and pitfalls of the Immunochip. Arthritis Res Ther 13 (1):101. https://doi.org/10.1186/ar3204
11. Naitza S, Porcu E, Steri M et al (2012) A genome-wide association scan on the levels of markers of inflammation in Sardinians reveals associations that underpin its complex regulation. PLoS Genet 8(1):e1002480. https://doi.org/10.1371/journal.pgen.1002480
12. Sudmant PH, Rausch T, Gardner EJ et al (2015) An integrated map of structural variation in 2,504 human genomes. Nature 526 (7571):75–81. https://doi.org/10.1038/nature15394
13. Yang J, Lee SH, Goddard ME et al (2013) Genome-wide complex trait analysis (GCTA): methods, data analyses, and interpretations. Methods Mol Biol 1019:215–236. https://doi.org/10.1007/978-1-62703-447-0_9
14. Maller JB, McVean G, Wellcome Trust Case Control Consortium et al (2012) Bayesian refinement of association signals for 14 loci in 3 common diseases. Nat Genet 44 (12):1294–1301. https://doi.org/10.1038/ng.2435
15. Benner C, Spencer CC, Havulinna AS et al (2016) FINEMAP: efficient variable selection using summary data from genome-wide association studies. Bioinformatics 32 (10):1493–1501. https://doi.org/10.1093/bioinformatics/btw018
16. Li YI, van de Geijn B, Raj A et al (2016) RNA splicing is a primary link between genetic

variation and disease. Science 352 (6285):600–604. https://doi.org/10.1126/science.aad9417

17. GTEx Consortium (2015) Human genomics. The genotype-tissue expression (GTEx) pilot analysis: multitissue gene regulation in humans. Science 348 (6235):648–660. doi: https://doi.org/10.1126/science.1262110
18. Wallace C, Rotival M, Cooper JD et al (2012) Statistical colocalization of monocyte gene expression and genetic risk variants for type 1 diabetes. Hum Mol Genet 21 (12):2815–2824. https://doi.org/10.1093/hmg/dds098
19. Hormozdiari F, Bunt MVD, Segre AV et al (2016) Colocalization of GWAS and eQTL signals detects target genes. Am J Hum Genet 99(6):1245–1260. https://doi.org/10.1101/065037
20. ENCODE Project Consortium (2012) An integrated encyclopedia of DNA elements in the human genome. Nature 489 (7414):57–74. https://doi.org/10.1038/nature11247
21. Zheng HF, Forgetta V, Hsu YH et al (2015) Whole-genome sequencing identifies EN1 as a determinant of bone density and fracture. Nature 526(7571):112–117. https://doi.org/10.1038/nature14878
22. Plenge RM, Scolnick EM, Altshuler D (2013) Validating therapeutic targets through human genetics. Nat Rev Drug Discov 12 (8):581–594. https://doi.org/10.1038/nrd4051
23. Cohen J, Pertsemlidis A, Kotowski IK et al (2005) Low LDL cholesterol in individuals of African descent resulting from frequent nonsense mutations in PCSK9. Nat Genet 37 (2):161–165. https://doi.org/10.1038/ng1509
24. Giugliano RP, Desai NR, Kohli P et al (2012) Efficacy, safety, and tolerability of a monoclonal antibody to proprotein convertase subtilisin/kexin type 9 in combination with a statin in patients with hypercholesterolaemia (LAPLACE-TIMI 57): a randomised, placebo-controlled, dose-ranging, phase 2 study. Lancet 380(9858):2007–2017. https://doi.org/10.1016/S0140-6736(12)61770-X
25. Raal F, Scott R, Somaratne R et al (2012) Low-density lipoprotein cholesterol-lowering effects of AMG 145, a monoclonal antibody to proprotein convertase subtilisin/kexin type 9 serine protease in patients with heterozygous familial hypercholesterolemia: the reduction of LDL-C with PCSK9 inhibition in heterozygous familial hypercholesterolemia disorder (RUTHERFORD) randomized trial. Circulation 126(20):2408–2417. https://doi.org/10.1161/CIRCULATIONAHA.112.144055
26. Sevigny J, Chiao P, Bussiere T et al (2016) The antibody aducanumab reduces Abeta plaques in Alzheimer's disease. Nature 537 (7618):50–56. https://doi.org/10.1038/nature19323
27. Ramirez A, van der Flier WM, Herold C et al (2014) SUCLG2 identified as both a determinator of CSF Abeta1-42 levels and an attenuator of cognitive decline in Alzheimer's disease. Hum Mol Genet 23(24):6644–6658. https://doi.org/10.1093/hmg/ddu372
28. Lambert JC, Ibrahim-Verbaas CA, Harold D et al (2013) Meta-analysis of 74,046 individuals identifies 11 new susceptibility loci for Alzheimer's disease. Nat Genet 45 (12):1452–1458. https://doi.org/10.1038/ng.2802
29. Lek M, Karczewski KJ, Minikel EV et al (2016) Analysis of protein-coding genetic variation in 60,706 humans. Nature 536(7616):285–291. https://doi.org/10.1038/nature19057
30. Samocha KE, Robinson EB, Sanders SJ et al (2014) A framework for the interpretation of de novo mutation in human disease. Nat Genet 46(9):944–950. https://doi.org/10.1038/ng.3050
31. Hurle MR, Nelson MR, Agarwal P et al (2016) Trial watch: impact of genetically supported target selection on R&D productivity. Nat Rev Drug Discov 15(9):596–597. https://doi.org/10.1038/nrd.2016.164
32. Ramanan VK, Risacher SL, Nho K et al (2014) APOE and BCHE as modulators of cerebral amyloid deposition: a florbetapir PET genome-wide association study. Mol Psychiatry 19(3):351–357. https://doi.org/10.1038/mp.2013.19
33. Loh PR, Danecek P, Palamara PF et al (2016) Reference-based phasing using the haplotype reference consortium panel. Nat Genet 48 (11):1443–1448. https://doi.org/10.1038/ng.3679

INDEX

Evangelos Evangelou (ed.), *Genetic Epidemiology: Methods and Protocols*, Methods in Molecular Biology, vol. 1793, https://doi.org/10.1007/978-1-4939-7868-7, © Springer Science+Business Media, LLC, part of Springer Nature 2018

D

E

R

S

CPSIA information can be obtained
at www.ICGtesting.com
Printed in the USA
LVHW061530020521
686264LV00005B/333

9 781493 978670